Heart Disease: A Collection of Cases

Heart Disease: A Collection of Cases

Editor: Jordyn Cooper

AMERICAN
MEDICAL PUBLISHERS
www.americanmedicalpublishers.com

AMERICAN
MEDICAL PUBLISHERS
www.americanmedicalpublishers.com

Cataloging-in-Publication Data

Heart disease: a collection of cases / edited by Jordyn Cooper.
p. cm.
Includes bibliographical references and index.
ISBN 979-8-88740-641-1
1. Heart--Diseases--Pathophysiology. 2. Heart--Pathophysiology. 3. Heart--Diseases.
4. Physiology, Pathological. I. Cooper, Jordyn.
RC682 .P38 2023
616.12--dc23

American Medical Publishers,
41 Flatbush Avenue,
1st Floor, New York,
NY 11217, USA

ISBN 979-8-88740-641-1 (Hardback)

Contents

Preface

The set of conditions that affect the cardiovascular system are referred to as heart diseases. Congenital heart defects, dilated cardiomyopathy, heart failure, mitral valve regurgitation, aortic stenosis, coronary artery disease, arrhythmia, myocardial infarction, hypertrophic cardiomyopathy and mitral valve prolapse, are the common types of heart diseases. There are several risk factors of heart diseases such as family history, high blood pressure, diabetes, unhealthy diet, high cholesterol, and smoking. Heart diseases may lead to potentially fatal conditions or diseases such as heart attack, peripheral artery disease, and sudden cardiac arrest. Heart diseases can be diagnosed by examining the medical history of a person and by performing test such as heart tests and blood tests. Heart diseases are not curable or reversible, but they can be managed with the help of medications, surgery or invasive procedures, and lifestyle changes. This book contains case studies related to all the contemporary topics relevant for studying heart diseases. It will help new researchers by foregrounding their knowledge in these conditions.

This book unites the global concepts and researches in an organized manner for a comprehensive understanding of the subject. It is a ripe text for all researchers, students, scientists or anyone else who is interested in acquiring a better knowledge of this dynamic field.

I extend my sincere thanks to the contributors for such eloquent research chapters. Finally, I thank my family for being a source of support and help.

Editor

1

Right-Sided Subcutaneous Implantable Cardioverter Defibrillator System Implantation in a Patient with Complex Congenital Heart Disease and Dextrocardia

Bandar Al-Ghamdi[1,2]

[1]*Heart Centre, King Faisal Specialist Hospital and Research Centre (KFSH&RC), Riyadh, Saudi Arabia*
[2]*Alfaisal University, Riyadh, Saudi Arabia*

Correspondence should be addressed to Bandar Al-Ghamdi; balghamdi@kfshrc.edu.sa

Academic Editor: Assad Movahed

Patients with complex congenital heart disease (CHD) and low left ventricular ejection fraction are at an increased risk of sudden cardiac death (SCD). Prevention of SCD by subcutaneous implantable cardioverter defibrillator (S-ICD) implantation may represent a valuable option in certain CHD patients. Patients with CHD and dextrocardia pose a challenge in S-ICD system implantation, and nonstandard device placement may be required. Furthermore, electrocardiogram (ECG) screening prior to S-ICD implantation in CHD patients has significant limitations. This case represents the placement of a S-ICD system on the right side of the chest in a 26-year-old male with severe biventricular failure and nonsustained ventricular tachycardia following multiple corrective surgeries of situs inversus totalis, double-outlet right ventricle with a ventricular septal defect, and pulmonary atresia. The use of S-ICDs in a CHD population and in particular CHD patients with dextrocardia and right-sided S-ICD implantation is briefly discussed.

1. Introduction

Patients with complex congenital heart disease (CHD) and low left ventricular ejection fraction are at an increased risk of sudden cardiac death (SCD) [1–3]. Prevention of SCD by subcutaneous implantable cardioverter defibrillator (S-ICD) implantation may represent a valuable option in certain CHD patients. Patients with CHD and dextrocardia pose a challenge in S-ICD system implantation, and nonstandard device placement may be required.

The placement of a S-ICD system on the right side of the chest in a patient with complex CHD with dextrocardia and advanced heart failure is presented here.

The use of S-ICDs in a CHD population and in particular CHD patients with dextrocardia and right-sided S-ICD implantation is briefly discussed.

2. Case Presentation

The patient is a 26-year-old male with a history of situs inversus totalis, double-outlet right ventricle with a ventricular septal defect, and pulmonary atresia, a type of tetralogy of Fallot (TOF). He underwent multiple corrective surgeries including biventricular repair in 1993 and tricuspid valve repair, residual ventricular septal defect (VSD) closure, and right ventricle (RV) to pulmonary artery (PA) homograft in 1997. Subsequently, he underwent a redo replacement of the pulmonary valve utilizing a cryopreserved pulmonary homograft with a size of 29 mm due to dysfunctional pulmonary homograft in 2010. A small residual ventricular septal defect with a restrictive left to right shunt (peak end -systolic gradient of 42 mmHg) and moderate tricuspid regurgitation with a peak gradient of 27 mmHg were

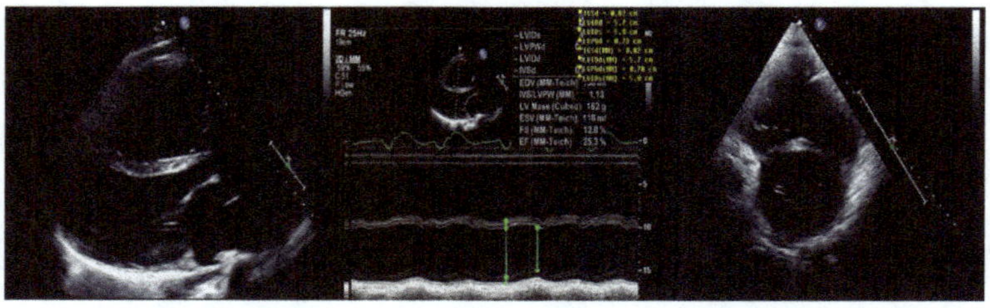

(a) (b) (c)

FIGURE 1: Echocardiogram: (a) parasternal long axis view showing right and left ventricular dilatation, (b) M-mode with left ventricular measurements, and (c) parasternal short axis view at mitral valve level with biventricular enlargement.

noted in the echocardiogram. He had severe biventricular dysfunction (left ventricular ejection fraction < 25%, Figure 1) with frequent heart failure admissions requiring intermittent inotropic support, and he was on the waiting list for heart transplantation.

The right heart catheterization showed low resistance (pulmonary vascular resistance index (PVRI) 1.3 Wood units (WU)), and shunt calculation showed a normal pulmonary flow (Qp) to systemic flow (Qs) ratio (Qp : Qs was 1 : 1). Both the inferior vena cava (IVC) and superior vena cava (SVC) were draining to the left-sided atrium. He also had intra-atrial reentry tachycardia with a ventricular rate of 117 beats per minute in 2012 and had external synchronized cardioversion once. He was considered for an electrophysiology study and ablation of the intra-atrial reentry tachycardia, but there was no significant change in his LVEF after cardioversion, and later on, he went into atrial fibrillation (AF) with a controlled ventricular rate. He was on anticoagulation with warfarin. An electrocardiogram (ECG) showed AF and right bundle branch block with a QRS duration of 164 milliseconds (ms) (Figure 2). He had premature ventricular complexes (PVCs) and runs of nonsustained ventricular tachycardia (VT) up to 5 beats at 187 beats per minute documented in telemetry and 24-hour Holter monitoring (Figure 3).

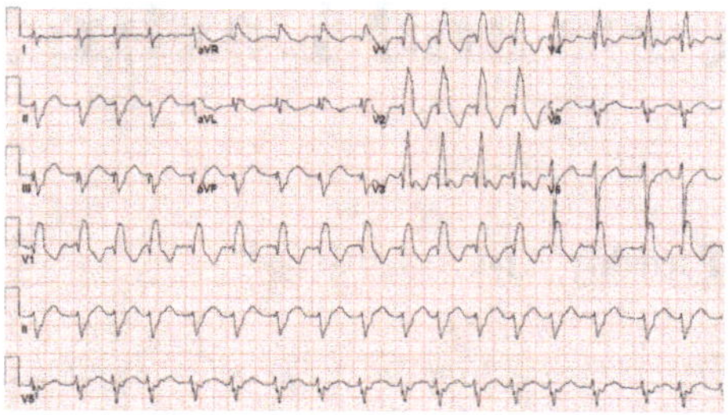

FIGURE 2: 12-lead electrocardiogram showing atrial fibrillation with a ventricular rate of 104 beats per minute and right bundle branch block.

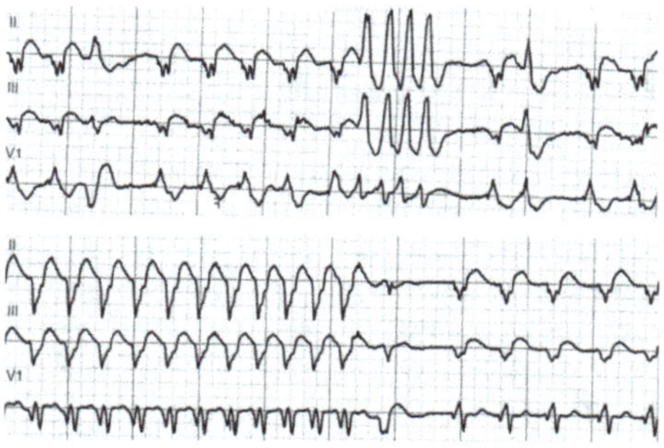

FIGURE 3: Nonsustained ventricular tachycardia on telemetry with two different morphologies.

His other medical problems included acquired perforating dermatosis, folliculitis (hair follicle abscess), and bilateral lower limb varicose veins. His skin swab was positive for a methicillin-resistant *Staphylococcus aureus* (MRSA).

The case was discussed in the cardiology meeting, and it was felt that he has a high risk of ventricular arrhythmias and SCD. It was also decided that S-ICD would be the best option for him considering his anatomy with residual VSD and a high risk of infection due to folliculitis and positive MRSA which may put him at risk of infective endocarditis with a transvenous implantable cardioverter defibrillator (TV-ICD). The S-ICD ECG screening showed only an alternate vector to be acceptable in the supine and sitting positions (Figure 4(a)).

The risks, benefits, and alternative of the procedure were all discussed with the patient including the risk of inappropriate ICD shocks. He agreed to the procedure, and informed consent was obtained.

The patient underwent S-ICD implantation (Emblem S-ICD (model A209) and S-ICD electrode (lead) (model 3401), Boston Scientific, Marlborough, MA) on the right side of the chest in December 2016. The pulse generator was placed at the right midaxillary line between the 5th and 6th intercostal spaces, and the S-ICD electrode was placed on the right parasternal area utilizing the standard intermuscular three-incision technique. Careful attention was made to avoid sternal wire contact with the S-ICD electrode.

The S-ICD analysis at the end of the procedure revealed acceptable three sensing factors (primary, secondary, and alternate) (Figure 4(b)). Defibrillation threshold testing was not performed due to the concern of severe biventricular dysfunction. There was no T-wave oversensing with a limited exercise test on the first-day post device implantation. The chest X-ray showed an acceptable lead and device position (Figure 5). The patient made a good recovery with no complication related to the procedure.

During the follow-up period of 22 months, he had no sustained ventricular arrhythmia, and he did not have any appropriate or inappropriate ICD shocks.

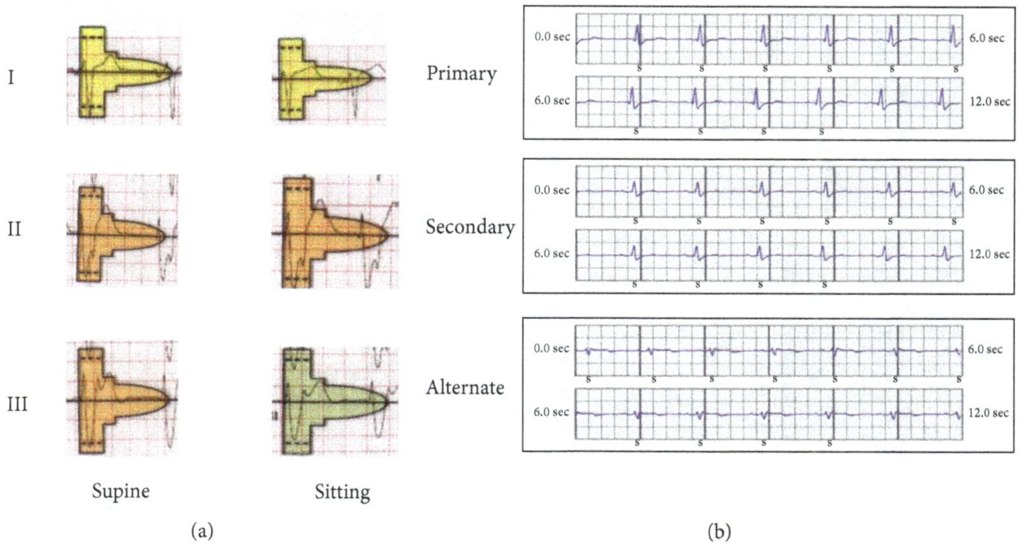

FIGURE 4: (a) Manual ECG screening test showing only lead I (alternate vector) in supine and sitting positions as acceptable vector at 10 mm/mV. (b) Postimplantation S-ECG sensing with gain setting 1X showing adequate sensing in the primary, secondary, and alternate vectors. The primary vector was automatically selected. S: subcutaneous.

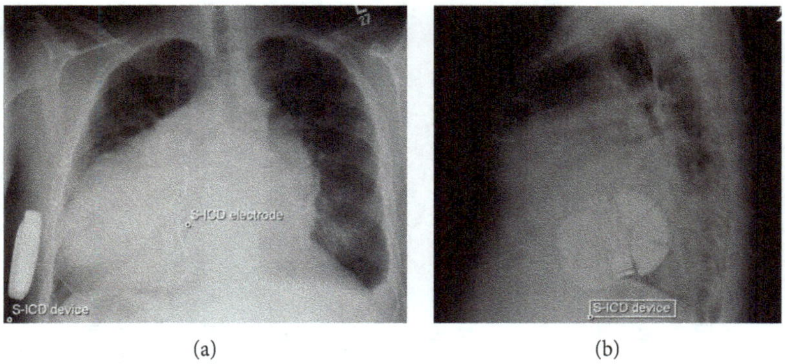

FIGURE 5: Posteroanterior (a) and lateral (b) chest x-rays showing situs inversus totalis, pectus excavatum, sternal wires from previous cardiac surgeries, and the S-ICD device and electrode. Note the presence of cardiomegaly, small left pleural effusion, and basilar atelectasis. S-ICD: subcutaneous implantable cardioverter defibrillator.

3. Discussion

Implantation of a TV-ICD may be challenging or even impossible in patients with CHD due to complex cardiac and vascular anatomy. Furthermore, implantation of transvenous or epicardial systems in these patients is associated with short- and long-term risks. The incidence of venous occlusion, inappropriate shocks, and lead fractures is higher in CHD patients compared to non-CHD patients [4–6].

S-ICD represents an attractive alternative to TV-ICD in CHD patients. However, there is limited data on the S-ICD use in these patients' population. In the EFFORTLESS (Evaluation of Factors Affecting the Clinical Outcome and Cost-Effectiveness) registry, only thirty-three patients (7%) had CHD [7].

The analysis of the CHD cohort in the pooled data from the IDE (investigational device exemption) study and the EFFORTLESS registry including 19 out of 865 patients, after exclusion of patients with hypertrophic cardiomyopathy or cardiac channelopathies (Brugada syndrome, arrythmogenic right ventricular cardiomyopathy, and long QT syndrome), shows that S-ICD is a safe option in CHD patients at risk of SCD [8]. It has similar complication rates for the CHD versus non-CHD groups (10.5 vs. 9.6% [$p = 0.89$]) and similar rate of inappropriate shocks for both groups (10.5% vs. 10.9% [$p = 0.96$]). Successful defibrillation testing at 80 J was comparable for the two groups (100% in CHD vs. 98.5% in non-CHD, $p = 0.62$), but there was a significant difference found with threshold testing at 65 J with lower success in CHD patients (88.2% in CHD vs. 94.6% in non-CHD, $p = 0.26$) [8]. In another study that looked at the long-term experience with S-ICD in teenagers (<20 years of age) and young adults (20 to 26 years of age), thirty-one patients were included: thirteen were teenagers, and eighteen were young adults with a comparison to an age-matched control group with TV-ICDs. However, only four patients with CHD were included in this study. Ventricular arrhythmias were adequately terminated in eight patients (25.8%), and oversensing

Table 1: Comparison of the reported cases with right-sided S-ICD implantation and current case.

Study year, author	Diagnoses	Surgeries/procedures	Reason to implant S-ICD	Device	Follow-up
2015, Waller et al. [13]	A 31-year-old female with TGA, situs inversus with dextrocardia Out-of-hospital VF arrest	Mustard procedure aged 18 months Transvenous dual chamber pacemaker in situ for bradycardia Atrial lead revision due to failure to capture of the original lead	Potential risk of baffle stenosis and superior vena cava obstruction with transvenous system	Boston Scientific SQ-RX S-ICD	—
2014, Ceresnak et al. [14]	A 21-year-old man with a history of dextrocardia, TOF, and Klinefelter syndrome History of VT and easily inducible VF in the EPS.	Multiple cardiac surgeries including placement of a right modified BT shunt in the newborn period, complete repair of TOF at age 1 year, PV replacement with intraoperative cryoablation of the RV/RVOT due to VT, TV annuloplasty, and modified RA maze procedure because of recurrent atrial flutter Left-sided transvenous ICD at the of age 14 years with placement of a subcutaneous coil due to failed DFT Repeat PV replacement, TV replacement for severe TR and PR, RVOT patch augmentation, and partial removal of the transvenous ICD system	Epicardial ICD system could be not implanted due to abdominal compartment syndrome and recurrent fever and the concern for infection	Boston Scientific SQ-RX S-ICD	—
Current case	A 26-year-old male situs inversus totalis, double-outlet RV with a VSD, and pulmonary atresia (a type of TOF). Severe biventricular dysfunction, on the waiting list for heart transplantation Nonsustained VT	Multiple corrective surgeries including biventricular repair in 1993 and TV repair, residual VSD closure, and RV to PA homograft in 1997 redo replacement of the PV utilizing a cryopreserved pulmonary homograft due to dysfunctional pulmonary homograft in 2010	A small residual VSD	Boston Scientific Emblem A209 S-ICD	22 months

BT: Blalock–Taussig; DFT: defibrillation threshold testing; EPS: electrophysiology study; ICD: implantable cardioverter defibrillator; PA: pulmonary artery; PR: pulmonary regurgitation; PV: pulmonary valve; RA: right atrial; RV: right ventricle; RVOT: right ventricular outflow tract; S-ICD: subcutaneous implantable cardioverter defibrillator; TOF: tetralogy of Fallot; TGA: transposition of the great arteries; TV: tricuspid valve; VF: ventricular fibrillation; VSD: ventricular septal defect; VT: ventricular.

was observed in five patients (16.1%), resulting in at least one inappropriate shock. Younger age was an independent predictor of inappropriate shocks in S-ICD (hazard ratio: 0.56; 95% confidence interval: 0.34 to 0.92; $p < 0.05$) [9]. However, the rates of inappropriate shocks were comparable to those in patients with TV-ICDs [9].

Our patient has only one acceptable sensing vector with manual ECG screening. An automated screening tool was not available at the time of device implantation. However, during implantation procedure, all sensing vectors were acceptable. Patients with CHD commonly have conduction system disease with prolonged QRS duration which is a predictor of failed screening [10]. However, there were no significant differences observed in S-ICD eligibility between complex CHD patients and controls in a study that evaluated ECG vector screening in thirty patients with CHD and ten control subjects [11]. The alternate and primary vectors were most suitable in the complex CHD patients (tetralogy of Fallot (TOF), transposition of great arteries (TGA), Fontan circulation, and single ventricle physiology (SVP)). Furthermore, no significant impact of the postural change was observed for S-ICD eligibility compared to morphologically normal heart patients [11].

ECG screening may not be very accurate, and preprocedure screening with an external S-ICD to evaluate sensing at rest and during exercise in all three sensing vectors (algorithm-based screening) was shown in a small study to improve patients' selection and reduce the number of false-positive and false-negative ECG screening of the standard screening method [12]. There is no study with algorithm-based screening in CHD patients.

Effective implantation of S-ICD on the right side of the chest in patients with dextrocardia and CHD was described in two previous case reports [13, 14]. However, our patient has more advanced heart failure compared to the previously reported cases and on the heart transplant list, and we have about two years of follow-up with no problems. Table 1 summarizes the reported cases with right-sided S-ICD and comparison to the current patient. Patients with CHD may require bradycardia or cardiac resynchronization therapy pacing. The S-ICD system can be used in conjunction with a transvenous pacing system if bradycardia pacing is needed [14].

Coordinating S-ICD with a leadless pacemaker is another novel approach that may convert arrhythmias with anti-tachycardia pacing (ATP) instead of a shock and provide bradycardia pacing at the same time. An early animal study with this approach is encouraging. However, studies in humans are still awaited [15, 16].

4. Conclusions

A S-ICD system is an attractive option for CHD patients with a risk of SCD and vascular access problems and intracardiac shunts at a high risk of device infection with a risk of bacteremia and infective endocarditis. In patients with dextrocardia, right-sided S-ICD implantation is feasible and effective.

Consent

Although in this case report the patient's personal identifiable information is sufficiently anonymized, a written informed consent has been obtained from the patient.

References

[1] M. J. Silka, B. G. Hardy, V. D. Menashe, and C. D. Morris, "A population-based prospective evaluation of risk of sudden cardiac death after operation for common congenital heart defects," *Journal of the American College of Cardiology*, vol. 32, no. 1, pp. 245–251, 1998.

[2] A. Ghai, C. Silversides, L. Harris, G. D. Webb, S. C. Siu, and J. Therrien, "Left ventricular dysfunction is a risk factor for sudden cardiac death in adults late after repair of tetralogy of Fallot," *Journal of the American College of Cardiology*, vol. 40, no. 9, pp. 1675–1680, 2002.

[3] J. W. Roos-Hesselink, F. J. Meijboom, S. E. Spitaels et al., "Decline in ventricular function and clinical condition after Mustard repair for transposition of the great arteries (a prospective study of 22–29 years)," *European Heart Journal*, vol. 25, no. 14, pp. 1264–1270, 2004.

[4] C. I. Berul, G. F. van Hare, N. J. Kertesz et al., "Results of a multicenter retrospective implantable cardioverter-defibrillator registry of pediatric and congenital heart disease patients," *Journal of the American College of Cardiology*, vol. 51, no. 17, pp. 1685–1691, 2008.

[5] E. B. Fortescue, C. I. Berul, F. Cecchin, E. P. Walsh, J. K. Triedman, and M. E. Alexander, "Patient, procedural, and hardware factors associated with pacemaker lead failures in pediatrics and congenital heart disease," *Heart Rhythm*, vol. 1, no. 2, pp. 150–159, 2004.

[6] J. D. R. Thomson, M. E. Blackburn, C. van Doorn, A. Nicholls, and K. G. Watterson, "Pacing activity, patient and lead survival over 20 years of permanent epicardial pacing in children," *The Annals of Thoracic Surgery*, vol. 77, no. 4, pp. 1366–1370, 2004.

[7] P. D. Lambiase, C. Barr, D. A. M. J. Theuns et al., "Worldwide experience with a totally subcutaneous implantable defibrillator: early results from the EFFORTLESS S-ICD registry," *European Heart Journal*, vol. 35, no. 25, pp. 1657–1665, 2014.

[8] B. A. D'Souza, A. E. Epstein, F. C. Garcia et al., "Outcomes in patients with congenital heart disease receiving the subcutaneous implantable-cardioverter defibrillator: results from a pooled analysis from the IDE study and the EFFORTLESS S-ICD registry," *JACC: Clinical Electrophysiology*, vol. 2, no. 5, pp. 615–622, 2016.

[9] M. Bettin, R. Larbig, B. Rath et al., "Long-term experience with the subcutaneous implantable cardioverter-defibrillator in teenagers and young adults," *JACC: Clinical Electrophysiology*, vol. 3, no. 13, pp. 1499–1506, 2017.

[10] L. R. A. Olde Nordkamp, J. L. F. Warnaars, K. M. Kooiman et al., "Which patients are not suitable for a subcutaneous ICD: incidence and predictors of failed QRS-T-wave morphology screening," *Journal of Cardiovascular Electrophysiology*, vol. 25, no. 5, pp. 494–499, 2014.

[11] M. Zeb, N. Curzen, G. Veldtman et al., "Potential eligibility of congenital heart disease patients for subcutaneous implantable cardioverter defibrillator based on surface electrocardiogram mapping," *Europace*, vol. 17, no. 7, pp. 1059–1067, 2015.

[12] T. F. Brouwer, K. M. Kooiman, L. R. Olde Nordkamp, V. P. van Halm, and R. E. Knops, "Algorithm-based screening may improve patient selection for the subcutaneous implantable defibrillator," *JACC: Clinical Electrophysiology*, vol. 2, no. 5, pp. 605–614, 2016.

[13] J. R. Waller, A. P. Salmon, and P. R. Roberts, "A right-sided subcutaneous implantable cardioverter defibrillator in a patient with congenital heart disease," *Europace*, vol. 17, no. 1, p. 77, 2014.

[14] S. R. Ceresnak, K. S. Motonaga, I. S. Rogers, and M. N. Viswanathan, "Right-sided subcutaneous implantable cardioverter-defibrillator placement in a patient with dextrocardia, tetralogy of Fallot, and conduction disease," *HeartRhythm Case Reports*, vol. 1, no. 4, pp. 186–189, 2015.

[15] F. V. Y. Tjong, T. F. Brouwer, B. Koop et al., "Acute and 3-month performance of a communicating leadless antitachycardia pacemaker and subcutaneous implantable defibrillator," *JACC: Clinical Electrophysiology*, vol. 3, no. 13, pp. 1487–1498, 2017.

[16] B. Al-Ghamdi, "Subcutaneous implantable cardioverter defibrillators: an overview of implantation techniques and clinical outcomes," *Current Cardiology Reviews*, vol. 15, no. 1, pp. 38–48, 2018.

2

A Case Report of Cardiac Amyloidosis Highlighting the Importance of Strain Analysis

Andres Cordova Sanchez,[1] Ryan Murphy,[2] Suman Rao,[1] Fidel Martinez,[3] Stephanie Bryant,[4] and Debanik Chaudhuri[3]

[1]*Department of Medicine, SUNY Upstate Medical University, Syracuse, NY 13210, USA*
[2]*College of Medicine, SUNY Upstate Medical University, Syracuse, NY 13210, USA*
[3]*Division of Cardiology, SUNY Upstate Medical University, Syracuse, NY 13210, USA*
[4]*Department of Pathology, SUNY Upstate Medical University, Syracuse, NY 13210, USA*

Correspondence should be addressed to Andres Cordova Sanchez; cordovaa@upstate.edu

Academic Editor: Yigit Canga

Cardiac involvement in light-chain (AL) amyloidosis has a high mortality. Once cardiac symptoms are present, it is important to make a diagnosis as there is an inverse relationship between mortality and time of diagnosis. Echocardiography is usually one of the first tests performed. But strain analysis, which can provide important clues, is not routinely performed. This is a case of AL amyloidosis presenting with heart failure in which echocardiographic strain analysis was vital for its diagnosis.

1. Introduction

Amyloidosis consists of the accumulation of misfolded beta-pleated proteins anywhere in the body leading to organ dysfunction. Primary amyloidosis or AL amyloidosis is the result of a plasma cell dyscrasia that produces kappa or lambda monoclonal light chains which are deposited as amyloid fibrils in the body [1].

AL amyloidosis is the most common type of amyloid. It represents approximately half of the diagnosed amyloid disorders. In 2015, the prevalence of AL amyloidosis had more than doubled compared to 2007, with a prevalence of 50.1 cases per million in 2015, with a somewhat similar incidence [2]. Due to chemotherapy advances, survival of AL amyloidosis has increased drastically from 18 months before 2005 to more than 5 years [3].

Symptomatology depends on the affected organ. The most common associated conditions are nephrotic syndrome, heart failure, and peripheral neuropathy. This wide variety of nonspecific symptoms make the diagnosis of AL amyloidosis challenging. Patients are usually diagnosed once severe organ damage is present [4].

Due to the frequent cardiac involvement seen with AL amyloidosis, an echocardiogram is likely to be part of the initial workup. Missing the signs of amyloidosis in this test can result in poor outcomes. Early diagnosis is of vital importance given the inverse relationship between time after the onset of cardiac symptoms and survival [5].

Here, we present a case of a patient who had approximately 4 months of heart failure with preserved ejection fraction and years of polyneuropathy in whom the echocardiogram findings during strain analysis were vital in identifying amyloidosis. Highlighting the importance of cardiac imaging in its diagnosis. The purpose of this case report is to raise awareness about the importance of strain analysis in the early recognition of AL amyloidosis.

2. Case Report

A 72-year-old male is with a past medical history of pulmonary embolism, factor V Leiden deficiency, atrial fibrillation, and a 9-year history of unspecified/undiagnosed muscle weakness and pain of the lower extremities. For 4 months, our patient experienced progressive dyspnea, generalized

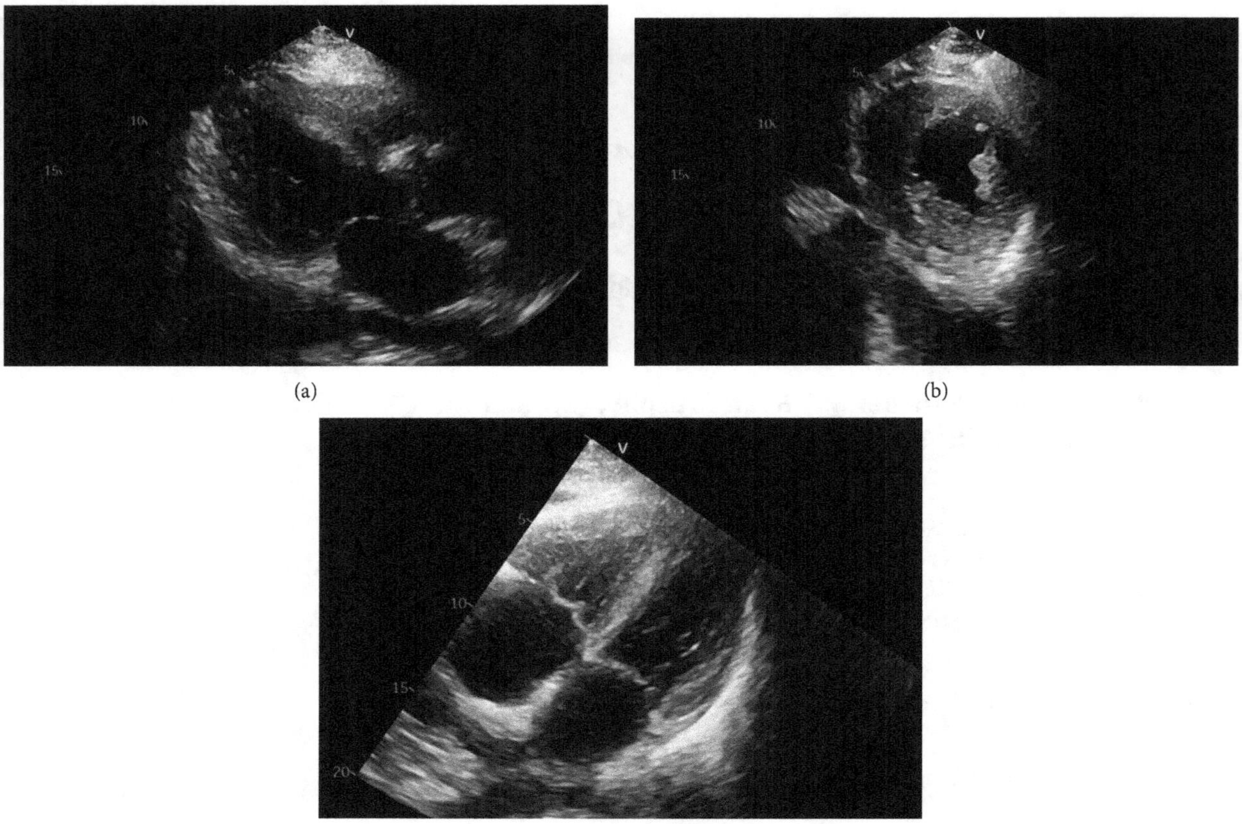

(a) (b) (c)

Figure 1: Previous echocardiogram (a). Parasternal long axis (b). Parasternal short axis (c). Apical four-chamber showing moderate concentric left ventricular hypertrophy, right ventricular dilation, and moderately dilated atria.

edema, bilateral pleural effusions, and recurrent syncope that was diagnosed as heart failure with preserved ejection fraction.

Previous echocardiograms (Figure 1) had shown moderate concentric left ventricular hypertrophy, normal ejection fraction, hypokinesis of basoseptal left ventricular wall, with right ventricular dilation, moderately dilated atria, and pulmonary hypertension at around 40 mmHg; tissue Doppler was not performed. Our patient presented with monthly episodes of dyspnea and syncope which were managed as heart failure exacerbation.

During this admission, he came after another syncopal episode which happened while walking associated with presyncopal nausea, dizziness, and a sensation of heat all over the body. He had a witnessed loss of consciousness of 2 minutes, with no postsyncopal symptoms.

On arrival, he was hemodynamically stable, his laboratory results were significant for a pro-BNP of 13,458 and high sensitivity troponin T of 0.16, the electrocardiogram showed atrial fibrillation with a ventricular rate of 90 beats per minute, and a chest X-ray shows bilateral pleural effusion.

Cardiac catheterization showed normal left ventricular systolic function with an ejection fraction of 55%, without wall motion abnormalities, elevated left ventricular end-diastolic pressure at 25 mmHg, elevated mean pulmonary artery pressure of 37 mmHg, and a capillary wedge pressure of 30 mmHg. There was no significant coronary artery disease.

An echocardiogram was repeated, this time with tissue Doppler and strain analysis (Figures 2 and 3) which was significant for a cherry on top appearance with relative basal sparing, increased E/e' ratio at 23.6, decreased e' at 2 cm/s, severe concentric hypertrophy, and an ejection fraction of 37%.

Cardiac magnetic resonance imaging confirmed an ejection fraction of 37% with diffuse hypokinesis of both ventricles, diffusely thickened left ventricle, and abnormal nulling of the myocardium (Figure 4).

Serum and urine electrophoresis did not show an M spike, and no paraproteins were found in immunofixation. However, increased kappa and lambda free light chains with a decreased kappa/lambda ratio were found on serum-free immunoglobulin analysis. Subsequent bone marrow biopsy showed 4.2% clonal plasma cells. Fat pad and two bone marrow biopsies were negative for Congo red staining. Finally, a cardiac biopsy was positive for amyloid with Congo red staining (Figure 5) and demonstrated AL amyloid on mass spectrometry.

Chemotherapy with daratumumab, bortezomib, cyclophosphamide, and dexamethasone was started, and normalization of kappa and lambda chain levels was achieved after the second cycle.

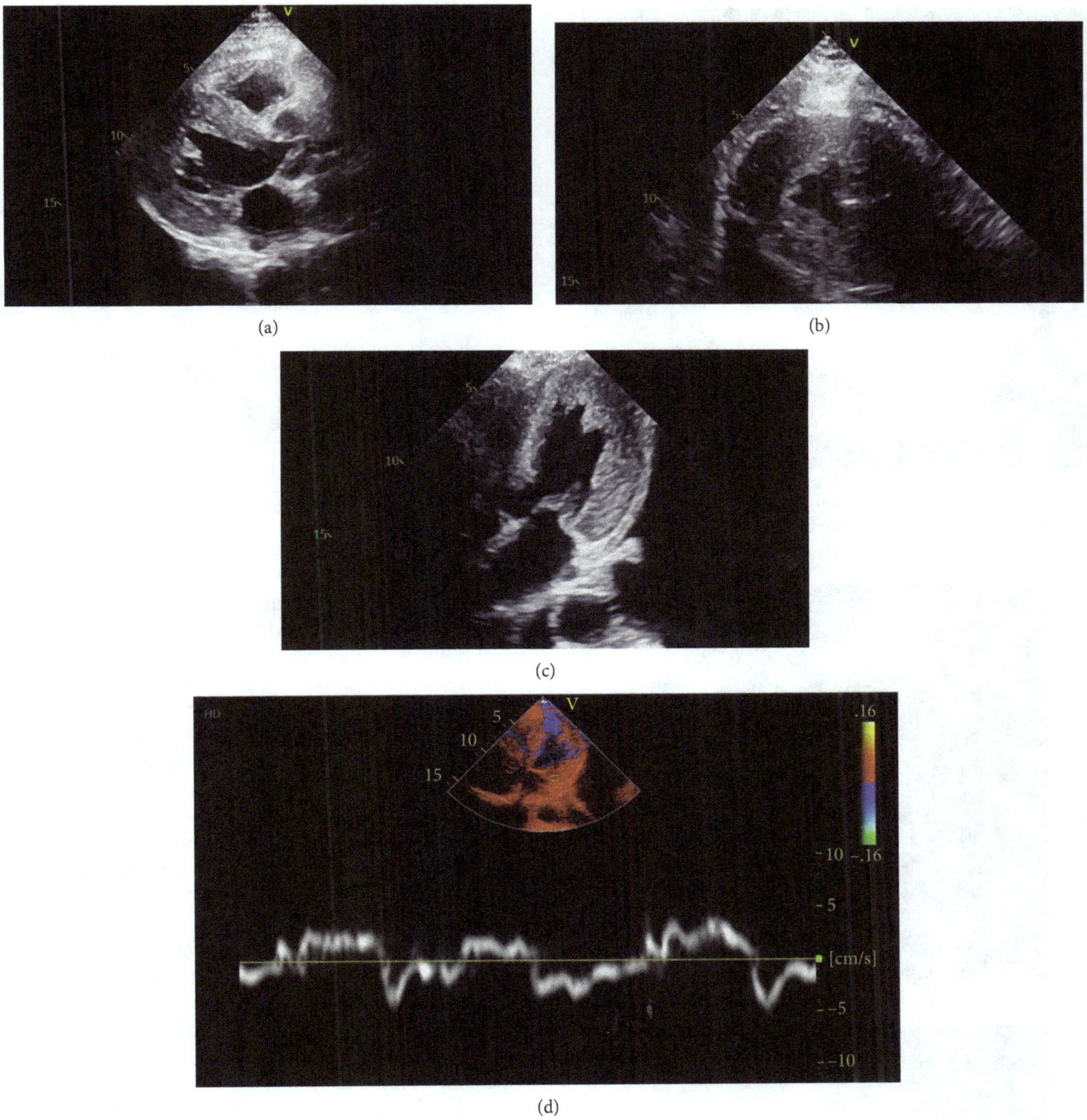

Figure 2: Echocardiogram (a). Parasternal long axis (b). Parasternal short axis (c). Apical two-chamber of left ventricle and (d) tissue Doppler showing severe left ventricular hypertrophy and diastolic dysfunction.

3. Discussion

Cardiac involvement in AL amyloidosis presents with arrhythmias and/or rapidly progressing heart failure. Amyloid fibrils cause stiffening of the heart which explains restrictive physiology found on the echocardiogram. Once a patient develops cardiac symptoms, they usually have a large amount of amyloid in the heart [6]. Amyloid deposit in the atrium causes an irregular surface that makes these patients prone to thrombus formation, irrespective of atrial fibrillation development [6].

Oubari et al. found a significant inverse relationship between time of diagnosis after the onset of cardiac symptoms and 5-year survival. Survival ranged from 79% if diagnosed during the first 6 months to 19% after 19 months [5]. This difference was statistically significant when using a 1-year cutoff, indicating there is a 1-year window for diagnosis after the onset of cardiac symptoms. Heart function in patients with AL amyloidosis does not appear to recover after treatment [7]. The main cause for delayed diagnosis is insufficient physician awareness [5].

Initial workup for AL amyloidosis includes immunofixation, serum and urine electrophoresis, and immunoglobulin free light chains assay. Serum and urine protein electrophoresis can be negative in half of the patients. Immunofixation and serum-free light chain are more sensitive tests. Serum-

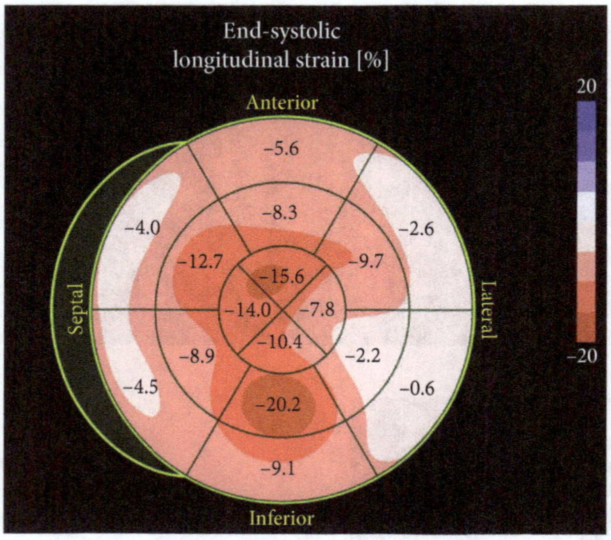

FIGURE 3: Echocardiographic strain analysis showing a relative sparing of the apex compared to the bases.

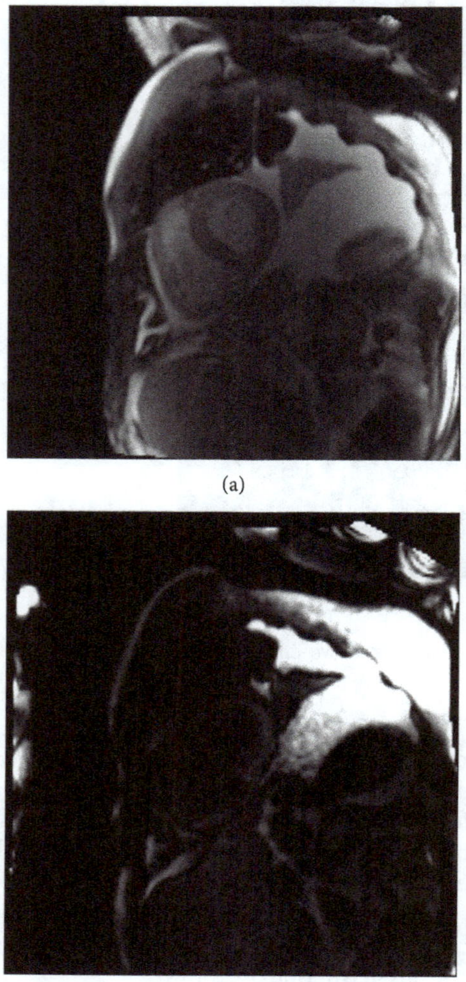

(a)

(b)

FIGURE 4: Cardiac magnetic resonance; (a) left ventricle hypertrophy, (b) abnormal nulling of the myocardium.

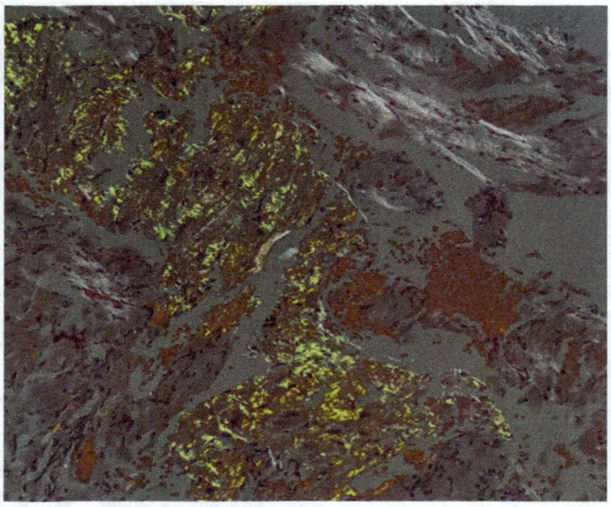

FIGURE 5: Cardiac biopsy with Congo red stain, demonstrating apple green birefringence in polarized light, consistent with amyloidosis.

free light chain immunoglobulin can be seen in >90% of the cases. However, it is important to remember that a negative immunofixation does not rule out the disease [6].

Definitive diagnosis requires identification of amyloid with Congo red staining and identification of the type of misfolded protein [3, 8]. Specific organ biopsy is required only 15% of the time [3]. Fat pad and bone marrow biopsy are diagnostic 67% and 72% of the time, respectively. Cardiac and renal biopsies are positive 100% of the time [9]. In our case, fat pad and two different bone marrow biopsies were negative. However, due to high suspicion, we confirmed the diagnosis of AL amyloidosis with endomyocardial biopsy.

Due to the frequent cardiac involvement, the first signs suggestive of AL amyloidosis will often be found during cardiac workup. Pro-BNP and troponin levels are typically elevated [6]; classically low amplitude QRS is found on electrocardiogram [10].

Echocardiogram will likely be part of the work-up ordered early in the course of the disease. Accurately identifying the echocardiographic signs of amyloidosis can expedite diagnosis and increase life expectancy. Severe ventricular wall thickening, heart failure with preserved ejection fraction, and restrictive pattern on Doppler are typical signs seen in cardiac amyloidosis. In tissue Doppler, E/e' can be >15 due to the elevated filling pressures; transmitral A wave can be absent with atrial involvement [6]. Strain analysis showing relative apical sparing with a "cherry on top" appearance seems to be the most sensitive and specific finding of amyloidosis [11].

Cardiac magnetic resonance is another important diagnostic tool; classic signs of amyloidosis are difficult nulling of the myocardium after gadolinium administration and late gadolinium enhancement in ventricles and atria [6]. In AL amyloidosis, this delayed enhancement is typically global, subendocardial, and does not follow a specific arterial distribution [12].

^{99m}Tectetium pyrophosphate uptake is seen with TTR amyloidosis but not with AL amyloid and can help differentiate between these two [6] but is not a test used when there is high suspicion for AL amyloidosis.

Management of AL amyloidosis consists of medical optimization of the organs involved and chemotherapy to eliminate the plasma cells responsible for the abnormal free light chain in the body.

Our patient had sudden onset, rapidly progressive heart failure, associated with syncope, difficult to control atrial fibrillation, and a long history of undiagnosed lower extremity pain and weakness. Initially, the suspicion for cardiac amyloidosis was low. However, once severe left ventricular hypertrophy, biatrial enlargement, restrictive physiology, and global longitudinal strain with relative apical sparing were found on echocardiogram, our suspicion for it was very high. We consider that his history of undiagnosed muscular weakness was a peripheral neuropathy and was part of the systemic involvement of AL amyloidosis. The diagnosis was confirmed with an endomyocardial biopsy, and chemotherapy was started.

4. Conclusion

This case highlights the importance of echocardiography in the diagnosis of AL amyloidosis. The characteristic result from strain analysis was strongly indicative of cardiac amyloidosis. We believe that tissue Doppler with strain should be included in all patients with heart failure as it has the potential to provide vital information to perform an accurate diagnosis.

References

[1] M. Rosenzweig and H. Landau, "Light chain (AL) amyloidosis: update on diagnosis and management," *Journal of Hematology and Oncology*, vol. 4, no. 1, 2011.

[2] T. P. Quock, T. Yan, E. Chang, S. Guthrie, and M. S. Broder, "Epidemiology of AL amyloidosis: a real-world study using US claims data," *Blood Advances*, vol. 2, no. 10, 2018.

[3] S. Ravichandran, H. J. Lachmann, and A. D. Wechalekar, "Epidemiologic and survival trends in amyloidosis, 1987–2019," *New England Journal of Medicine*, vol. 382, no. 16, pp. 1567-1568, 2020.

[4] S. Law, M. Fontana, and J. D. Gillmore, "Advances in diagnosis and treatment of cardiac and renal amyloidosis," *Cardiology Clinics*, vol. 39, no. 3, pp. 389–402, 2021.

[5] S. Oubari, E. Naser, M. Papathanasiou et al., "Impact of time to diagnosis on Mayo stages, treatment outcome, and survival in patients with AL amyloidosis and cardiac involvement," *European Journal of Haematology*, vol. 107, no. 4, pp. 449–457, 2021.

[6] R. H. Falk, K. M. Alexander, R. Liao, and S. Dorbala, "AL (light-chain) cardiac amyloidosis: a review of diagnosis and therapy," *Journal of the American College of Cardiology*, vol. 68, no. 12, pp. 1323–1341, 2016.

[7] S. Dubrey, L. Mendes, M. Skinner, and R. H. Falk, "Resolution of heart failure in patients with AL amyloidosis," *Annals of Internal Medicine*, vol. 125, no. 6, pp. 481–484, 1996.

[8] G. Merlini, A. Dispenzieri, V. Sanchorawala et al., "Systemic immunoglobulin light chain amyloidosis," *Nature Reviews Disease Primers*, vol. 4, no. 1, 2018.

[9] M. A. Gertz, M. Q. Lacy, A. Dispenzieri et al., "Autologous stem cell transplant for immunoglobulin light chain amyloidosis: a status report," *Leukemia and Lymphoma*, vol. 51, no. 12, pp. 2181–2187, 2010.

[10] R. Mussinelli, F. Salinaro, A. Alogna et al., "Diagnostic and prognostic value of low QRS voltages in cardiac AL amyloidosis," *Annals of Noninvasive Electrocardiology*, vol. 18, no. 3, pp. 271–280, 2013.

[11] D. Phelan, P. Collier, P. Thavendiranathan et al., "Relative apical sparing of longitudinal strain using two-dimensional speckle-tracking echocardiography is both sensitive and specific for the diagnosis of cardiac amyloidosis," *Heart*, vol. 98, no. 19, pp. 1442–1448, 2012.

[12] M. Fontana, R. Chung, P. N. Hawkins, and J. C. Moon, "Cardiovascular magnetic resonance for amyloidosis," *Heart Failure Reviews*, vol. 20, no. 2, pp. 133–144, 2015.

3

The Full Spectrum of Infective Endocarditis

Aniket S. Rali,[1] Mejalli Al-Kofahi,[2] Nilay Patel,[1] Benjamin Wiele,[1] Zubair Shah,[1] and Jayant Nath[1]

[1]*Department of Cardiovascular Diseases, University of Kansas Medical Center, Kansas City, KS, USA*
[2]*Department of Internal Medicine, University of Kansas Medical Center, Kansas City, KS, USA*

Correspondence should be addressed to Jayant Nath; jnath@kumc.edu

Academic Editor: Kathleen Ngu

Over the past five decades, the incidence of intravenous drug use- (IVDU-) associated infective endocarditis (IE) has been on the rise in North America. Classically, IVDU has been thought to affect right-sided valves. However, in recent times a more variable presentation of IVDU-associated IE has been reported. Here, we report a case of a patient with a known history of IVDU who presented with clinical symptoms concerning for right- as well as left-sided endocarditis. In addition, we also discuss what should be considered adequate evaluation for patients with suspected endocarditis, and more specifically, what should be the role of transesophageal echocardiography in patients with IE noted on transthoracic echocardiography.

1. Introduction

Extended intravenous drug use (IVDU) is a known risk factor for infective endocarditis (IE) [1]. Over the last five decades, the incidence of IE-related hospitalizations in North America has continued to increase with increasing IVDU. *Staphylococcus aureus* is the most common causative microorganism [2, 3]. Classically, IVDU has been thought to be the main cause of right-sided valvular IE. However, the incidence of specific valvular site involvement in patients with a history of IVDU is reported to be variable [3, 4]. A prospective, randomized clinical trial noted a higher incidence of right-sided lesions with IVDU. Two out of twenty patients had bilateral involvement [5]. In a sample population of patients with a history of IVDU who suffered death from IE, 16% were noted to have bilateral vegetations [6]. Another retrospective cohort study showed that left-sided lesions were more common than right-sided ones and that concurrent involvement was rare [7]. Older studies reported equal frequencies of right- and left-sided lesions [8].

Here, we report a case of a patient with a known history of IVDU who presented with clinical symptoms concerning for right- as well as left-sided endocarditis.

2. Case Report

A 56-year-old male presented with a 3-day history of altered mental status and weakness. His past medical history was significant for long-standing IVDU, chronic purulent cellulitis of bilateral lower extremities, osteomyelitis of bilateral tibiae, latent tuberculosis treated eleven years prior to presentation, and previously treated hepatitis C infection. The current hospitalization was his second within eight months, as he was previously hospitalized for methicillin-sensitive *Staphylococcus aureus* (MSSA) bacteremia due to cellulitis and osteomyelitis attributed to extensive ongoing intravenous drug injections through lower extremity veins. A transthoracic echocardiogram (TTE) performed during that hospitalization was negative for endocarditis.

During the current admission, the patient's Glasgow coma scale was 13 on presentation. Physical examination was limited by the patient's inability to cooperate, but the patient was noted to have left lower quadrant abdominal tenderness, bilateral lower extremity and right upper extremity wounds, and a large tender sacrocoxal erythematous ulcerated lesion. Presenting vital signs included a blood

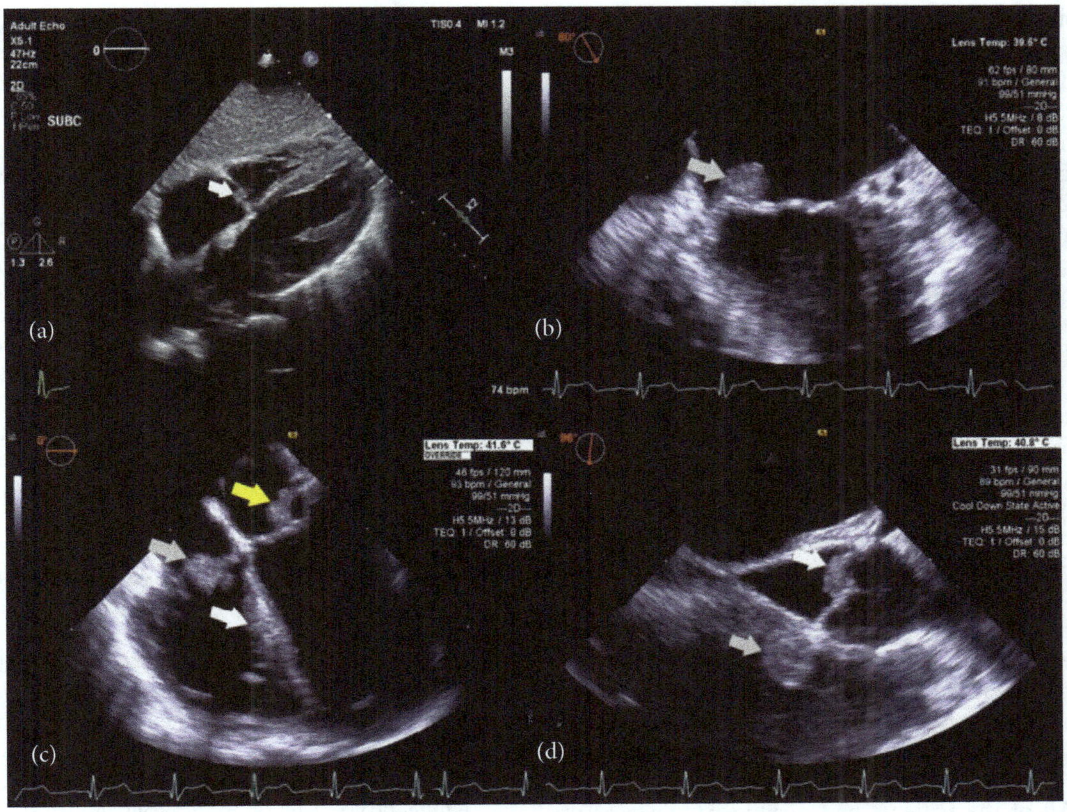

FIGURE 1: (a) Tricuspid valve vegetation on TTE (white arrow). (b) Mitral valve vegetation on TEE (grey arrow). (c) TEE showing mitral valve vegetation (grey arrow), RV outflow tract vegetation (white arrow), and tricuspid valve vegetation (yellow arrow) from left to right. (d) TEE showing RV outflow tract vegetation (grey arrow) and aortic valve vegetation (white arrow) from left to right.

pressure of 140/79 mm Hg, temperature of 36.4 Celsius, heart rate of 114 beats per minute, respiratory rate of 28 breaths per minute, and oxygen saturation of 95% on 3 liters of supplemental oxygen. Laboratory studies were concerning for leukocytosis of 25.6 K/μL (4.5–11.0 K/μL), hemoglobin of 5.7 gm/dL (13.5–16.5 gm/dL), and platelet count of 129 K/μL (150–400 K/μL). Iron studies were suggestive of anemia of chronic inflammation. Other laboratory abnormalities included serum creatinine of 1.25 mg/dL (0.4–1.24 mg/dL), serum sodium of 127 mmol/L (137–147 mmol/L), and albumin of 2.0 g/dL (3.5–5.0 g/dL). Creatine kinase was 1288 U/L (35–232 U/L), lactic acid was 3.1 mmol/L (0.5–2.0 mmol/L), and troponin was 0.18 ng/mL (0–0.05 ng/mL). Blood as well as urine cultures were positive for MSSA. Furthermore, urine drug screening returned positive for cocaine and opioids. Soon after presentation, the patient developed acute hypoxic respiratory failure, hemodynamic shock, and worsening encephalopathy. He was admitted to the medical intensive care unit (MICU) for pressor support and mechanical ventilation.

Pan-computed tomography (CT) scans revealed bilateral multiple pulmonary nodular opacities, some of which were cavitary in nature concerning for multifocal pneumonia, acute hematomas in the abdominal wall musculature, and multiple subacute to chronic left cerebellar and left occipital infarcts, all concerning for septic emboli. These brain lesions were confirmed on subsequent brain MRI. Cultures from the bronchoalveolar lavage were positive for MSSA, negative fungal culture, and acid-fast stain. Further laboratory testing showed negative results in a fourth generation HIV1/2 immunoassay and in T-spot tuberculosis screening.

A transthoracic echocardiogram (TTE) revealed a 0.5 cm mobile mass, consistent with vegetation, in the atrial aspect of the septal leaflet of the tricuspid valve without any valvular dysfunction (Figure 1(a)). Although the other valves were not well visualized on this study, the patient's left ventricular ejection function was noted to be normal. Given concerns for left-sided endocarditis, a transesophageal echocardiogram (TEE) was pursued. TEE showed vegetations on the tricuspid, mitral, and aortic valves, as well as in the right ventricular outflow tract. The tricuspid valve had a 1.0 × 1.0 cm vegetation on the anterior leaflet and a 0.5 × 0.5 cm vegetation on the septal leaflet. The mitral valve had a 1.2 × 1.1 cm vegetation on the P3 segment. There was also a 0.8 cm vegetation on the noncoronary cusp of the aortic valve with only mild aortic insufficiency. The pulmonic valve itself was without vegetations, but there was a 1.1 × 1.1 cm vegetation in the right ventricle outflow tract (RVOT) (Figure 1(b–d)).

The patient continued to receive medical care in the MICU for 2 weeks with a progressive decline in his condition. The patient was deemed to be a poor unstable surgical candidate by the cardiothoracic surgery team, and hence, the patient was transitioned to comfort care measures only after detailed discussions with the family. The patient passed away shortly thereafter from multiorgan failure. An autopsy was declined by the family.

3. Discussion

Our report discusses a rather unusual presentation of infective endocarditis and hence leads into the discussion of an adequate work-up for suspected endocarditis. The American Heart Association (AHA) and the European Society of Cardiology (ECS) both recommend TTE as the modality of choice for the initial evaluation of suspected IE [9, 10]. TTE is a noninvasive diagnostic modality with a reported sensitivity ranging between 44 and 70% for the detection of native valve vegetation and a sensitivity of 50% for the detection of abscesses [11, 12]. The ease of this test makes it the obvious choice for initial evaluation. However, the question begets if further evaluation is recommended if IE is already confirmed on initial TTE.

In our case, multiple bilateral vegetations leading to pulmonic and systemic septic emboli were noted on TEE, only one of which was diagnosed on initial TTE. Those bilateral vegetations ultimately guided the patient's goals of care discussion. TEE is well known to have much greater sensitivity for the detection of infective endocarditis. TEE has greater than 90% sensitivity for native valve vegetation and 90% sensitivity for paravalvular abscess. Specificity on both modalities is similar and is greater than 90% [11, 12].

To the best of our knowledge, only five previous cases have been reported where patients with IVDU had bilateral cardiac IE. All of the patients had positive *Staphylococcus aureus* bacteremia [13–16], except one who had negative blood cultures but vegetations with gram positive cocci on autopsy [17]. Among these cases, left-sided manifestations included paravalvular abscess with aortico-left atrial fistula [13], isolated mitral valve vegetations [14], aortic and mitral valve vegetations [15], extension of tricuspid vegetation through patent foramen ovale [16], and vegetation in the left ventricular outflow tract and mitral valve found on autopsy [17]. Only one prior case had more than two concurrent bilateral vegetations such as ours, with vegetations on pulmonic, tricuspid, and aortic valves with a perforation of the anterior leaflet of the mitral valve [15].

In conclusion, patients with a history of IVDU are at an increased risk for IE that could be right-sided, left-sided, or bilateral. Even though a TEE is logistically harder to obtain in the acute setting, physicians should generally be encouraged to obtain it early in the clinical course to allow for a more thorough evaluation. As was the case with our patient, this additional information can be pivotal in recommending the appropriate plan for care for patients.

Authors' Contributions

Aniket S. Rali and Mejalli Al-Kofahi contributed equally to the manuscript.

References

[1] S. Larney, A. Peacock, B. M. Mathers, M. Hickman, and L. Degenhardt, "A systematic review of injecting-related injury and disease among people who inject drugs," *Drug and Alcohol Dependence*, vol. 171, pp. 39–49, 2017.

[2] S. Pant, N. J. Patel, A. Deshmukh et al., "Trends in infective endocarditis incidence, microbiology, and valve replacement in the United States from 2000 to 2011," *Journal of the American College of Cardiology*, vol. 65, no. 19, pp. 2070–2076, 2015.

[3] R. Moss and B. Munt, *Injection Drug Use and Right Sided Endocarditis*, May 2018, https://www-ncbi-nlm-nih-gov.proxy.kumc.edu/pmc/articles/PMC1767660/pdf/hrt08900577.pdf.

[4] J. San Román, I. Vilacosta, J. Zamorano, C. Almería, and L. Sánchez-Harguindey, "Transesophageal echocardiography in right-sided endocarditis," *Journal of the American College of Cardiology*, vol. 21, no. 5, pp. 1226–1230, 1993.

[5] E. Ruotsalainen, K. Sammalkorpi, J. Laine et al., "Clinical manifestations and outcome in *Staphylococcus aureus* endocarditis among injection drug users and nonaddicts: a prospective study of 74 patients," *BMC Infectious Diseases*, vol. 6, no. 1, 137 pages, 2006.

[6] F. A. Dressler and W. C. Roberts, "Infective endocarditis in opiate addicts: analysis of 80 cases studied at necropsy," *The American Journal of Cardiology*, vol. 63, no. 17, pp. 1240–1257, 1989.

[7] M. K. Graves and L. Soto, "Left-sided endocarditis in parenteral drug abusers: recent experience at a large community hospital," *Southern Medical Journal*, vol. 85, no. 4, pp. 378–380, 1992.

[8] J. Mathew, T. Addai, A. Anand, A. Morrobel, P. Maheshwari, and S. Freels, "Clinical features, site of involvement, bacteriologic findings, and outcome of infective endocarditis in intravenous drug users," *Archives of Internal Medicine*, vol. 155, no. 15, pp. 1641–1648, 1995.

[9] G. Habib, P. Lancellotti, and B. Iung, "2015 ESC guidelines on the management of infective endocarditis: a big step forward for an old disease," *Heart*, vol. 102, no. 13, pp. 992–994, 2016.

[10] L. M. Baddour, W. R. Wilson, A. S. Bayer et al., "Infective endocarditis in adults: diagnosis, antimicrobial therapy, and management of complications," *Circulation*, vol. 132, no. 15, pp. 1435–1486, 2015.

[11] A. Mügge, W. G. Daniel, G. Frank, and P. R. Lichtlen, "Echocardiography in infective endocarditis: reassessment of prognostic implications of vegetation size determined by the transthoracic and the transesophageal approach," *Journal of the American College of Cardiology*, vol. 14, no. 3, pp. 631–638, 1989.

[12] A. Evangelista and M. T. González-Alujas, "Echocardiography in infective endocarditis," *Heart*, vol. 90, no. 6, pp. 614–617, 2004.

[13] F. Seghatol and I. Grinberg, "Left-sided endocarditis in intravenous drug users: a case report and review of the literature," *Echocardiography*, vol. 19, no. 6, pp. 509–511, 2002.

[14] M. Oylumlu, S. Ercan, F. Basanalan, and V. Davutoglu, "Both-sided native valve endocarditis in an intravenous drug misuser," *BML Case Reports*, vol. 2013, article bcr2013201980, 2013.

[15] S. Piran, P. Rampersad, D. Kagal, L. Errett, and H. Leong-Poi, "Extensive fulminant multivalvular infective endocarditis," *JACC: Cardiovascular Imaging*, vol. 2, no. 6, pp. 787–789, 2009.

[16] A. M. Johri, K. A. Kovacs, and H. Kafka, "An unusual case of infective endocarditis: extension of a tricuspid valve vegetation into the left atrium through a patent foramen ovale," *The Canadian Journal of Cardiology*, vol. 25, no. 7, pp. 429–431, 2009.

4

ST-Segment Elevation Myocardial Infarction from Septic Emboli Secondary to Infective Endocarditis by Abiotrophia Defectiva

Bashar Khiatah[1], **Sam Jazayeri**[1], **John Wilde**[1], **Mathew Westfall**[1], **Thomas Q. Kong Jr.**[2] **and Amanda Frugoli**[3]

[1]*Department of Internal Medicine, Community Memorial Hospital, 147 N Brent St, Ventura, CA 93003, USA*
[2]*Ventura Cardiology Consultants, 100 North Brent Street, Suite 301, Ventura, CA 93003, USA*
[3]*Department of GME Internal Medicine, GME Internal Medicine of Community Memorial Hospital of Ventura, 147 N Brent St, Ventura, CA 93003, USA*

Correspondence should be addressed to Bashar Khiatah; bkhiatah@cmhshealth.org

Academic Editor: Ertugrul Ercan

This article showcases a young patient who presented with STEMI secondary to septic emboli due to endocarditis with Abiotrophia Defectiva in the setting of a congenital bicuspid aortic valve. We aim to discuss current considerations for STEMI in young individuals including embolism due to IE, especially in patients with known or suspected congenital heart valve disease.

1. Introduction

Bicuspid aortic valve "BAV" is the most common congenital cardiac defect and is the most common valvular malformation. Several studies have shown that bicuspid aortic valve (BAV) has a higher incidence of IE than the general population; thus, it is currently considered intermediate-risk cardiac conditions for IE. Infective endocarditis "IE" prevalence has been increasing drastically due to expansion of at-risk persons including a generally aging population, an increase in intravenous drug users (IVDU), increased need for hemodialysis, and an increase in cardiac devices. IE can occur on any single valve or, in rarer cases, may include all valves. It has a wide range of complications that can occur, including prolonged bacteremia, valvular regurgitation, or dehiscence leading to pulmonary edema and heart failure, interruption in the cardiac electrical system, development of metastatic infection focus, and cardioembolic events causing MI or stroke. These are some of the most common findings but others can develop such as mycotic aneurysm, perivalvular abscess, and free wall rupture.

In this case report, we present a unique case of a healthy young male sustaining sudden onset STEMI secondary to infectious endocarditis from Abiotrophia Defectiva in the setting of a congenital bicuspid aortic valve.

2. Clinical Case

A 22-year-old healthy male presented to the hospital with complaints of sudden onset substernal chest pain and shortness of breath. Shortly after arrival, ventricular fibrillation occurred and he was defibrillated immediately. ECG (Figure 1) showed ST-segment elevation in the inferior leads, and he was transferred for an urgent angiogram which demonstrated total occlusion of the proximal RCA for which a bare metal stent was placed that successfully restored blood flow (Figures 2(a) and 2(b)).

2.1. Differential Diagnosis. STEMI among the young is often divided into the following categories including atheromatous CAD, nonatheromatous CAD (e.g., Kawasaki), sympathomimetic abuse, spontaneous coronary artery or aortic dissection, hypercoagulable states, and cardioembolism.

2.2. Investigation. ECG showed ST-elevation MI in the distribution area of the RCA with elevated troponin I. He was found to have an elevated leukocyte count, creatinine (minor), and BNP levels with mild normocytic anemia. Other basic labs such as TSH, lipid panel, and urine drug screen were within normal limits. Further history investigation after stabilizing

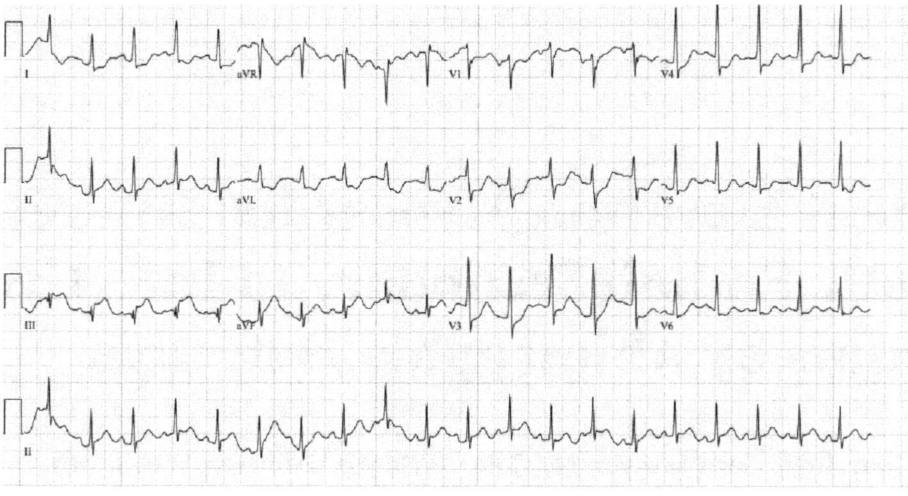

FIGURE 1: Sinus tachycardia with fusion complexes, ST elevation in lead II, III, AVF, ST depression in V2-V4.

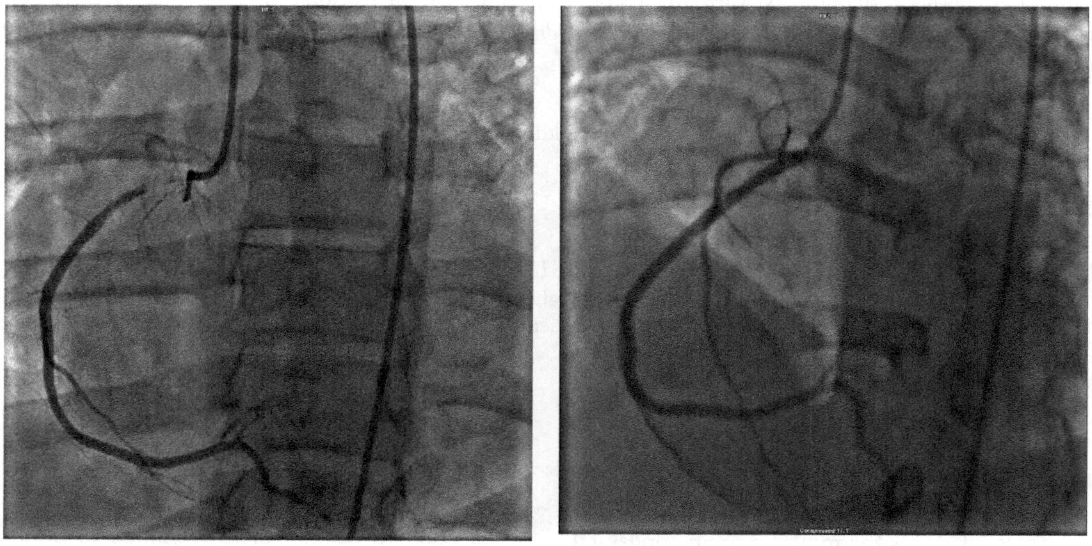

(a) (b)

FIGURE 2: (a) Occlusive septic embolism of the proximal RCA. (b) RCA post stenting.

the patient revealed weight loss, occasional hemoptysis, and night sweats for the last month for which he was prescribed antibiotics for presumed community-acquired pneumonia. He denied any drug abuse, recent invasive surgery, or recent trauma. His family history was negative for early MI or familial hyperlipidemia. A 2D transthoracic echocardiogram demonstrated left atrial enlargement, a bicuspid aortic valve with a large mobile echodensity measuring 0.9×1.7 cm, severe aortic insufficiency, and a malcoaptation of the anterior mitral valve leaflet with moderate to severe eccentric mitral insufficiency and turbulent flow in the left inferior pulmonary vein (Figures 3(a)–3(d)). CTA (Figure 4) was negative for aortic aneurysm or dissection but revealed perihilar pulmonary infiltrates with pulmonary edema, mediastinal adenopathy, and splenomegaly. Blood cultures grew Abiotrophia defectiva from two different bottles. Workup for hypercoagulable disorders was performed and found to be within normal limits. These tests included JAK2, APAS, Factor V Leiden, prothrombin mutation, and DIC panel. Infectious workup for HIV, syphilis, and tuberculosis testing was also negative.

2.3. Management. He was treated with empiric antibiotics pending cultures and experienced refractory heart failure due to severe aortic insufficiency and mitral regurgitation. He subsequently underwent successful aortic and mitral valve replacement with bioprosthetic valves and was discharged with an extended course of IV antimicrobials.

3. Discussion

ST-segment elevation myocardial infarction in very young patients (≤35 years) is most likely related to illicit or prescribed drug use or to hypercoagulable status such as antiphospholipid, nephrotic syndrome, and factor V Leiden.

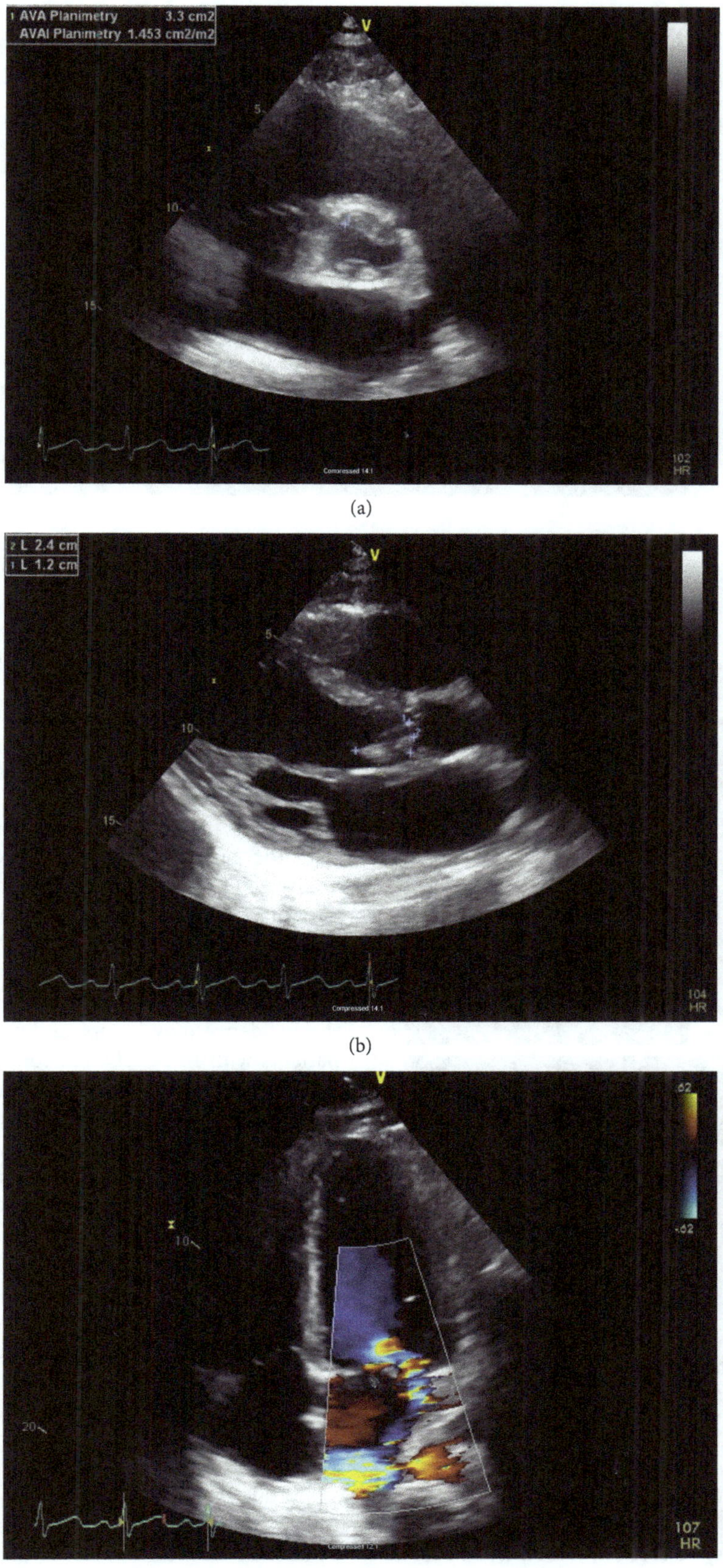

(a)

(b)

(c)

Figure 3: Continued.

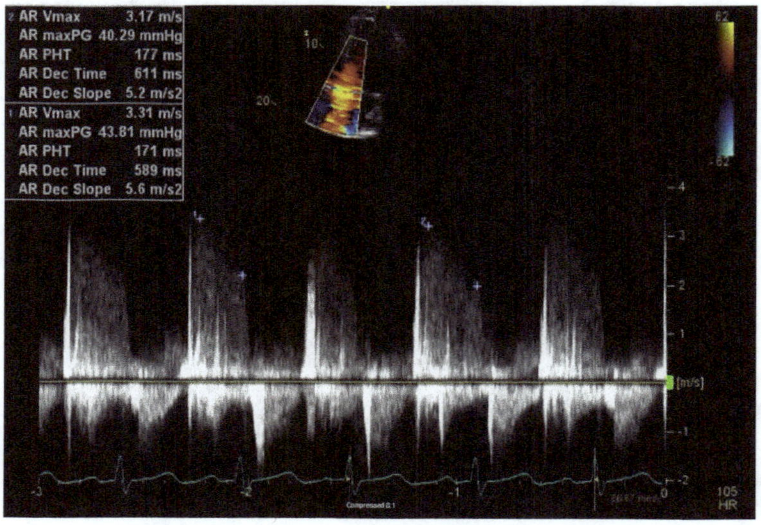

(d)

Figure 3: (a) Bicuspid aortic valve. (b) Vegetation on the Aortic valve. (c) Moderate to severe eccentric mitral regurgitation. (d) Severe Aortic valve insufficiency.

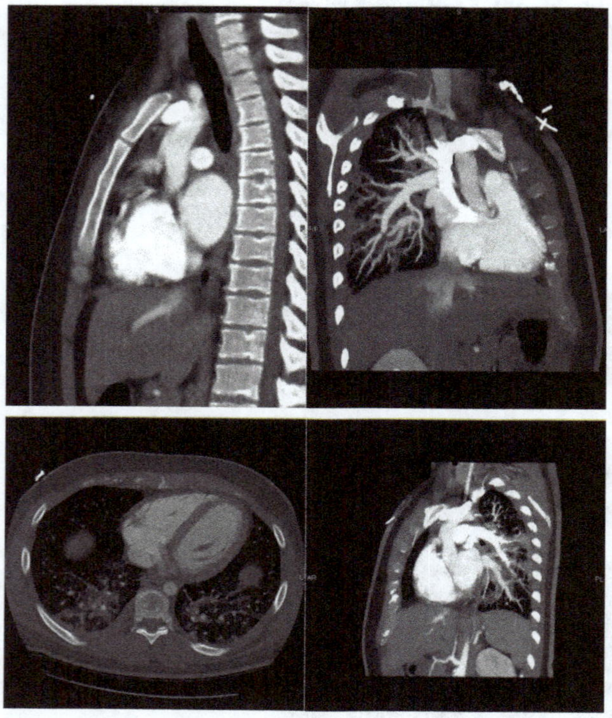

Figure 4: CT Angiography showed perihilar pulmonary infiltrates with ground-glass opacities, mediastinal adenopathy, and splenomegaly.

Smoking, dyslipidemia, and family history remain the most significant traditional risk factors for atheromatous CAD. Spontaneous coronary artery dissection, vasculitis, and septic emboli from an infected valve are also causes of nonatheromatous STEMI. Physicians providing care for such patients are less likely to consider nontraditional cardiac etiologies for myocardial ischemia which may result in delaying diagnosis. The pattern of care and outcomes of the very young with ST-segment elevation myocardial infarction is therefore not well defined [1, 2].

The incidence of IE in the United States is 15 per 100,000 population; however, it is much higher in those with congenital bicuspid aortic heart valves (about one percent of the population) [3]. The incidence of IE among this group is 14 per 10,000 patient-years, which is almost 11 times higher than the general population [4, 5]. Only 0.4% of IE cases are caused by Abiotrophia defectiva, which is a nutritionally variant streptococcus and part of normal oral, urogenital, and intestinal flora [6]. Despite the low incidence rate of IE by Abiotrophia defectiva, it has been reported in the literature in multiple case reports and series demonstrating that the incidence may be uptrending [6]. Notably, 10.5% of all patients with IE by AD had congenital heart disease including bicuspid aortic valve [4]. Among all the patients with IE, only 3% have the complication of acute coronary syndrome [7]. The pathophysiology of ACS in IE could be caused by obstructive coronary embolism, pseudoaneurysm formation, large vegetation blocking the coronary ostia, or compression of the coronary artery by an abscess [7]. It has been reported that a septic embolism of the coronary artery causing a cardioembolic myocardial infarction is a very rare complication of bacterial IE, accounting for <1% of IE complications. Risk factors for embolism in IE include the presence of a mobile vegetation, infection with staphylococci or nonviridans streptococci, vegetation size >10 mm, and previous embolic events [8]. It has been reported that the embolic events were more frequent at early stages [9].

While guidelines for treating infectious endocarditis remain the same [8], the best practices for management of STEMI in IE are not known, and the data is controversial due to the rarity of cases. Although thrombolytic agents have been used successfully in a few cases, the data militate against the use of such agents due to increased risk of severe intracranial hemorrhage, which is thought to be attributed to the high prevalence of silent cerebral infarctions and mycotic aneurysms [10]. Despite limited evidence on the efficacy of PCI, there appears to be a trend in using recanalization as a treatment for STEMI in IE. It has been reported, however, that balloon inflation at the site of the occlusion might cause a displacement of the vegetation and increase the risk of further embolic phenomena and coronary artery mycotic aneurysms [11]. Recently, Nazir S et al. have reported the success rate of each intervention as follows: 56% in balloon angioplasty, 68% in aspiration thrombectomy, and 81% in coronary stenting [10].

Surgery remains indicated in patients who have large vegetations associated with severe valvular disease, those presenting with moderate to severe HF, or in patients with uncontrolled infection. Surgical timing [i.e., urgent versus early (within 48 hours) versus delayed] should be based on individual risk-benefit analysis, with early surgery being strongly indicated when benefits exceed operative risks. Surgery is usually delayed in patients with intracerebral hemorrhage and patients with large cerebral infarction as surgery may pose a significant risk of neurological deterioration and preoperative cerebral bleeding [12].

The choice of replacement with mechanical or tissue prosthesis valves in IE of a native aortic valve remains based on the patient's factors, especially given similar survival and endocarditis recurrence rate in both bioprosthetic and mechanical valves [13]. It has been reported that there is a national trend in using bioprosthetic rather than mechanical valves for aortic valve replacement in IE patients [14]. This is juxtaposed to IE of a native mitral valve, when repair is not an option, replacement with a prosthetic valve is the only choice as there are no established alternatives yet. [13]

In our case, the patient presented with a STEMI requiring urgent angiography and PCI due to occlusive septic embolism of the proximal RCA. Early mitral and aortic valve replacement were indicated due to the large size of the vegetation, severe mitral regurgitation, severe aortic insufficiency, and refractory heart failure in an otherwise young, healthy male with a congenital bicuspid aortic valve.

4. Follow-Up

One month postdischarge and after completing a course of six weeks antibiotics regimen, the patient was recovering well.

5. Conclusion

Increasing the awareness of the differential diagnosis for STEMI in young patients, especially given the increased incidence of septic coronary artery emboli from infective endocarditis, and determining the most appropriate treatment (thrombolysis vs PCI vs surgery), which itself remains a subject of debate, may help to clarify the standard of care in such patients. Furthermore, given the disparity of evidence and practice, further studies to substantiate the use of PCI in STEMI patients during IE is warranted. Lastly, the consideration of normal flora as a cause of infective endocarditis in a healthy young patient should be considered and further evaluation for undiagnosed congenital heart defect should be pursued.

Abbreviations

STEMI: ST-elevation myocardial infarction
ROSC: Return of spontaneous circulation
CAD: Coronary artery disease
ECG: Electrocardiogram
RCA: Right coronary artery
DIC: Diffuse intravascular coagulation
CTA: Computed tomography angiography
ACS: Acute coronary syndrome
PCI: Percutaneous coronary intervention
IE: Infective endocarditis.

Additional Points

Learning Objectives. (i) Review the differential diagnosis for STEMI in very young patients. (ii) Treatment options for STEMI secondary to IE.

References

[1] S. Bangalore, G. C. Fonarow, E. D. Peterson et al., "Age and gender differences in quality of care and outcomes for patients with ST-segment elevation myocardial infarction," *The American Journal of Medicine*, vol. 125, no. 10, pp. 1000–1009, 2012.

[2] M. Egred, G. Viswanathan, and G. K. Davis, "Myocardial infarction in young adults," *Postgraduate Medical Journal*, vol. 81, no. 962, pp. 741–745, 2005.

[3] S. Pant, N. J. Patel, A. Deshmukh et al., "Trends in infective endocarditis incidence, microbiology, and valve replacement in the United States from 2000 to 2011," *Journal of the American College of Cardiology*, vol. 65, no. 19, pp. 2070–2076, 2015.

[4] H. I. Michelena, O. Katan, R. M. Suri, L. M. Baddour, and M. Enriquez-Sarano, "Incidence of infective endocarditis in patients with bicuspid aortic valves in the community," *Mayo Clinic Proceedings*, vol. 91, no. 1, pp. 122-123, 2016.

[5] J. I. E. Hoffman and S. Kaplan, "The incidence of congenital heart disease," *Journal of the American College of Cardiology*, vol. 39, no. 12, pp. 1890–1900, 2002.

[6] A. Téllez, J. Ambrosioni, J. Llopis et al., "Epidemiology, clinical features, and outcome of infective endocarditis due to Abiotrophia species and Granulicatella species: report of 76 cases, 2000-2015," *Clinical Infectious Diseases*, vol. 66, no. 1, pp. 104–111, 2018.

[7] M. C. Manzano, I. Vilacosta, J. A. San Román et al., "Acute Coronary Syndrome in Infective Endocarditis," *Revista Española de Cardiología*, vol. 60, no. 1, pp. 24–31, 2007.

[8] G. Habib, P. Lancellotti, M. J. Antunes et al., "2015 ESC guidelines for the management of infective endocarditis: the task force for the management of infective endocarditis of the European Society of Cardiology (ESC). Endorsed by: European Association for Cardio-Thoracic Surgery (EACTS), the European Association of Nuclear Medicine (EANM)," *European Heart Journal*, vol. 36, no. 44, pp. 3075–3128, 2015.

[9] J. Fabri Jr., V. S. Issa, P. M. A. Pomerantzeff, M. Grinberg, A. C. P. Barretto, and A. J. Mansur, "Time-related distribution, risk factors and prognostic influence of embolism in patients with

left-sided infective endocarditis," *International Journal of Cardiology*, vol. 110, no. 3, pp. 334–339, 2006.

[10] S. Nazir, E. Elgin, R. Loynd, M. Zaman, and A. Donato, "ST-elevation myocardial infarction associated with infective endocarditis," *The American Journal of Cardiology*, vol. 123, no. 8, pp. 1239–1243, 2019.

[11] F. Khan, R. Khakoo, and C. Failinger, "Managing embolic myocardial infarction in infective endocarditis: current options," *The Journal of Infection*, vol. 51, no. 3, pp. e101–e105, 2005.

[12] D. Kang, "*Timing of surgery in infective endocarditisHeart,*" *Heart*, vol. 101, pp. 1786–1791, 2015.

[13] G. B. Pettersson, J. S. Coselli, G. B. Pettersson et al., "2016 The American Association for Thoracic Surgery (AATS) consensus guidelines: Surgical treatment of infective endocarditis: Executive summary," *The Journal of Thoracic and Cardiovascular Surgery*, vol. 153, no. 6, pp. 1241–1258.e29, 2017.

[14] E. B. Savage, P. Saha-Chaudhuri, C. R. Asher, J. M. Brennan, and J. S. Gammie, "Outcomes and prosthesis choice for active aortic valve infective endocarditis: analysis of the Society of Thoracic Surgeons adult cardiac surgery database," *The Annals of Thoracic Surgery*, vol. 98, no. 3, pp. 806–814, 2014.

5

Acute Myocardial Infarction of the Left Main Coronary Artery Presenting with Cardiogenic Shock and Pulmonary Edema during Noncardiac Surgery

Sakae Takenaka,[1] Takao Konishi,[1] Tomoya Sato,[1] Atsushi Tada,[1] Takuya Koizumi,[1] Yoshifumi Mizuguchi,[1] Takahide Kadosaka,[1] Ko Motoi,[1] Yuta Kobayashi,[1] Hirokazu Komoriyama,[1] Yoshiya Kato,[1] Miwa Sarashina,[1] Kazunori Omote,[1] Shingo Tsujinaga,[1] Takuma Sato,[1] Rui Kamada,[1] Kiwamu Kamiya,[1] Hiroyuki Iwano,[1] Toshiyuki Nagai,[1] Tatsuya Orimo,[2] Hirofumi Kamachi,[2] Akinobu Taketomi,[2] and Toshihisa Anzai[1]

[1]*Department of Cardiovascular Medicine, Faculty of Medicine and Graduate School of Medicine, Hokkaido University, Sapporo, Japan*
[2]*Department of Gastroenterological Surgery I, Faculty of Medicine and Graduate School of Medicine, Hokkaido University, Sapporo, Japan*

Correspondence should be addressed to Takao Konishi; takaokonishi0915@gmail.com

Academic Editor: Kathleen Ngu

Acute myocardial infarction (AMI) caused by severe stenosis of left main coronary artery (LMCA) presenting with cardiogenic shock and pulmonary edema during noncardiac surgery is uncommon, but a catastrophic event. A 77-year-old male with cholangiocarcinoma underwent hepatectomy. During the surgery, he presented with cardiogenic shock, which did not respond to infusion administration or vasopressor. A transesophageal echocardiogram revealed anterior, septal, and lateral severe hypokinesia and impaired left ventricular function. Emergent coronary angiogram showed severe stenosis of LMCA. The patient underwent primary percutaneous coronary intervention (PCI) under the support of intra-aortic balloon pump, followed by extracorporeal membrane oxygenation. The chest roentgenogram showed pulmonary edema. Two days after PCI, he successfully underwent hepatectomy and bile duct resection. Early identification of the cause of hemodynamic instability during noncardiac surgery and invasive strategy are important for minimizing the myocardial injury and improving clinical outcomes in AMI of LMCA.

1. Background

Acute myocardial infarction (AMI) of the left main coronary artery (LMCA) is a rare, but critical event [1]. Furthermore, AMI during noncardiac surgery is extremely rare [2]. As the LMCA provides three-fourth of the myocardial blood supply [3], acute stenosis or occlusion of the LMCA without sufficient collateral arteries is often complicated by cardiogenic shock or pulmonary edema. Early diagnosis and reperfusion therapy are associated with improved clinical outcomes in patients with AMI complicated with shock [2]. We report a case of AMI of the LMCA presenting with cardiogenic shock and pulmonary edema during noncardiac surgery.

2. Case Presentation

A 77-year-old man with a history of hypertension and smoking underwent hepatectomy for cholangiocarcinoma. He had no angina symptoms prior to the surgery. In preoperative examination, a twelve-lead electrocardiogram (ECG) was normal, and no wall motion abnormality was detected on echocardiography. During the hepatectomy, his systolic blood pressure dropped to 40 mmHg and was not improved by rapid infusion administration and a vasopressor. He was referred to our department for identification of the cause of his refractory hypotension. On physical examination, he was intubated with body temperature 36.0° C, systemic blood pressure 40/- mmHg, and heart rate 120 bpm. His percutaneous oxygen saturation on artificial respirator (FiO_2 100%) was 90%. Laboratory tests revealed a $7.2 \times 10^3/mm^3$ white blood cell count, $10.4 \times 10^4/mm^3$ platelet count, 10.1 g/dL hemoglobin concentration, 170 IU/L creatine kinase, 22 IU/L MB fraction, 273 ng/L troponin-I, 3.09 μg/mL d-dimer, 1.2 mg/dL total bilirubin, 1757 IU/L AST, 2647 IU/L ALT, 5158 IU/L LDH, and 0.06 mg/dL C-reactive protein serum concentration. The ECG showed ST depression in lead II, and a transesophageal echocardiogram (TEE) revealed severe hypokinesia of the anteroseptal and lateral wall, left ventricular ejection fraction (LVEF) of 20%, and severe mitral regurgitation (Figures 1(a)–1(c); see video 1 and 2 in Supplementary Material available online at https://drive.google.com/file/d/1RdC-7s-jwodX6bldxCBS1Kba2cS1DIjS/view and https://drive.google.com/file/d/1KsyF4WTUgB0X9wdrhtMetjzbgzYSdaSC/view, respectively). After abdominal closure, he was transferred to a near hybrid operation room. Coronary angiography (CAG) revealed severe stenosis of the left main coronary artery (LMCA) with a thrombolysis in myocardial infarction (TIMI) flow of grade II and moderate stenosis of the proximal segment of the left circumflex artery and ramus intermediate branch (Figure 2(a); see video 3 in Supplementary Material available online at https://drive.google.com/file/d/1LO67IkfRkyN1SEi9XlvNDTMhEjtHeG75/view). After the insertion of an intra-aortic balloon pump (IABP), emergent percutaneous coronary intervention (PCI) was performed. An intravascular ultrasound study (IVUS) of the LMCA revealed the presence of an attenuation plaque around the entire circumference of the mid portion of the LMCA (Figure 2(b); see video 4 in Supplementary Material available online at https://drive.google.com/file/d/1Iwo7m03maLjClM5FUgyT8rMfzQH3xj8o/view). The IVUS also showed ulceration and positive remodeling, suggesting an unstable plaque. The minimum lumen area of the LMCA lesion was 1.50 mm^2. After IVUS, a predilatation was performed using a 2.5×15 mm semicompliant balloon. A drug-eluting stent (XIENCE Sierra® 3.0×33 mm, Abbott Vascular, Santa Clara, CA, USA) was implanted between the LMCA and the proximal left anterior descending artery. The final CAG showed optimal dilatation of the LMCA stent and a TIMI flow of grade III (Figure 2(c)). Extracorporeal membrane oxygenation (ECMO) was initiated to improve hypooxygenation due to severe pulmonary edema demonstrated by a chest roentgenogram (Figure 3). After the initiation of ECMO, the right heart catheterization showed that right atrial pressure, mean pulmonary arterial pressure, and pulmonary capillary wedge pressure were 9 mmHg, 24 mmHg, and 14 mmHg, respectively, suggesting the hemodynamic improvement. On the next day, ECMO was extracted due to the improvement of pulmonary edema. As the bile duct resection was not completed during the initial surgery, he had a high risk of intra-abdominal infection, which meant that it might be preferable to resume the hepatic surgery as early as possible. Two days after PCI, he successfully underwent hepatectomy and bile duct resection under the support of an IABP. The peak CK and CK-MB were 4296 IU/L and 438 IU/L, respectively. One month after PCI, LVEF was improved to 64% and mitral regurgitation was ameliorated from severe to mild. He remained free from chest pain or coronary ischemic events during hospitalization on a regimen of aspirin 100 mg/day and clopidogrel 75 mg/day until he died of sepsis three months after the surgery.

3. Discussion

This case illustrates the rare characteristics of AMI of the LMCA complicated by cardiogenic shock and pulmonary edema during a noncardiac surgery, which were successfully treated by PCI under the support of IABP and ECMO. AMI in the LMCA is a rare clinical event, with incidences of 0.9% to 5.2% according to previous studies of patients with AMI undergoing CAG [1, 4]. Among AMI patients with cardiogenic shock undergoing PCI, the prevalence of the LMCA as the culprit vessel is 1.3% to 9.5% [5–7]. Smilowitz et al. reported that perioperative AMI was observed in 84,093 (0.88%) of 9,566,277 patients who underwent noncardiac surgery and more than half of them were associated with vascular or orthopedic surgery [2]. Therefore, intraoperative AMI of the LMCA, complicated by cardiogenic shock and pulmonary edema, during hepatectomy for cholangiocarcinoma is extremely rare.

The etiology of AMI in this case might be due to a thrombotic cause, classified as a type 1 MI, while the dominant mechanism of perioperative acute coronary syndrome is demand ischemia, which is classified as a type 2 MI [8]. Helwani et al. showed that most perioperative AMIs were adjudicated as type 2 MI (73%) compared to type 1 MI (25%) from CAG findings [8]. In this case, the IVUS showed a stenotic lesion with ulceration in the midportion of the LMCA (Figure 2(b)). Persistent pain due to surgical invasion might have caused increased sympathetic nervous system activity, leading to increased cardiac afterload. Bleeding and hypovolemia during surgery could have caused anemia and tachycardia. In addition to these hemodynamic and physiological changes, acute inflammation and a prothrombotic state during surgery might have caused plaque rupture and acute thrombotic events in this case.

Early diagnosis and interventional strategies are needed to improve the prognosis of AMI of the LMCA presenting with cardiogenic shock and/or pulmonary edema. In addition to electrocardiographic monitoring, TEE might be useful, although not routinely used, for detecting myocardial ischemia by identifying regional wall motion abnormalities, even in a noncardiac surgery [9]. Because twelve-lead ECG is often not available due to operative positions or sterile fields, TEE could reveal abnormal wall motion in response to persistent intraoperative hemodynamic instability. Actually, in this case, twelve-lead ECG and transthoracic echocardiography could not be performed because the precordial lead placement and echocardiographic windows were in the proximity of the sterile fields. Smilowitz et al. showed that

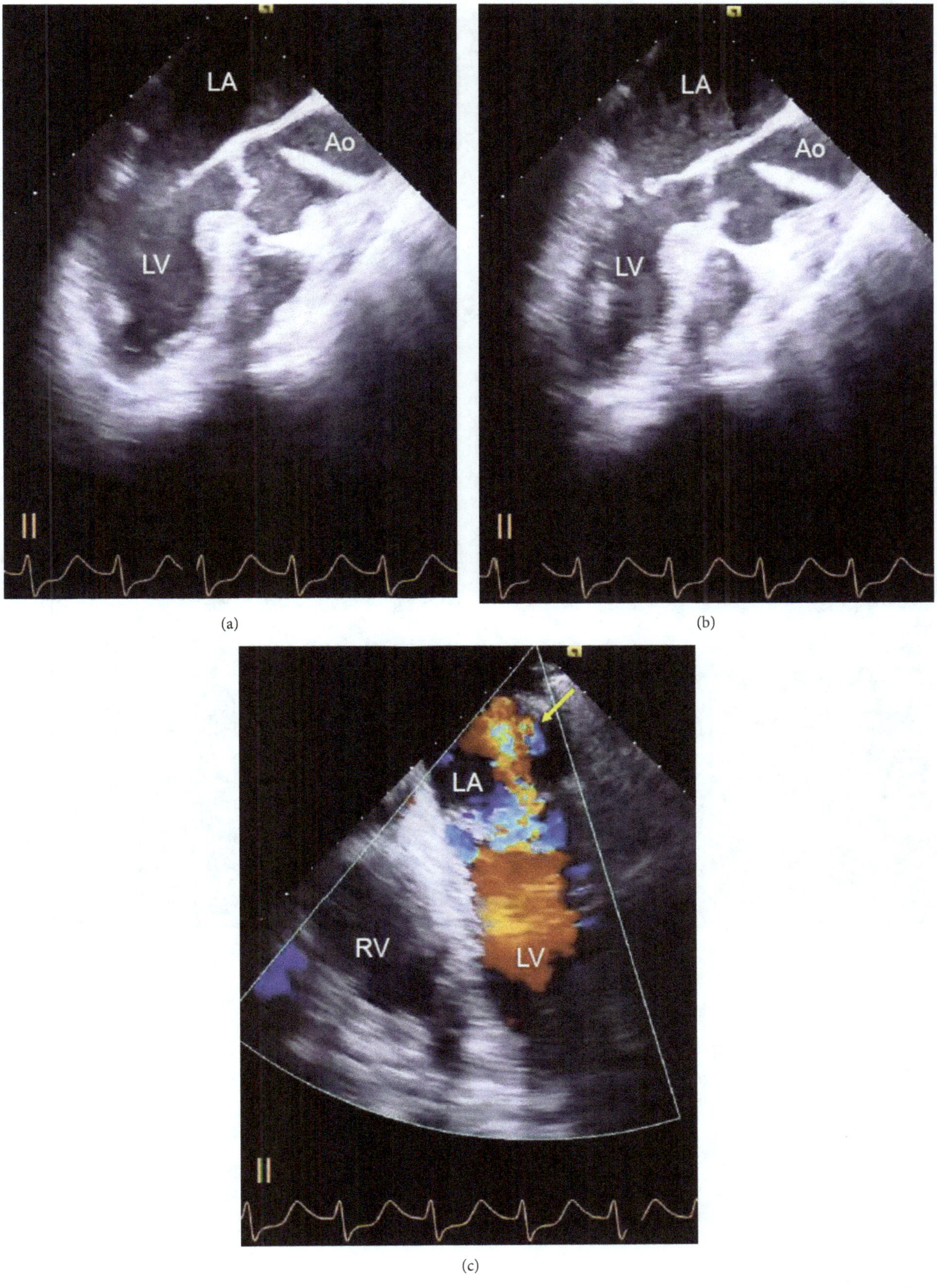

Figure 1: Transesophageal echocardiography. (a, b) Severe hypokinesis of the anteroseptal wall was observed at a 130° angle in a (diastole) and b (systole). Left ventricular ejection fraction was measured as 20%. LA: left atrium; LV: left ventricle; Ao: aorta; RV: right ventricle. (c) Severe mitral regurgitation at a 0° angle (arrow).

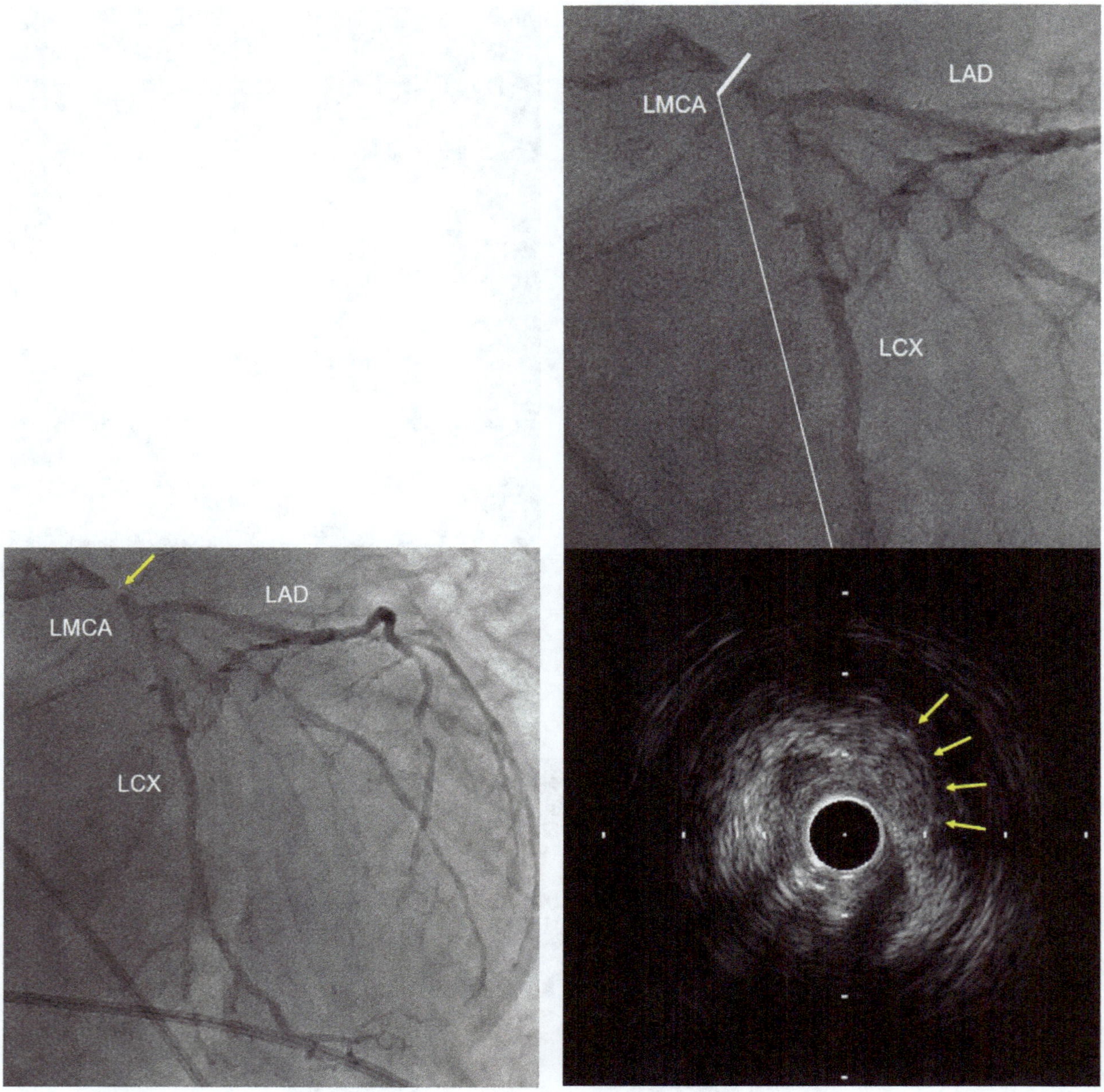

(a) (b)

Figure 2: Continued.

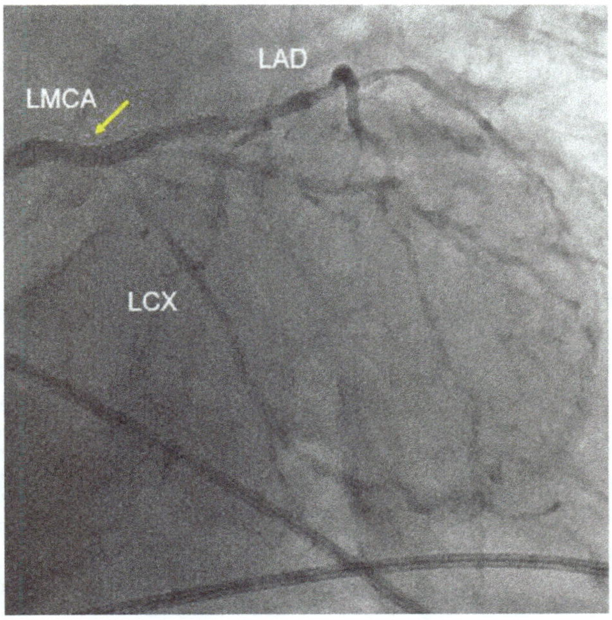

(c)

Figure 2: (a) Emergent coronary angiography. Right anterior oblique caudal view showing a severe stenosis of mid LMCA (arrow). LMCA: left main coronary artery; LAD: left anterior descending artery; LCX: left circumflex artery. (b) Intravascular ultrasound study. The section at the white line showing low attenuation plaque around the entire circumference of the vessel with ulceration (arrows) in the mid LMCA. LMCA: left main coronary artery; LAD: left anterior descending artery; LCX: left circumflex artery. (c) Final coronary angiography. Right anterior oblique caudal view showing no significant LMCA stenosis with grade 3 TIMI flow after stent implantation (arrow). LMCA: left main coronary artery; LAD: left anterior descending artery; LCX: left circumflex artery.

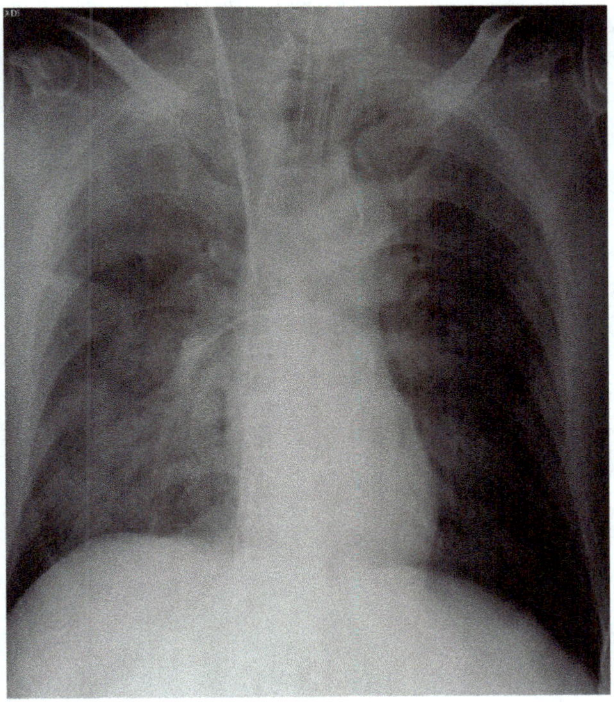

Figure 3: Chest roentgenogram. Chest X-ray showed a severe pulmonary edema.

invasive management, such as PCI or coronary artery bypass grafting, was associated with lower in-hospital mortality than conservative management in a propensity-matched cohort of 34,650 patients with perioperative AMI (8.9% vs. 18.1%, $P < 0.001$) [2]. Furthermore, delays to reperfusion were associated with larger infarct size and 1-year mortality in patients with large anterior myocardial infarction [10]. Therefore, emergent primary PCI in a hybrid operation room, located near the original operation room, might be a reasonable treatment for patients with AMI of LMCA during noncardiac surgery.

A bleeding is one of the major concerns particularly in liver surgery because a lot of blood passes through the liver. Previous studies have shown that a hemorrhage and the need for a transfusion not only adversely affect perioperative outcomes but also the long-term prognosis in patients undergoing a hepatectomy for primary or secondary malignancies [11, 12]. If this case had undergone hepatectomy under the management of ECMO, adequate heparin would have been needed to prevent thrombotic complications within the circuit of ECMO. Due to the systemic anticoagulation, the volume of blood loss and volume of blood transfusions would have been increased during and after the operation. Although the vessel occlusion technique reduces blood loss during the operation, it is directly correlated with a high risk of postoperative hepatic failure [13]. In this case, the LVEF was improved from 20% to 40% two days after the emergent PCI and the roentgenogram also showed the improvement of pulmonary edema. These improvements of hemodynamic and respiratory conditions enabled the resumption of hepatectomy without ECMO. For these reasons, the hepatectomy and bile duct resection were performed two days after emergent PCI.

4. Conclusions

Early identification of the cause of hemodynamic instability during noncardiac surgery and emergent primary PCI might minimize myocardial injury and improve clinical outcomes in AMI of the LMCA.

Acknowledgments

We thank Ms. Kaori Okamoto for her contribution in acquiring the clear IVUS images.

Supplementary Materials

Supplementary 1. Video 1: two-dimensional transesophageal echocardiography, three-chamber view showing a severe hypokinesia of the anteroseptal wall.

Supplementary 2. Video 2: two-dimensional transesophageal echocardiography, four-chamber view showing severe mitral regurgitation.

Supplementary 3. Video 3: emergent coronary angiography, left anterior oblique cranial view showing a severe stenosis of the mid portion of the left main coronary artery.

Supplementary 4. Video 4: intravascular ultrasound study showing low attenuation plaque with ulceration and positive remodeling in the mid portion of the left main coronary artery.

References

[1] A. Pappalardo, M. A. Mamas, F. Imola et al., "Percutaneous coronary intervention of unprotected left main coronary artery disease as culprit lesion in patients with acute myocardial infarction," *JACC. Cardiovascular Interventions*, vol. 4, no. 6, pp. 618–626, 2011.

[2] N. R. Smilowitz, N. Gupta, Y. Guo, J. S. Berger, and S. Bangalore, "Perioperative acute myocardial infarction associated with non-cardiac surgery," *European Heart Journal*, vol. 38, no. 31, pp. 2409–2417, 2017.

[3] J. J. Mahmarian, C. M. Pratt, T. M. Boyce, and M. S. Verani, "The variable extent of jeopardized myocardium in patients with single vessel coronary artery disease: quantification by thallium-201 single photon emission computed tomography," *Journal of the American College of Cardiology*, vol. 17, no. 2, pp. 355–362, 1991.

[4] G. B. Pedrazzini, D. Radovanovic, G. Vassalli et al., "Primary Percutaneous Coronary Intervention for Unprotected Left Main Disease in Patients With Acute ST-Segment Elevation Myocardial Infarction: The AMIS (Acute Myocardial Infarction in Switzerland) Plus Registry Experience," *JACC. Cardiovascular Interventions*, vol. 4, no. 6, pp. 627–633, 2011.

[5] S. A. Wayangankar, S. Bangalore, L. A. McCoy et al., "Temporal trends and outcomes of patients undergoing percutaneous coronary interventions for cardiogenic shock in the setting of acute myocardial infarction: a report from the CathPCI registry," *JACC. Cardiovascular Interventions*, vol. 9, no. 4, pp. 341–351, 2016.

[6] U. Zeymer, K. Werdan, G. Schuler et al., "Editor's Choice-Impact of immediate multivessel percutaneous coronary intervention versus culprit lesion intervention on 1-year outcome in patients with acute myocardial infarction complicated by cardiogenic shock: results of the randomised IABP-SHOCK II trial," *European Heart Journal Acute Cardiovascular Care*, vol. 6, no. 7, pp. 601–609, 2017.

[7] J. S. Park, K. S. Cha, D. S. Lee et al., "Culprit or multivessel revascularisation in ST-elevation myocardial infarction with cardiogenic shock," *Heart*, vol. 101, no. 15, pp. 1225–1232, 2015.

[8] M. A. Helwani, A. Amin, P. Lavigne et al., "Etiology of acute coronary syndrome after noncardiac surgery," *Anesthesiology*, vol. 128, no. 6, pp. 1084–1091, 2018.

[9] A. Fayad and S. K. Shillcutt, "Perioperative transesophageal echocardiography for non-cardiac surgery," *Canadian Journal of Anaesthesia*, vol. 65, no. 4, pp. 381–398, 2018.

[10] A. Guerchicoff, S. J. Brener, A. Maehara et al., "Impact of delay to reperfusion on reperfusion success, infarct size, and clinical outcomes in patients with ST-segment elevation myocardial infarction: the INFUSE-AMI Trial (INFUSE-Anterior Myocardial Infarction)," *JACC. Cardiovascular Interventions*, vol. 7, no. 7, pp. 733–740, 2014.

[11] D. A. Kooby, Y. Fong, A. Suriawinata et al., "Impact of steatosis on perioperative outcome following hepatic resection," *Journal of Gastrointestinal Surgery*, vol. 7, no. 8, pp. 1034–1044, 2003.

[12] D. Gomez, H. Z. Malik, G. K. Bonney et al., "Steatosis predicts postoperative morbidity following hepatic resection for colorectal metastasis," *The British Journal of Surgery*, vol. 94, no. 11, pp. 1395–1402, 2007.

[13] F. Romano, M. Garancini, R. Caprotti et al., "Hepatic resection using a bipolar vessel sealing device: technical and histological analysis," *HPB: The Official Journal of the International Hepato Pancreato Biliary Association*, vol. 9, no. 5, pp. 339–344, 2007.

6

A Unique and Rare Presentation of Adult Congenital Heart Disease: Common Atrium Associated with Coronary Aneurysms and Fistula

Muhammad Shabbir Rawala,[1] Alex Munoz,[2] and Mohammad Hassan Pervaiz[3]

[1]*Department of Internal Medicine, WVU-Charleston Division, Charleston, WV, USA*
[2]*Department of Radiology, University of Kentucky, Louisville, KY, USA*
[3]*Department of Cardiology, WVU-Charleston Division, Charleston, WV, USA*

Correspondence should be addressed to Muhammad Shabbir Rawala; muhammad_rawala@hotmail.com

Academic Editor: Alfredo E. Rodriguez

An atrial septal defect is the second most common congenital heart disease found in adults with a female to male ratio of 4 : 1. However, it is rare to have a complete absence of the interatrial septum (IAS) to be diagnosed in an elderly patient associated with other coexisting anomalies. We present a case of a 60-year-old female presenting with common atrium, coronary arteriovenous fistula, and coronary artery aneurysms. This case highlights rare adult congenital cardiac anomalies and the importance of thorough workup to evaluate for the intracardiac shunt in a patient who has right heart enlargement and development of pulmonary disease in adulthood without a significant history of chronic smoking. A 60-year-old female patient presented with substernal chest pain. The nuclear stress test showed no reversible ischemia; however, right ventricle (RV) dilation was present. The patient underwent further evaluation for RV dilation with a transthoracic echocardiogram that demonstrated a complete absence of IAS and was confirmed by a positive bubble study. The patient had an invasive angiography that showed severely elevated RV pressure. Oxygen saturation in the right atrium was higher than in the inferior vena cava. Hence, an intracardiac shunt with a 10% increase in oxygen saturation was identified. It also identified aneurysmal coronary arteries (measuring 0.8 to 1.0 cm). Cardiac computed tomography angiogram was performed that identified all coronary arteries to be ectatic/aneurysmal measuring up to 8-10 mm, an absence of IAS, and a possible fistula between the distal left anterior descending and a coronary vein. To our knowledge, this is the first-ever presentation of a complete congenital absence of IAS in a patient who has survived into adulthood with the development of severe pulmonary hypertension without Eisenmenger syndrome. It is unclear at this point if surgical treatment to correct the anatomical defect (which would be probably palliative) would be superior to conservative medical therapy. Besides, the presence of coronary arteriovenous fistula would make the decision-making process more complex regarding surgical versus conservative management.

1. Introduction

Single or common atrium (CA) is a rare congenital abnormality arising due to a complete absence of the interatrial septum (IAS). It was initially thought to be an entity accompanied with endocardial cushion defect and was first described by Young and Robinson [1]. The CA can occur as part of skeletal and muscular malformation syndromes such as the Ellis-van Creveld syndrome [2]. There are few isolated cases of CA that have been reported in young adults; however, we report a case of an elderly woman with a single atrium accompanied with coronary arteriovenous fistula and coronary artery aneurysm.

2. Case Report

We present a case of a 60-year-old female who presented to the hospital with complaints of dull substernal chest pain. She had chronic atrial fibrillation, chronic obstructive pulmonary disease with home oxygen, osteoarthritis, and

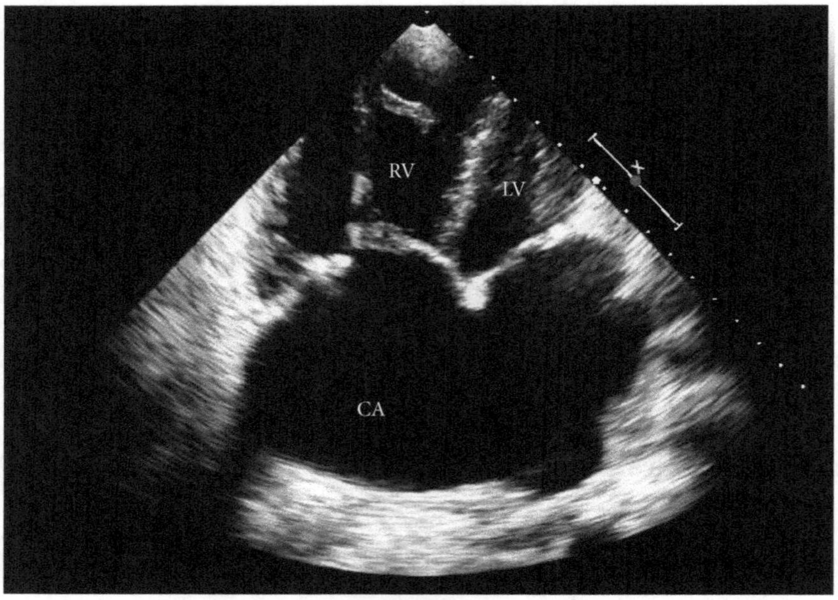

(a) TTE: absence of atrial septum; CA = common atrium; LV = left ventricle; RV = right ventricle

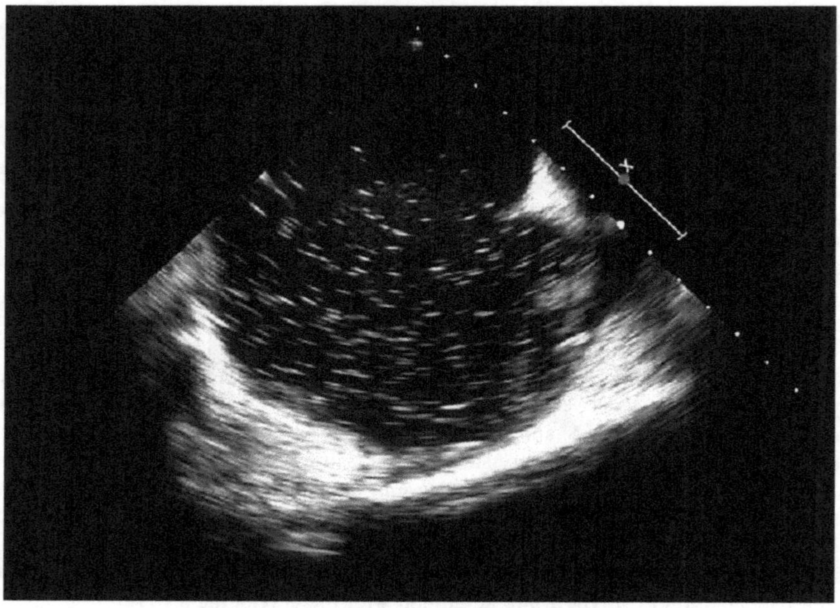

(b) TEE: absence of atrial septum confirmed by positive bubble study

FIGURE 1: Echocardiography images revealing common atrium. (a) TTE: absence of interatrial septum. (b) TEE: positive bubble study.

anxiety disorder as her comorbid conditions. On examination, she did have chronic dyspnea and was on home oxygen. She did not have any cyanosis, palpitations, paroxysmal nocturnal dyspnea, or orthopnea.

She was initially evaluated with a nuclear stress test that did not show any reversible ischemia but dilation of the right ventricle (RV); ejection fraction was identified to be 54%. The patient was further evaluated by a transthoracic echocardiogram (TTE) in order to evaluate the RV dilatation. TTE identified a complete absence of IAS and a CA (Figure 1(a)). The findings were confirmed with a positive bubble study (Figure 1(b)). Transesophageal echocardiogram (TEE) was performed that confirmed the absence of IAS, demonstrated free mixing of color flow, moderate to severe tricuspid regurgitation, normal mitral valve structure, normal left ventricular ejection fraction, and enlarged right atrium (RA) and RV.

The patient was evaluated with cardiac computed tomography angiogram (CCTA) that demonstrated the right coronary artery to be the dominant artery, all coronary arteries to be ectatic/aneurysmal and measuring up to 8-10 mm, a complete absence of IAS, marked dilation of CA and both ventricles, a coronary arteriovenous fistula (CAF) between the distal left anterior descending and coronary sinus, massive dilation of pulmonary arteries, and no mitral or aortic valvular abnormalities; left ventricular ejection fraction was measured to be 59% (Figures 2(a)–2(d)).

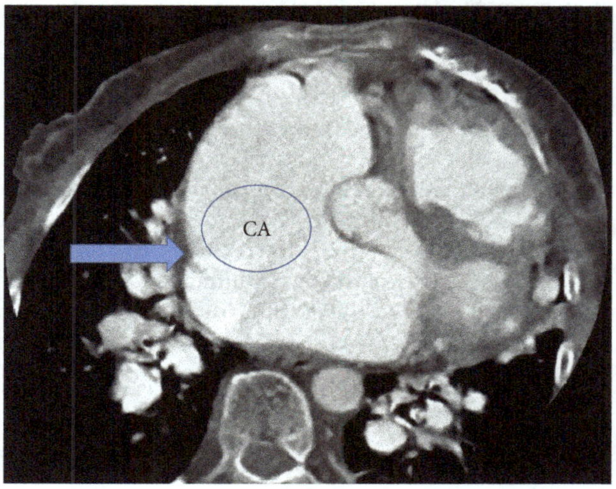

(a) CCTA: absence of atrial septum (arrow); CA = common atrium

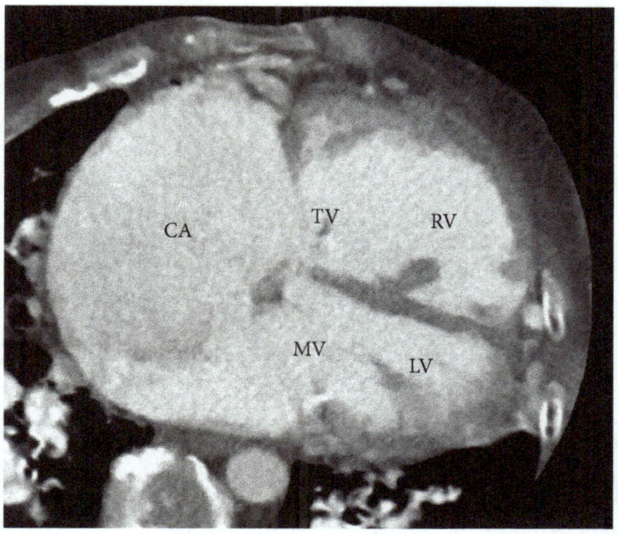

(b) CCTA: absence of IAS, free mixing of blood and contrast present in the right atrium; CA = common atrium; LV = left ventricle; RV = right ventricle; MV = mitral valve; TV = tricuspid valve

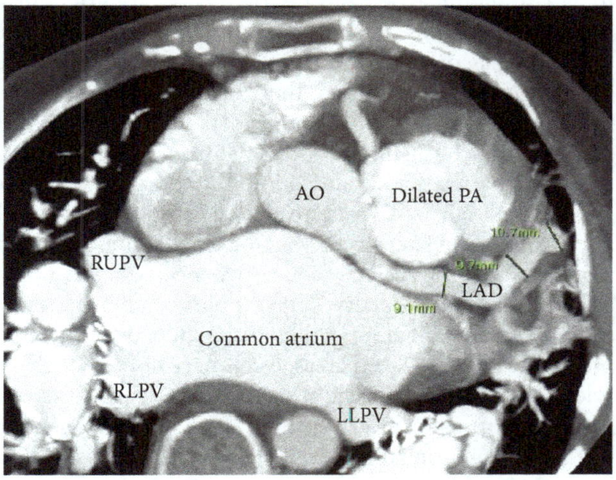

(c) CCTA: common atrium with normal pulmonary connections, dilated pulmonary artery, and ectatic/aneurysmal LAD; AO = aortic orifice; PA = pulmonary artery; LAD = left anterior descending; RUPV = right upper pulmonary vein; RLPV = right lower pulmonary vein; LLPV = left lower pulmonary vein

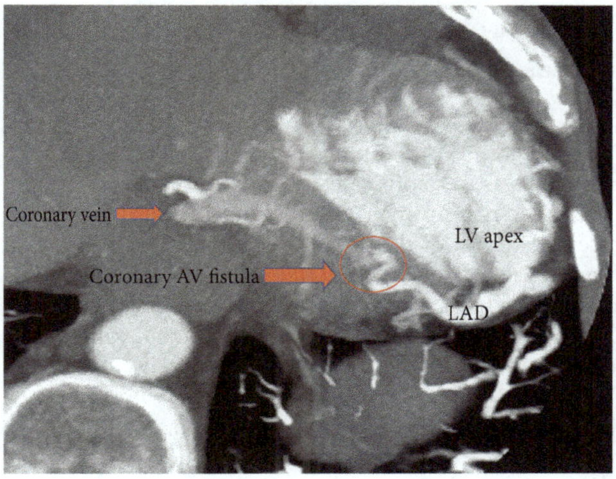

(d) CCTA: identifying fistula between the coronary artery (LAD) and the coronary vein; LV = left ventricle; AV = arteriovenous; LAD = left anterior descending

FIGURE 2: Cardiac computed tomography angiography images. (a) Absence of the atrial septum (arrow). (b) Absence of interatrial septum showing free mixing of blood and contrast present in the atrium. (c) Common atrium with normal pulmonary connections, dilated pulmonary artery, and ectatic/aneurysmal left anterior descending artery. (d) Identifying fistula between the coronary artery and the coronary vein.

The patient underwent an invasive angiography (IA) which demonstrated many abnormal findings. It showed that the patient had coronary artery aneurysms measuring 0.7 cm to 1 cm (Figure 3). IA was instrumental in taking measurements regarding oxygen saturation and pressure at multiple levels identifying a large interatrial shunt with a 10% increase in oxygen saturation from IVC to RA. IA measured RV pressure to be 98/5 mmHg denoting severe pulmonary hypertension, RV end-diastolic pressure at 12 mmHg, mean RA pressure as 10 mmHg, and left ventricular (LV) end-diastolic pressure as 6 mmHg; oxygen saturation in the inferior vena cava (IVC) was 68.3%; oxygen saturation in RA was 79.8%; oxygen saturation in RV was 79.1%, and oxygen saturation in the femoral artery was 88%.

The patient had survived into adulthood with these congenital abnormalities. The patient did not have any muscular, skeletal, ophthalmologic, or vascular abnormalities to signify that her abnormalities were part of any congenital syndrome. Cardiothoracic surgery had been consulted; however, due to the technical implications of surgery, the patient was managed conservatively with no intervention to correct the congenital abnormalities. The patient was not considered for a transcatheter approach of fixing the atrial septal defect as there was a complete absence of the septum. The decision to approach

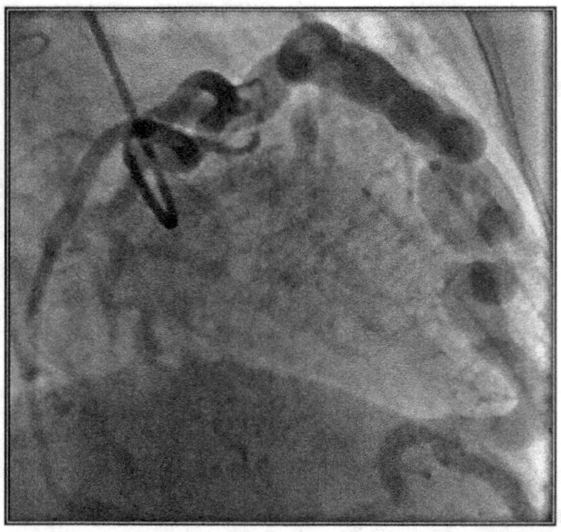

FIGURE 3: Invasive angiography revealing ectatic/aneurysmal arteries.

conservatively also included factors such as the age of the patient, comorbid conditions, and the ability of the patient to tolerate this defect (without Eisenmenger syndrome).

3. Discussion

The CA is a rare entity that has been classified as being part of the endocardial cushion defect. Rastelli et al. [3] described it as (1) complete absence of the atrial septum or its representation by a small strand of tissue present in the cephalad wall of the common chamber, (2) absence of interventricular communication, and (3) an accompanying cleft in the anterior leaflet of the mitral valve. Our case did not demonstrate any abnormality of the mitral valve and was confirmed with TEE.

Levy et al. [4] reported CA as a specific and individual entity. They recommended that the term single or common atrium should be used to denote the condition characterized by (1) complete absence of the atrial septum, (2) absence of malformation of the AV valves, and (3) absence of interventricular communication.

Patients who present with CA usually report symptoms that are related to the large atrial septal defect. They can present with dyspnea on exertion, hypoxia, cyanosis, and developmental delay. Patients mostly are diagnosed during early years; however, few case reports described patients progressing to young adulthood before being diagnosed with CA [5–10]. Echocardiography is usually the first step in diagnosing CA [10]. IA and further investigative methods do help in the evaluation of coexistent congenital abnormalities. Our case had a coronary arteriovenous fistula and coronary artery aneurysms. Our case had survived to 60 years of age before this congenital abnormality was discovered to be the cause of her chronic dyspnea. The patient had not been assessed by echocardiogram or any cardiologist prior to her current presentation for evaluation of intracardiac shunt even though she had developed pulmonary disease in adulthood without a significant history of chronic smoking.

Coronary artery aneurysm (CAA) had been previously reported in 1.4% of postmortem examinations [11]. Due to routine use of IA, more cases of CAA have been diagnosed and reported. The incidence of coronary artery aneurysm has been reported to be 0.3% to 4.9% [12]. Atherosclerotic coronary artery disease accounts to be the etiology in the majority of cases [13]. Most of the patients remain asymptomatic; however, CAA does behave as arterial aneurysms elsewhere in the body and can lead to complications such as rupture, thrombus formation, and embolization. To the best of our knowledge, case reports in the literature have described the rupture of CAA if 3 cm or greater but no major case series or guidelines are established. There is also no significant consensus regarding the treatment of CAA due to the rarity of this condition and associated congenital abnormalities. Some cases in literature recommend antiplatelet along with anticoagulation to prevent thrombus formation whereas others recommend surgical resection and bypass graft surgery to prevent the risk of rupture [14].

CAF is quite rare with an incidence of 0.13% to 0.22% in patients undergoing invasive coronary angiography [15, 16]. Common etiologies of CAF are congenital, trauma, cardiac surgery, and angioplasty. It is thought that fistulas more commonly arise from the right coronary artery or left anterior descending artery [17]. Approximately 40% of coronary fistulas drain to the right ventricle, 25%–48% to the right atrium, 17%–38% to the pulmonary artery, 7% to the coronary sinus, and 3%-8% to the left heart [15–20]. In our case, the fistula was arising from the left anterior descending artery and draining into the coronary sinus. Most of the cases remain asymptomatic during infancy and childhood but present later in adulthood due to complications arising from fistulas such as congestive heart failure (due to arterialization of coronary sinus), pulmonary hypertension, angina, or myocardial infarction arising due to coronary steal phenomenon [18]. The increased coronary flow through a fistulous artery adds to the shear stress which causes atherosclerosis. Atherosclerosis can further give rise to aneurysms further complicating the presentation of CAF. IA usually diagnoses CAF; however, multidimensional CCTA is evolving as a reliable noninvasive method of identifying CAF [21]. There is no clear guideline on the management of CAF; some recommend an observation policy for benign fistulas as there are reports of spontaneous closure; however, it is uncommon. Some suggest surgical therapy in order to prevent fistula-related complications [19].

The overall prognosis of CA and absence of IAS is poor as patients who are unable to receive corrective surgery can develop pulmonary hypertension, hypoxia, heart failure, and arrhythmia. The primary objective of surgery is to reconstruct the atrial septum and correct associated congenital abnormalities. Early diagnosis is crucial as the development of Eisenmenger syndrome is a contraindication to surgery [10, 22].

4. Conclusion

To the best of our knowledge, this is the first-ever case presentation of a complete absence of the atrial septum diagnosed at 60 years and accompanied with congenital malformations such as coronary artery aneurysm and coronary arteriovenous fistula.

The mainstay therapy is surgery to correct the underlying congenital abnormality; however, due to other associated comorbidities and accompanied malformations, surgery can be challenging. As in our case, it is uncertain whether surgery is of any clear benefit versus conservative measures as the patient did survive till 60 years of age without any corrective measures.

This case also highlights the importance of thorough workup to evaluate for the intracardiac shunt in a patient who has right heart enlargement and development of pulmonary disease in adulthood without a significant history of chronic smoking.

Disclosure

This case has been presented at the State ACC Meeting 2014 at Charleston, WV.

Acknowledgments

The case was done at the Department of Internal Medicine, Charleston Area Medical Center–WVU, Charleston, WV.

References

[1] A. H. Young and A. Robinson, "Some malformations of the human heart," *Med Chron*, vol. 47, pp. 96–106, 1907-1908.

[2] D. Gorani, L. Kamberi, and N. Gorani, "Common atrium associated with polydactily and dwartfism in middle age male patient," *Medical Archives*, vol. 65, no. 3, pp. 170–172, 2011.

[3] G. C. Rastelli, S. H. Rahimtoola, P. A. Ongley, and D. C. McGoon, "Common atrium: anatomy, hemodynamics, and surgery," *The Journal of Thoracic and Cardiovascular Surgery*, vol. 55, no. 6, pp. 834–841, 1968.

[4] M. J. Levy, J. Salomon, and B. A. Vidne, "Correction of single and common atrium, with reference to simplified terminology," *Chest*, vol. 66, no. 4, pp. 444–446, 1974.

[5] A. N. Ray and J. Mukhopadhyay, "42 years old male with single atrium," *The Journal of the Association of Physicians of India*, vol. 59, pp. 671–673, 2011.

[6] F. Fu, J. Yang, J. Zhang, and Y. Feng, "Crossed pulmonary arteries associated with single atrium in an adult: a case report," *BMC Cardiovascular Disorders*, vol. 16, no. 1, p. 172, 2016.

[7] S. Hirai, Y. Hamanaka, N. Mitsui, M. Isaka, and T. Mizukami, "Surgical repair of a common atrium in an adult," *Annals of Thoracic and Cardiovascular Surgery*, vol. 9, no. 2, pp. 130–133, 2003.

[8] A. Grimaldi, F. Figini, E. Ammirati et al., "Giant single atrium," *International Journal of Cardiology*, vol. 177, no. 1, pp. e37–e38, 2014.

[9] S. Avula, M. Salazar, N. Alturk, S. Kukafka, S. Ritter, and R. S. Grodman, "Cor triatriatum with single atrium presenting in adulthood," *Echocardiography*, vol. 22, no. 10, pp. 839–843, 2005.

[10] S. Demirelli, S. Firtina, E. Ermis, and S. Inci, "Common atrium: a rare congenital heart anomaly," *Turk Kardiyoloji Dernegi Arsivi-Archives of the Turkish Society of Cardiology*, vol. 43, no. 6, p. 579, 2015.

[11] A. S. Daoud, D. Pankin, H. Tulgan, and R. A. Florentin, "Aneurysms of the coronary artery. Report of ten cases and review of literature," *The American Journal of Cardiology*, vol. 11, no. 2, pp. 228–237, 1963.

[12] R. Vijayanagar, E. Shafii, M. DeSantis, R. S. Waters, and A. Desai, "Surgical treatment of coronary aneurysms with and without rupture," *The Journal of Thoracic and Cardiovascular Surgery*, vol. 107, no. 6, pp. 1532–1535, 1994.

[13] S. Wan, J. L. LeClerc, J. L. Vachiery, and J. L. Vincent, "Cardiac tamponade due to spontaneous rupture of right coronary artery aneurysm," *The Annals of Thoracic Surgery*, vol. 62, no. 2, pp. 575-576, 1996.

[14] S. Kimura, K. Miyamoto, and Y. Ueno, "Cardiac tamponade due to spontaneous rupture of large coronary artery aneurysm," *Asian Cardiovascular and Thoracic Annals*, vol. 14, no. 5, pp. 422–424, 2006.

[15] D. L. C. Cheung, W.-K. Au, H. H. C. Cheung, C. S. W. Chiu, and W.-T. Lee, "Coronary artery fistulas: long-term results of surgical correction," *The Annals of Thoracic Surgery*, vol. 71, no. 1, pp. 190–195, 2001.

[16] C. Gillebert, R. Van Hoof, F. Van de Werf, J. Piessens, and H. De Geest, "Abnormal wall movements of the right ventricle and both atria in patients with pericardial effusion as indicators of cardiac tamponade," *European Heart Journal*, vol. 7, no. 5, pp. 437–443, 1986.

[17] R. M. Gowda, B. C. Vasavada, and I. A. Khan, "Coronary artery fistulas: clinical and therapeutic considerations," *International Journal of Cardiology*, vol. 107, no. 1, pp. 7–10, 2006.

[18] S. C. Urrutia, G. Falaschi, D. A. Ott, and D. A. Cooley, "Surgical management of 56 patients with congenital coronary artery fistulas," *The Annals of Thoracic Surgery*, vol. 35, no. 3, pp. 300–307, 1983.

[19] H. Y. Karagoz, Y. I. Zorlutuna, K. M. Babacan et al., "Congenital coronary artery fistulas. Diagnostic and surgical considerations," *Japanese Heart Journal*, vol. 30, no. 5, pp. 685–694, 1989.

[20] U. Demirkilic, E. Ozal, H. Bingol et al., "Surgical treatment of coronary artery fistulas: 15 years' experience," *Asian Cardiovascular and Thoracic Annals*, vol. 12, no. 2, pp. 133–138, 2004.

[21] J. J. Lim, J. I. Jung, B. Y. Lee, and H. G. Lee, "Prevalence and types of coronary artery fistulas detected with coronary CT angiography," *American Journal of Roentgenology*, vol. 203, no. 3, pp. W237–W243, 2014.

[22] H. Jiang, H. Wang, Z. Wang, H. Zhu, and R. Zhang, "Surgical correction of common atrium without noncardiac congenital anomalies," *Journal of Cardiac Surgery*, vol. 28, no. 5, pp. 580–586, 2013.

7

Heart Block Initiated by Candlenut Ingestion

Osayi Lawani[1] and Mark Winter[2]

[1]*University of Houston College of Medicine/HCA Houston Healthcare, USA*
[2]*Southeast Texas Poison Center, University of Texas Medical Branch, USA*

Correspondence should be addressed to Osayi Lawani; osayimd@gmail.com

Academic Editor: Adrija Hajra

The candlenut tree is a tropical plant that has a vast number of uses which include fertilizer, dye, ink for tattooing, and fuel. The inner seed of the nut is the most utilized portion of the plant and is often sold as a food additive, natural laxative, or a weight loss supplement. Unfortunately, the seed itself is very toxic when consumed whole and in its raw state. Typical symptoms of toxicity include abdominal pain, vomiting, and diarrhea. Rarely, it can cause cardiac dysrhythmias, most commonly bradycardia and atrioventricular heart block. We present a case of a young adult female with no significant past medical history who developed typical symptoms of toxicity, as well as atrioventricular heart block following ingestion of a candlenut. Most documented cases describe complete resolution of gastrointestinal and cardiac symptoms about one week following ingestion; however, treatment while inpatient can consist of inotropes or vasopressor support, intravenous fluid hydration, electrolyte replacement, and antiemetics. Although the mechanism of action remains unclear, this report provides physicians with an understanding of the risks of ingestion and the knowledge of typical management of the toxic effects of the candlenut.

1. Introduction

Aleurites moluccana, otherwise known as the kukui nut or candlenut tree, is a medium-sized tree that is distinctive by its silver-green leaves, and originates from the Indonesian-Malaysian region of Southeast Asia [1]. The plant is now widely found throughout the tropics which includes Hawaii, the Caribbean, and South America [1]. It has a vast number of uses which may depend on its overall local need and cultural significance. Almost every part of the tree (leaves, fruit, and seeds) can be repurposed. Examples of some of its uses include fuel, dye, ink for tattooing, waterproofing, and fertilizer, and it can be found in some traditional Asian medicines [2].

Many of the candlenut tree's uses are found from its nut or the inner seed [1]. The candlenut is typically edible in small quantities when cooked; however, it is generally very toxic when ingested raw [1]. Although the popularity of the nut lies with its use as a weight loss supplement or laxative, symptoms of reported toxicity are commonly abdominal pain, vomiting, and diarrhea [2]. A rare complication that has been seen in those who have eaten a whole raw nut has been cardiac dysrhythmias. The most frequently seen arrhythmias reported were bradycardia and atrioventricular heart block [1]. Due to a chance incidence of morbidity and possible mortality, several countries have banned its use [3]. In this report, we present a case of a young female who was found to have these rare effects shortly following the ingestion of a candlenut.

2. Case History

A 21-year-old female with no significant past medical history presented to the emergency department with complaints of nausea and vomiting. The vomitus was nonbloody and nonbilious, and she stated that she experienced five intermittent episodes for about two hours before coming to the emergency department. Laboratory tests were taken, and results were all within normal range. The patient was administered antiemetics and one liter of intravenous fluids which improved her symptoms, and she was consequently discharged home. The following day, the patient returned to the emergency department with generalized malaise and continued nausea and vomiting that increased in frequency to about every 30 minutes. Additionally, the patient noted a decrease in her heart rate per her smart watch and a new sensation of numbness and tingling in her extremities while she was vomiting.

Vital signs were stable upon arrival. The physical exam was negative for any abnormalities. Laboratory results were again unremarkable. Urinalysis was negative for any illicit drug use. A chest X-ray was also unremarkable. An electrocardiogram (ECG) was performed and showed a first-degree atrioventricular (AV) heart block with a PR interval of 0.354 seconds and a heart rate of 86 beats per minute (Figure 1). The patient stated that the only recent change in her diet was the ingestion of a candlenut the day of her first emergency room visit, which she had obtained from her uncle who had recently returned from Latin America. She intended to take the nut as a weight loss supplement and ingested a whole nut with one can of an energy drink. About 45 minutes afterward she began experiencing nausea, vomiting, and abdominal pain. Poison control was contacted and it was suggested that the patient may have toxicity similar to what is seen with yellow oleander (*Thevetia peruviana*) poisoning. As per poison control, the patient was empirically administered three vials of digoxin immune Fab, one ampule of bicarbonate to increase her venous pH from 7.40 to 7.45, and started on 20% fat emulsion intravenously. The patient was later admitted to the intensive care unit (ICU) for further evaluation.

A peripherally inserted central catheter line was placed in the right arm, and the patient was continued on the infusion of 20% fat emulsion per poison control recommendations. The following day, the patient began to have complaints of dizziness with ambulation, and an abnormal rhythm was noticed on telemetry. A second ECG was performed and noted a new third-degree AV heart block with a ventricular rate of 45 beats per minute (Figure 2). Poison control recommended placement of a pacemaker. The patient was placed on intravenous dopamine, and cardiology was consulted for further evaluation.

It was advised by the poison center that the patient's potassium be kept greater than 4 mmol/L and magnesium greater than 2 mg/dL. A transthoracic echocardiogram was performed and showed no abnormalities. Per poison control recommendations, the fat emulsion therapy was stopped on day three of admission. On day four, the patient had reported improvement in her nausea and vomiting and was also able to be weaned off dopamine as her high-grade heart block resolved. However, she continued to display first-degree heart block with a heart rate of about 60 to 70 beats per minute. On day five, the patient was transferred from the ICU to a telemetry unit for further care and monitoring of her electrolytes. Ultimately, the patient showed marked improvement over the next two days with resolution of her first-degree heart block to normal sinus rhythm; she was then cleared by cardiology and the primary care team for discharge. The patient was instructed to refrain from ingesting candlenuts for weight loss or any other homeopathic use.

3. Discussion

Candlenuts are commonly marketed as a food additive, natural laxative, or a weight loss supplement [3]. Currently, the exact mechanism for its function within the body that leads to toxicity is unknown. The toxic component of the tree lies within the inner most part of the nut, the seed [3]. One known compound contained within the seed is phorbol esters, a chemical that produces a potent inflammatory response [4]. The gastrointestinal and cardiac systems are particularly affected by phorbol as it activates protein kinase C (PKC), which irreversibly inserts itself into the cell membrane of these two organ systems [4]. For the heart, phorbol can produce a negative inotropic effect on the myocytes, depress cell contractility by decreasing sarcolemma calcium influx, and also reduces the number of beta-adrenoceptors and their affinity for beta-agonists [1]. Additionally, activation of PKC can lead to phosphorylation and thus activation of calcium channels that can affect the function of the heart [5]. This could explain why patients may experience arrhythmias after ingestion of an undercooked candlenut.

Reports of cardiac dysfunction following the ingestion of the candlenut are rare; however, when cardiac abnormalities have been documented, they have included bradycardia, first-degree AV heart block, and second-degree AV heart block types 1 and 2 [6]. There are several causes of this disruption of impulse conduction within the heart, which include drug toxicity, hyperkalemia, ischemia, structural heart issues, and excessive vagal stimulation. Differential diagnoses include organophosphate poisoning, autoimmune disease in younger patients, and herbal medication overdose [1]. The abnormal electrical activity can be transient or permanent and can occur within the AV conduction system or originate from dysfunction below the system [6].

With first-degree AV block, the impulse is slowed to where the PR interval is greater than 300 milliseconds and the P-wave may be buried underneath the preceding T-wave [6]. This is a benign condition which usually does not require any treatment. With second-degree Mobitz type 1 AV heart block, the PR interval displays progressive prolongation with every beat until a nonconducted QRS occurs after a P-wave. This rhythm is also typically benign, and asymptomatic patients do not require treatment [6]. Symptomatic individuals will respond to atropine dosing, and, in rare instances, permanent pacemaker placement may be necessary [6]. Higher degrees of AV block have severe dysfunction of the conduction system and typically require urgent hospital admission and a permanent pacemaker [6].

One phenomenon that is also linked to candlenut ingestion is the change in ECG wave morphology. In a few reports, it was found that the ECG of those who consumed the seed displayed a characteristic scooping of the ST segment known as the *digitalis effect*, which is usually seen in patients taking the antiarrhythmic drug digoxin [7]. This was especially noted in adolescents and young adults that had ingested the seed as they were less likely to have taken digoxin [7]. The patient in this case was noted to have these effects and also did not take digoxin (Figures 1 and 2). This may be a result of the potential increased amount of

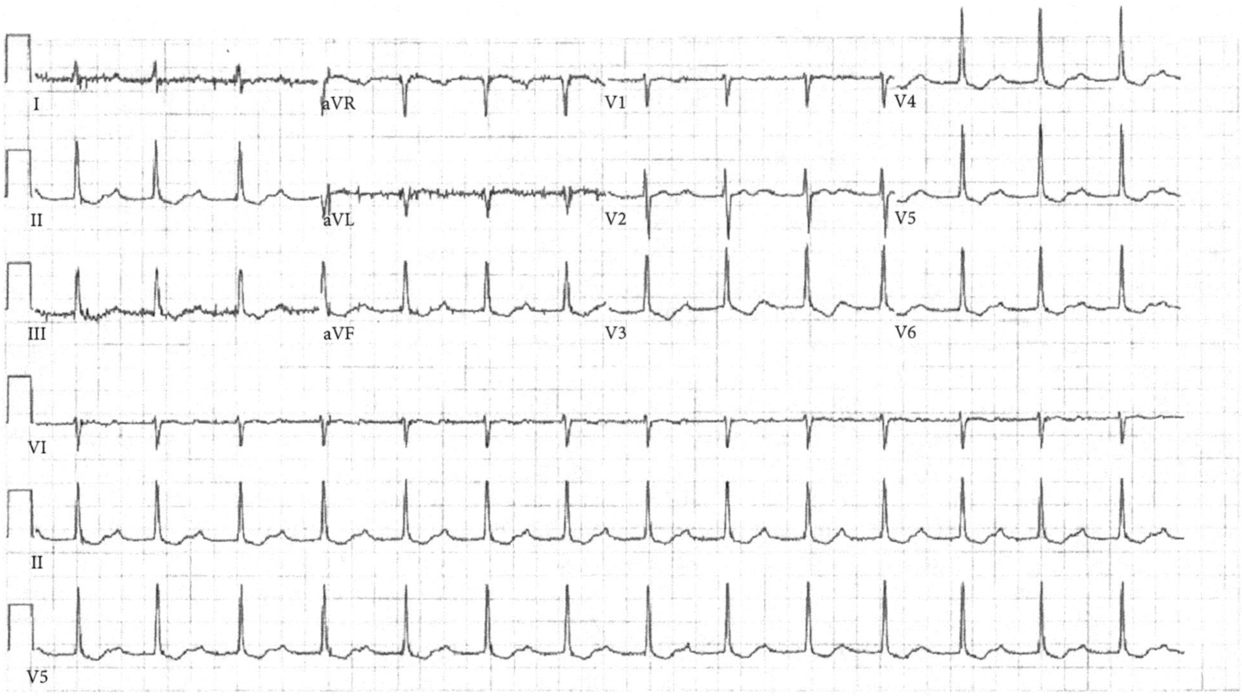

FIGURE 1: An electrocardiogram showing first-degree atrioventricular heart block two days following ingestion of a candlenut. Also noted is a characteristic scooping of the ST segment known as the *digitalis effect*.

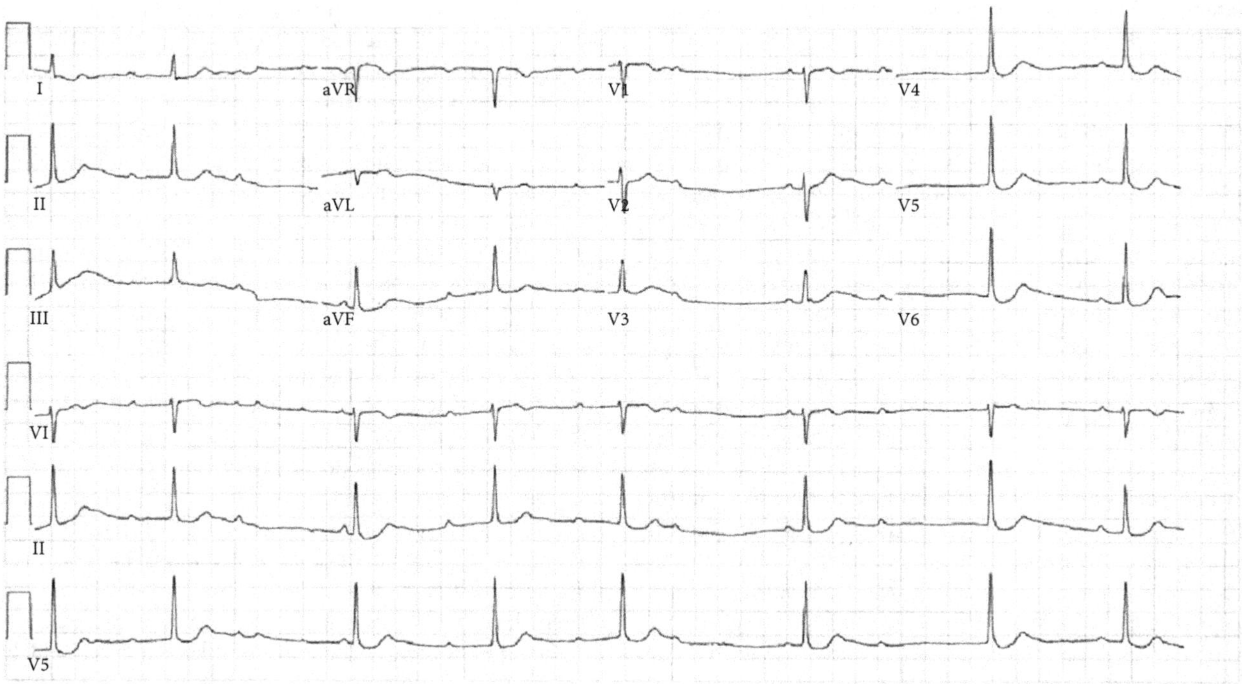

FIGURE 2: An electrocardiogram showing third-degree atrioventricular heart block three days following ingestion of a candlenut.

available calcium in the cardiac myocytes from phorbol's activation of PKC, as candlenuts have not been positively identified as a substance that contains cardiac glycosides. In a few cases, some patients were also noted to have elevated serum digoxin levels after candlenut ingestion, and each patient denied taking or being prescribed digoxin [2, 3]. It is unknown, however, if exposure to candlenuts could cause a falsely elevated serum digoxin level [3]. One paper suggests that possibly some individuals with arrhythmias that were thought to have eaten a candlenut may have mistakenly ingested a yellow oleander seed, which does contain cardiac glycosides [8]. This could be true in some instances; however, in this case, the patient was initially administered three vials of digoxin immune Fab which had no overall effect, and the patient eventually progressed to third-degree AV heart block a day later. Further studies will likely need to be performed to assess this unusual cardiac occurrence.

Although there was no specific sampling done to provide supportive evidence of candlenut ingestion other than the patients' subjective report, there was a temporal association between the reported ingestion and the related gastrointestinal and cardiac signs and symptoms that the patient experienced. The toxicity of this nut has not gone unnoticed. Similar to the ban placed on the herbal supplement ma huang (Ephedra species) by the United States in 2004 due to adverse cardiovascular events, the candlenut has also been banned in several countries, including Argentina, Spain, and Brazil [3, 9]. Unfortunately, the nut continues to be available for sale by small vendors and on select websites found on the Internet [2].

4. Conclusion

The candlenut has been advertised as a weight loss supplement and is sold worldwide [2]. Currently, there are only a limited number of documented cases of candlenut toxicity in humans, especially those leading to cardiovascular events. The recurring theme with all noted cases is that the cardiotoxic effects of AV heart block or bradycardia, as well as gastrointestinal disturbances, resolve on average of about six to seven days after nut ingestion. Treatment involves symptomatic management, which can comprise of inotropes or vasopressor support, intravenous fluid hydration, electrolyte replacement, and antiemetics [1]. Charcoal and gastric lavage may also be indicated in some cases [1]. Although the mechanism of action of the candlenuts' effects remains unclear, this report can provide physicians with an understanding of the risks of ingestion and the knowledge of typical management of the toxic effects of the candlenut.

Authors' Contributions

Osayi Lawani was responsible for the supervision, conceptualization, validation, resources, methodology, data curation, investigation, visualization, creation of the original draft, and review and editing. Mark Winter was responsible for the validation, resources, methodology, data curation, investigation, and review and editing of the original draft.

Acknowledgments

The authors would especially like to thank Dr. Syed Hasan and Cynthia Orpen for their support.

References

[1] M. Richman, T. Tong, R. Moss, A. Dym, M. Connolly, and A. Berman, "Food-induced hypotension and bradycardia: a case report," *Journal of Clinical Toxicology*, vol. 9, p. 417, 2019.

[2] A. E. González-Stuart and J. Ortíz-Rivera, "Toxicity of candlenut seed (*Aleurites moluccanus*), a purported herbal weight loss supplement," *Pharmacologia*, vol. 8, no. 1, pp. 25–31, 2017.

[3] A. L. Koons, L. T. Laubach, K. D. Katz, and G. A. Beauchamp, "Mobitz type II atrioventricular heart block after candlenut ingestion," *The Journal of the American Osteopathic Association*, vol. 120, no. 12, pp. 839–843, 2020.

[4] C. J. Limas and C. Limas, "Phorbol ester and diacylglycerol mediated desensitization of cardiac beta-adrenergic receptors," *Circulation Research*, vol. 57, no. 3, pp. 443–449, 1985.

[5] M. M. Hosey, F. C. Chang, C. M. O'Callahan, and J. Ptasienski, "L-Type calcium channels in cardiac and skeletal muscle," *Annals of the New York Academy of Sciences*, vol. 560, no. 1 Calcium Chann, pp. 27–38, 1989.

[6] A. H. Kashou, A. Goyal, T. Nguyen, and L. Chhabra, "Atrioventricular block. [Updated 2021 Aug 29]," in *StatPearls*, StatPearls Publishing, Treasure Island (FL), 2022, https://www.ncbi.nlm.nih.gov/books/NBK459147/.

[7] D. R. O'Brien, V. Szymczuk, and C. A. Albaro, "Weight loss supplement causing acute heart block in a child," *Cardiology in the Young*, vol. 30, no. 1, pp. 131–133, 2020.

[8] J. Cole and J. Corcoran, "Yellow oleander (Thevetia peruviana), a source of toxic cardiac glycosides, may be substituted for candlenuts (Aleurities moluccana) when taken as a weight-loss supplement," *Cardiology in the Young*, vol. 30, no. 11, pp. 1755-1756, 2020.

[9] P. A. Cohen and E. Ernst, "Safety of herbal supplements: a guide for cardiologists," *Cardiovascular Therapeutics*, vol. 28, 253 pages, 2010.

8

Myocardial Bridging Unmasks as an Acute Coronary Syndrome from Dehydration

Naji Maaliki,[1] Michael Omar,[1] Aleem Azal Ali,[1] Amy Roemer,[1] Jose Ruiz,[2] and Edin Sadic[2]

[1]*Internal Medicine, University of Florida College of Medicine, Jacksonville, USA*
[2]*Cardiology, University of Florida College of Medicine, Jacksonville, USA*

Correspondence should be addressed to Naji Maaliki; naji.maaliki@jax.ufl.edu

Academic Editor: Christopher S. Snyder

A 50-year-old male presented for loss of consciousness. He was initially treated with intravenous epinephrine and fluids, and an electrocardiogram (ECG) displayed an ST-segment elevation in lead aVR with global ST-segment depressions. A subsequent left heart catheterization revealed that the middle segment of the left anterior descending artery (LAD) demonstrated severe stenosis during systole but would become patent during diastole, which was suggestive of myocardial bridging. After stopping the epinephrine and increasing the fluid infusion, the ECG changes rapidly resolved. The patient had later admitted to significant dehydration all day. Myocardial bridging is a congenital anomaly in which a coronary artery segment courses through the myocardium instead of the usual epicardial surface. Occasionally, myocardial bridging may present similarly to acute coronary syndrome in severe dehydration or hyperadrenergic states. The diagnosis can be made through coronary angiography, which reveals a dynamic vessel obstruction pattern corresponding with the cardiac cycle. Long-term effects may also include accelerated atherosclerosis. Treatment consists of reversing precipitating causes during acute presentations and decreasing the risk of coronary artery disease on a chronic basis.

1. Introduction

New-onset ST-segment changes on electrocardiogram (ECG) are usually a cause of concern, with coronary artery occlusion among the lead differential diagnoses. Myocardial bridging is a peculiar condition that may lead to such changes, yet the vessel obstruction is mostly dynamic and dependent on the cardiac cycle. Though usually asymptomatic, it can manifest in emergent cases such as acute coronary syndrome when precipitated by some factors and long-term atherosclerosis.

2. Case Presentation

A 50-year-old male with a past medical history of hypertension presented for loss of consciousness. He was hypotensive with a mean arterial pressure of 55 mmHg, tachycardic with a heart rate around 140 bpm, and minimally arousable on initial evaluation while complaining of ill-defined chest pain. Physical exam showed a regular tachycardic rhythm, normal heart sounds, decreased bilateral air entry, and absent jugular venous distention or peripheral edema. Treatment started in the emergency department with intravenous fluids and epinephrine. The electrocardiogram (ECG) displayed an ST-segment elevation in lead aVR, along with global ST-segment depressions, most notably in the inferolateral leads (Figure 1(a)). Point of care troponin I was elevated at 0.42 ng/mL. An emergent left heart catheterization (LHC) revealed a smooth 99% filling defect at the middle segment of the left anterior descending artery (LAD) during systole (Figure 2(a)) that would rhythmically appear patent during diastole (Figure 2(b)), which was suggestive of myocardial bridging. The coronaries were otherwise angiographically normal. Epinephrine was discontinued, and after high-volume rehydration, blood pressure soon normalized.

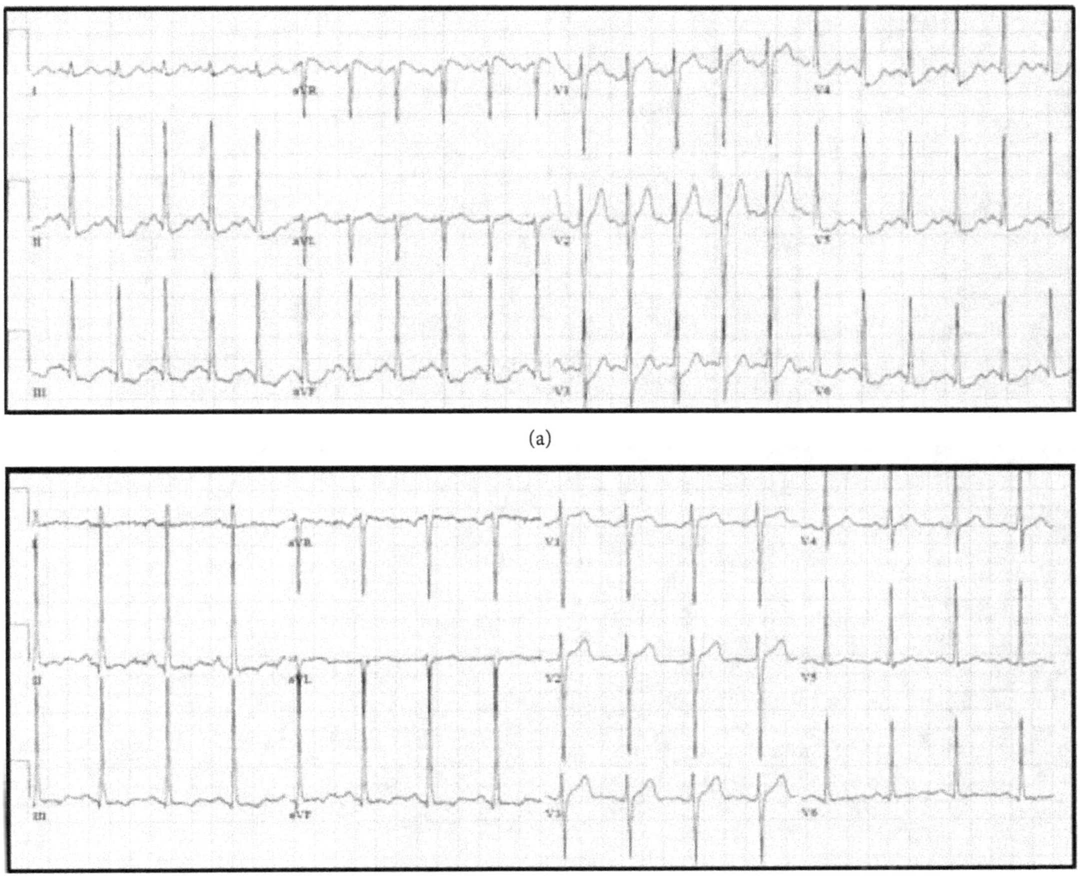

(a)

(b)

FIGURE 1: (a) Initial ECG displaying ST-segment elevation in lead aVR and diffuse ST-segment depressions. (b) ECG after aggressive hydration displaying normalization of ischemic changes.

Follow-up ECG demonstrated a complete resolution of the ischemic changes (Figure 1(b)), and the patient regained consciousness. Postprocedure cardiac echocardiography showed moderate concentric hypertrophy with a normal global systolic function. On reevaluation, he claimed that he was dehydrated after heavy alcohol drinking in the sun. He also attested to having a few episodes of mild, exertional, left-sided chest pressure in the past that spontaneously resolved with rest and that he never sought any medical care for it. He was then started on carvedilol and a low-intensity statin with instructions to avoid dehydration and adrenergic agents.

3. Discussion

Myocardial bridging is a congenital anomaly in which a segment of the coronary arteries courses through the myocardium, thus rendering it "bridged" by the overlying cardiac tissue. While often benign, it may lead to emergent clinical presentations and long-term vascular disease [1]. Myocardial bridging most commonly affects the middle segment of the LAD. The diagnosis can be made using coronary angiography, which demonstrates a characteristic "milking" obstruction of the bridged vessel [2]. The myocardial compression of the artery decreases anterograde blood flow during systole and can even extend into early diastole. During tachycardia, diastole becomes compromised, leading to a shortened time for myocardial relaxation; thus, a higher proportion of flow obstruction can be seen within the cardiac cycle. Additionally, increased inotropy can exacerbate the degree of vessel compression, further prolonging the obstructive effect [3]. These manifestations may become clinically significant in hyperadrenergic states such as dehydration, anemia, and the administration of adrenergic compounds. Long-term atherosclerosis has also been noted in the segment proximal to the bridge. Due to the increased shear wall stress and angulation at the bridged portion, there is increased flow turbulence in the upstream segment [4].

The treatment of myocardial bridging involves both avoiding the acute limitation of blood flow and the long-term decrease in symptoms and atherosclerosis incidence. Patients should refrain from conditions that may induce an adrenergic drive and dehydration. Beta-blockers have been the cornerstone of therapy as they increase the diastolic phase and decrease inotropy, in addition to nondihydropyridine calcium-channel blockers as an adjunct therapy or when beta-blockers are not tolerated [5]. As discussed above, hydration may be beneficial when hypovolemia is suspected.

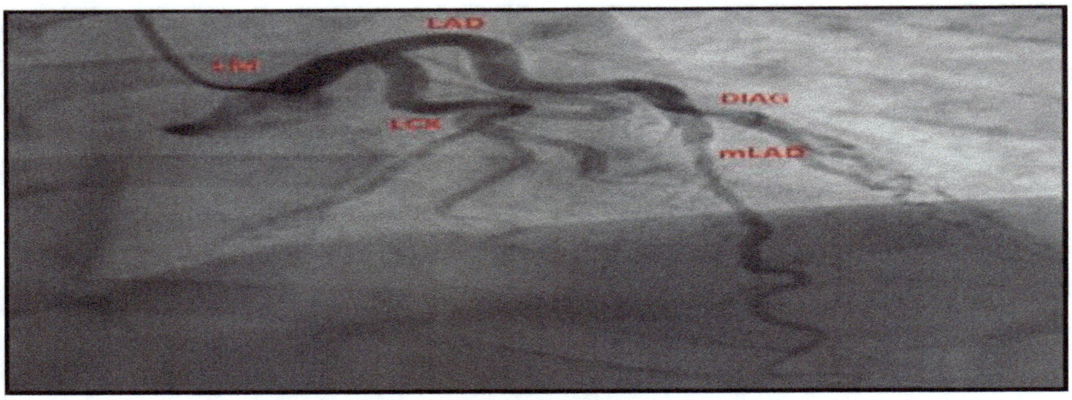

(a)

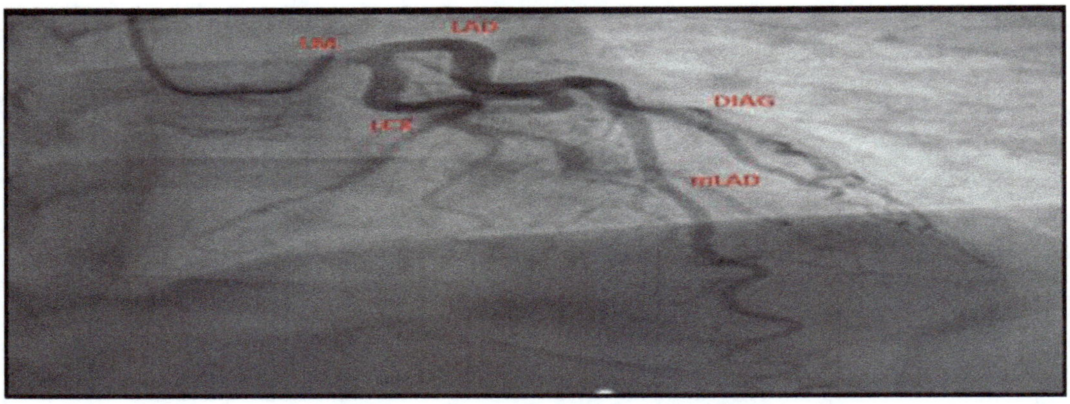

(b)

Figure 2: (a) RAO cranial LHC demonstrating significant middle-LAD stenosis during systole. (b) RAO cranial LHC demonstrating patent middle-LAD during diastole.

Conversely, nitroglycerin is contraindicated as it can cause reflex tachycardia and sympathetic response [5, 6]. When there is concurrent atherosclerosis, aspirin and statins are used to prevent accelerated atherosclerosis [1]. In symptomatic cases refractory to maximal medical therapy, surgical management with coronary artery bypass graft (CABG) or myotomy surgeries can be considered [2, 5, 6]. CABG commonly involves grafting the left internal mammary artery to the LAD, and results have shown substantial symptom relief, with the main complication being graft failure [5]. Myotomy is done by dissecting the muscle fibers surrounding the bridged vessel portions, but complications include ventricular wall perforation, uncontrolled bleeding, and ventricular aneurysm formation [5]. While limited reports have shown symptomatic relief with both techniques, further studies are needed to delineate each option's associated risks and benefits and compare outcomes [2, 5].

4. Conclusion

This case highlights the importance of identifying myocardial bridging as a potential cause of myocardial ischemia, especially in patients presenting with dehydration and hyperadrenergic states. Early recognition may guide proper treatment and avoid disease exacerbation.

Abbreviations

ECG: Electrocardiogram
LAD: Left anterior descending artery
LHC: Left heart catheterization
CABG: Coronary artery bypass grafting.

Additional Points

Limitations. Limitations of this case report include the lack of a control group for comparison, one study subject indicating a low sample size, and lack of long-term follow-up.

References

[1] M. Patel, B. Swofford, and E. Distler, "Myocardial bridge: bridging the differential diagnosis," *BMJ Case Reports*, vol. 2017, article bcr-2017, 2017.

[2] M. S. Lee and C. H. Chen, "Myocardial bridging: an up-to-date review," *The Journal of Invasive Cardiology*, vol. 27, no. 11, pp. 521–528, 2015.

[3] G. Tarantini, F. Migliore, F. Cademartiri, C. Fraccaro, and S. Iliceto, "Left anterior descending artery myocardial bridging: a clinical approach," *Journal of the American College of Cardiology*, vol. 68, no. 25, pp. 2887–2899, 2016.

[4] J. R. Alegria, J. Herrmann, D. R. Holmes Jr., A. Lerman, and C. S. Rihal, "Myocardial bridging," *European Heart Journal*, vol. 26, no. 12, pp. 1159–1168, 2005.

[5] M. T. Corban, O. Y. Hung, P. Eshtehardi et al., "Myocardial bridging: contemporary understanding of pathophysiology with implications for diagnostic and therapeutic strategies," *Journal of the American College of Cardiology*, vol. 63, no. 22, pp. 2346–2355, 2014.

[6] I. S. Rogers, J. A. Tremmel, and I. Schnittger, "Myocardial bridges: overview of diagnosis and management," *Congenital Heart Disease*, vol. 12, no. 5, pp. 619–623, 2017.

9

Cocaine and COVID-19 in ST-Elevation Myocardial Infarction

Florian Appenzeller, Meinrad Gawaz, and Iris Müller

University Hospital, Department of Cardiology and Cardiovascular Medicine, Eberhard Karls University Tübingen, 72076 Tübingen, Germany

Correspondence should be addressed to Florian Appenzeller; florian.appenzeller@med.uni-tuebingen.de

Academic Editor: Ertugurul Ercan

Both COVID-19 disease and cocaine consumption have prothrombotic and hypercoagulable effects and are associated with increased risk of cardiovascular events. We report the case of a patient with acute myocardial infarction in the setting of active COVID-19 disease and recent cocaine consumption. We hypothesize that COVID-19 and cocaine synergistically provoke cardiovascular events. Identifying COVID-19 disease and/or cocaine abuse as potential triggers of acute myocardial infarction can be crucial due to distinctive therapeutic consequences.

1. Introduction

Cocaine promotes acute myocardial ischemia and infarction by exerting various adverse effects on myocardium and coronary arteries: coronary vasoconstriction (increased levels of endothelin-1, impaired NO production, and alpha receptor stimulation), shift to a prothrombotic state (increased platelet activity and aggregation, elevated levels of fibrinogen, and von Willebrand factor), and increased myocardial oxygen demand (elevated heart rate, blood pressure, and myocardial contractility). The increase in risk for myocardial infarction after cocaine consumption has a volatile character with prompt onset and rapid decrease in the first two hours thereafter [1–6].

Myocardial perfusion impairment in COVID-19 underlies complex pathophysiological mechanisms including direct viral cellular toxicity and systemic hyperinflammation with cytokine-mediated damage leading to endothelial dysfunction, platelet hyperactivation, hypercoagulability, and atherosclerotic plaque destabilization predisposing towards micro- and macrovascular thrombotic occlusion, potentially resulting in myocardial infarction [7–9].

2. Case Presentation

A 38-year-old male presented to the emergency department with severe pain and tightness in his left chest without radiating into adjacent body parts. The symptoms had an acute onset approximately 45 minutes earlier while the patient was at rest. Upon arrival, we were informed about the patient's current COVID-19 infection diagnosed five days prior with previously mild course consisting of fever, shortness of breath, and fatigue. In addition, the patient conceded intranasal consumption of cocaine approximately one hour before onset of symptoms. Besides habitual nicotine and cocaine consumption, further cardiovascular risk factors were negated and no similar events have occurred to date. Medical history excluded other significant preconditions. Electrocardiogram showed ST-segment elevations in anterior and lateral leads implicating transmural myocardial infarction. Subsequently, intravenous acetylsalicylic acid and heparin were administered, and transportation to our catheterization laboratory was initiated. On the way, one episode of ventricular fibrillation occurred followed by cardiopulmonary resuscitation and external defibrillation with

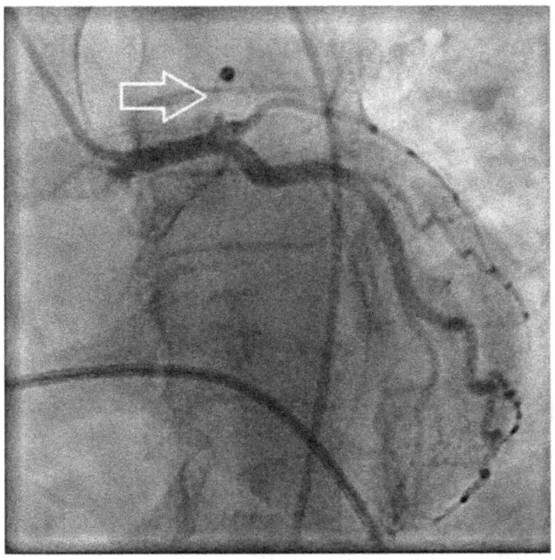

FIGURE 1: Angiography of the left coronary arteries revealing total occlusion of proximal LAD (arrow).

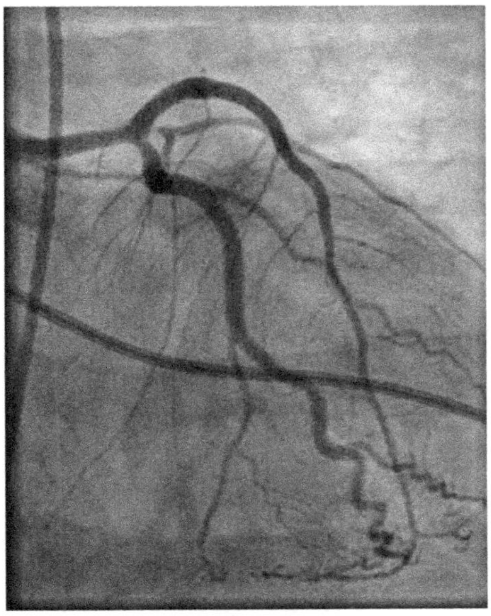

FIGURE 2: Restored perfusion established by percutaneous coronary angioplasty and stent implantation.

immediate return of spontaneous circulation. The patient arrived with spontaneous breathing and sufficient circulatory parameters. Coronary angiography was performed revealing total occlusion of the proximal left anterior descending (LAD) coronary artery in the setting of minor general coronary sclerosis (Figure 1). Coronary angioplasty and drug-eluting stent implantation fully restored perfusion of the LAD (Figure 2). Antithrombotic regime with acetylsalicylic acid was continued, and prasugrel was added. Initial echocardiography depicted extensive hypokinetic wall motion abnormality consistent with the culprit lesion. Laboratory results showed an initial troponin-I of 21,766 ng/l (<37 ng/l) and a peak in total creatine kinase at 3,065 U/l (<170 U/l) as well as elevated D-dimers of 2.1 μg/ml (<0.5 μg/ml) and IL-6 of 72 ng/l (<4 ng/l). COVID-19 infection was confirmed via reverse transcriptase-polymerase chain reaction. Consequently, the patient was isolated in our intensive care unit and received argatroban, remdesivir, and dexamethasone in accordance with current COVID-19 guidelines. There were no clinical signs of acute respiratory distress with a normal respiratory rate at rest and oxygen saturation on room air around 95%. Chest X-ray ruled out suspicious pulmonary opacities. Ultimately, former wall-motion abnormalities were regressive with residual minor systolic left ventricular impairment. The patient showed adequate clinical improvement and was discharged six days after admission. GRACE-score predicted a 6-month postdischarge mortality of 4%.

3. Discussion

Chest pain is the leading cause of cocaine-associated emergency department visits [10]. Acute coronary syndrome (ACS) associated with cocaine abuse differs from cocaine-unrelated ACS: myocardial infarction is considerably less likely to be confirmed [11], and suspected ST-elevation myocardial infarction (STEMI) is more likely to be revealed as false STEMI (i.e., nonocclusive myocardial infarction) [12]. Furthermore, these patients are more likely to be of younger age and male gender and to have lower socioeconomic status, while common cardiovascular risk factors such as diabetes and hypertension are less frequent [13].

COVID-19-associated ACS has been frequently described; however, data related to occlusive myocardial infarction are limited. Without differentiating between STEMI and non-STEMI, a register-based study estimated the incidence of acute myocardial infarction to be around five times higher in the first two weeks after COVID-19 diagnosis compared to a previous intraindividual control interval [14].

Here we describe the first case to our knowledge of STEMI in the unusual setting of both acute COVID-19 disease and prior cocaine consumption. Since both conditions exert various cardiovascular effects and are associated with thrombotic complications, a synergistic effect towards coronary events seems plausible. It remains speculative what proportion of cause is attributed to cocaine and/or COVID-19 in this case.

4. Conclusions

While laboratory screening for COVID-19 in every patient referred to our hospital is common practice, there is no routine assessment for illegal drug abuse in patients presenting with ACS. This is partially explained by the relatively low prevalence of cocaine consumption in our catchment area. Assessing illegal drug abuse by questioning and/or toxicological screening should be considered particularly in younger patients with a low to moderate cardiovascular risk profile presenting with ACS.

The underlying cause has neglectable consequence on guideline-recommended primary percutaneous coronary intervention and antiplatelet strategy in STEMI but there are therapeutic implications that should be considered, respectively: beta-blockers may aggravate cocaine-induced coronary spasm and should be avoided in the acute event while intravenous nitroglycerin and benzodiazepines were validated beneficial in this scenario [15]. In COVID-19 disease and STEMI, anticoagulation in addition to antiplatelet therapy should be carefully assessed in order to prevent thromboembolic complications depending on individual bleeding and thrombotic risk [16]. Current guidelines should be considered in order to do justice to the rapidly evolving pharmacological strategies in COVID-19 disease.

Consent

No written consent has been obtained from the patient as there is no patient identifiable data included in this case report.

Acknowledgments

This manuscript is financially supported by Open Access Publishing Fund of University of Tübingen.

References

[1] U. Wilbert-Lampen, C. Seliger, T. Zilker, and R. M. Arendt, "Cocaine increases the endothelial release of immunoreactive endothelin and its concentrations in human plasma and urine: reversal by coincubation with sigma-receptor antagonists," *Circulation*, vol. 98, no. 5, pp. 385–390, 1998.

[2] R. A. Lange, R. G. Cigarroa, C. W. Yancy Jr. et al., "Cocaine-induced coronary-artery vasoconstriction," *The New England Journal of Medicine*, vol. 321, no. 23, pp. 1557–1562, 1989.

[3] A. J. Siegel, J. H. Mendelson, M. B. Sholar et al., "Effect of cocaine usage on C-reactive protein, von Willebrand factor, and fibrinogen," *The American Journal of Cardiology*, vol. 89, no. 9, pp. 1133–1135, 2002.

[4] S. H. Rezkalla, J. J. Mazza, R. A. Kloner, V. Tillema, and S. H. Chang, "Effects of cocaine on human platelets in healthy subjects," *The American Journal of Cardiology*, vol. 72, no. 2, pp. 243–246, 1993.

[5] J. D. Boehrer, D. J. Moliterno, J. E. Willard et al., "Hemodynamic effects of intranasal cocaine in humans," *Journal of the American College of Cardiology*, vol. 20, no. 1, pp. 90–93, 1992.

[6] M. A. Mittleman, D. Mintzer, M. Maclure, G. H. Tofler, J. B. Sherwood, and J. E. Muller, "Triggering of myocardial infarction by cocaine," *Circulation*, vol. 99, no. 21, pp. 2737–2741, 1999.

[7] K. J. Clerkin, J. A. Fried, J. Raikhelkar et al., "COVID-19 and cardiovascular disease," *Circulation*, vol. 141, no. 20, pp. 1648–1655, 2020.

[8] G. Guagliumi, A. Sonzogni, I. Pescetelli, D. Pellegrini, and A. V. Finn, "Microthrombi and ST-segment-elevation myocardial infarction in COVID-19," *Circulation*, vol. 142, no. 8, pp. 804–809, 2020.

[9] Z. Varga, A. J. Flammer, P. Steiger et al., "Endothelial cell infection and endotheliitis in COVID-19," *Lancet*, vol. 395, no. 10234, pp. 1417-1418, 2020.

[10] E. H. Crane, "Highlights of the 2011 drug abuse warning network (DAWN) findings on drug-related emergency department visits," *The CBHSQ Report Rockville*, pp. 1–9, 2013.

[11] J. A. Feldman, S. S. Fish, J. R. Beshansky, J. L. Griffith, R. H. Woolard, and H. P. Selker, "Acute cardiac ischemia in patients with cocaine-associated complaints: results of a multicenter trial," *Annals of Emergency Medicine*, vol. 36, no. 5, pp. 469–476, 2000.

[12] I. Ifedili, T. Bob-Manuel, S. R. Kadire et al., "Cocaine positivity in ST-elevation myocardial infarction: a true or false association," *Perm J*, vol. 23, 2019.

[13] S. G. Shitole, N. Kayo, V. Srinivas et al., "Clinical profile, acute care, and middle-term outcomes of cocaine-associated ST-segment elevation myocardial infarction in an inner-city community," *The American Journal of Cardiology*, vol. 117, no. 8, pp. 1224–1230, 2016.

[14] D. Modin, B. Claggett, C. Sindet-Pedersen et al., "Acute COVID-19 and the incidence of ischemic stroke and acute myocardial infarction," *Circulation*, vol. 142, no. 21, pp. 2080–2082, 2020.

[15] J. E. Hollander, "The management of cocaine-associated myocardial ischemia," *The New England Journal of Medicine*, vol. 333, no. 19, pp. 1267–1272, 1995.

[16] G. N. Nadkarni, A. Lala, E. Bagiella et al., "Anticoagulation, bleeding, mortality, and pathology in hospitalized patients wit=h COVID-19," *Journal of the American College of Cardiology*, vol. 76, no. 16, pp. 1815–1826, 2020.

10

Feasibility and Safety of Sodium Glucose Cotransporter-2 Inhibitors in Adults with Heart Failure after the Fontan Procedure

Jun Muneuchi, Yuichiro Sugitani, Masaru Kobayashi, Hiroki Ezaki, Hiromu Yamada, and Mamie Watanabe

Department of Pediatrics, Kyushu Hospital, Japan Community Healthcare Organization, Kitakyushu, Japan

Correspondence should be addressed to Jun Muneuchi; jmune@msn.com

Academic Editor: Mihaela Mocan

Sodium glucose cotransporter-2 (SGLT-2) inhibitors have been widespread in patients with heart failure; however, there is little information regarding its feasibility and safety among patients after the Fontan procedure. We presented five adults after the Fontan procedure who were treated with SGLT-2 inhibitors. All patients reduced oedema and/or pleural effusion despite other conjunct medications were ineffective. Although we did not measure the urine volume in all patients, all patients themselves reported an increase in urinary output after the administration of a SGLT-2 inhibitor. In addition, administration of a SGLT-2 inhibitor resulted in weight loss (4/5), an increase in systemic oxygen saturation (4/5), an increase in serum albumin level (4/5), an increase in estimated glomerular filtration ratio (4/5), and a decrease in plasma brain natriuretic peptide level (4/5). Our case series supported the feasibility and safety of SGLT-2 inhibitors in patients with Fontan circulatory failure, although the exact changes in urinary output were unknown in all patients. Further investigation will be required to explore a diuretic effect by SGLT-2 in patients after the Fontan procedure.

1. Introduction

Future developing comorbidities, including heart failure, arrhythmias, protein-losing enteropathy, and liver disease, have been a concern in patients following the Fontan procedure. The Fontan circulation is characterized, not only by ventricular dysfunction owing to a functionally single ventricle but also by an increase in circulatory impedance and a decrease in circulatory capacitance owing to a lack of a subpulmonary ventricle. Regardless, the key sign of the Fontan circulatory failure is systemic congestion. Recent studies have suggested that sodium glucose cotransporter-2 (SGLT-2) inhibitors reduced the risk of hospitalization in patients with chronic congestive heart failure, irrespective of the presence of diabetes mellitus [1–3]. Although the precise pharmacological effects on heart failure remain unclear, a SGLT-2 inhibitor plays a role in natriuretic effect [4–6]. Therefore, this beneficial effect is posited to reduce systemic congestion in patients after the Fontan procedure. However, there is little information available in the literature regarding its feasibility and safety. We present a case series of five adults with heart failure who were treated with these agents long after the Fontan procedure.

2. Case Reports

2.1. Case 1. A 45-year-old male who had undergone the Fontan procedure was admitted due to oedema and dyspnoea on exertion. The patient had received enalapril, digoxin, furosemide, aspirin, and warfarin. However, he experienced 19 unexpected hospitalizations due to atrial fibrillation, resulting in exacerbated heart failure. Chest radiography on admission showed a bilateral pleural effusion. These findings suggest failed Fontan circulation. He was classified as New York Heat Association (NYHA) functional class III. After the administration of dapagliflozin, the urinary output increased, symptoms promptly disappeared, and he was subsequently discharged. During the follow-up of 4 months, there was no rehospitalization despite the occurrence of paroxysmal atrial fibrillation. No adverse events occurred.

2.2. Case 2. A 36-year-old male who had undergone the Fontan procedure was admitted due to oedema and dyspnoea on exertion. Due to the patient's existing comorbidities including hypertension, obesity, type 2 diabetes mellitus, cerebrovascular disease, and chronic kidney disease, there were 10 unexpected hospitalizations to date. He was classified as NYHA class III, receiving enalapril, digoxin, furosemide, spironolactone, aspirin, and apixaban. Urinalysis showed proteinuria and haematuria, while a renal biopsy revealed focal segmental glomerulosclerosis. Oral administration of empagliflozin was started for a sustained elevation of haemoglobin A1C level and subsequently caused increased urinary output and disappearance of oedema. Further urinalysis revealed that the proteinuria and haematuria disappeared. During the follow-up period of 24 months, he remained stable without unexpected rehospitalization. No adverse events occurred.

2.3. Case 3. A 35-year-old male who had undergone the Fontan procedure was admitted due to oedema of the lower extremities after viral infection. The patient was classified as NYHA class II with comorbidities including obesity, chronic kidney disease, type 2 diabetes mellitus, sleep apnoea syndrome, and Fontan-associated liver disease. To date, there have been two other unexpected hospitalizations. He had received carvedilol, enalapril, digoxin, furosemide, spironolactone, aspirin, and warfarin. Administration of dapagliflozin was started, and oedema in the lower extremities subsided following an increase in urinary output. During the follow-up of 16 months, he was stable in the outpatient clinic without rehospitalization. No adverse events occurred.

2.4. Case 4. A 24-year-old male after the Fontan procedure visited the outpatient clinic because of systemic oedema and headache. The patient had protein-losing enteropathy and plastic bronchitis due to Fontan circulatory failure and classified as NYHA class III. He had received carvedilol, digoxin, furosemide, spironolactone, tadalafil, aspirin, and warfarin. However, there were 29 unexpected hospitalizations due to these comorbidities. He had no history of hypertension, obesity, or diabetes. Urinary output increased with the commencement of dapagliflozin treatment, leading to improved clinical manifestations. During the follow-up of 3 months, there was no unexpected hospitalization except for hospitalization for a scheduled lower intestinal endoscopy. No adverse event occurred. Protein-losing enteropathy and plastic bronchitis were not improved.

2.5. Case 5. A 21-year-old male presented the deterioration of pleural effusion and oedema in the face and lower extremities after the Fontan procedure. The patient was classified as NYHA class III with comorbidities including chronic kidney disease, type 2 diabetes mellitus, and Fontan-associated liver disease. He had received β-blocker, enalapril, digoxin, furosemide, and warfarin. Urinalysis revealed neither proteinuria nor haematuria. The administration of dapagliflozin was initiated due to a sustained elevation of haemoglobin A1C levels. The increased urinary output caused by dapagliflozin reduced oedema. During the follow-up of 18 months, he was stable without rehospitalization and any adverse effects.

3. Discussion

In our case series (Table 1), three out of five patients initially received SGLT-2 inhibitors for glucose intolerance before the evidence of clinical trials were published. However, the agents improved cardiac manifestations as well as proteinuria and haematuria. Therefore, we prescribed a SGLT-2 inhibitor due to the development of heart failure despite conventional medical therapy in the other two patients as well. Although the usual dose of dapagliflozin was 10 mg, we cautiously prescribed an initial dose of 5 mg in 4 patients since clinical effects on patients with the Fontan circulation were still unclear. All patients had increased urinary output and reduced oedema and/or pleural effusion despite other conjunct medications were ineffective. Although we did not measure the urine volume in all patients, all patients themselves reported an increase in urinary output after the administration of a SGLT-2 inhibitor. In addition, administration of a SGLT-2 inhibitor resulted in weight loss (4/5), an increase in systemic oxygen saturation (4/5), an increase in serum albumin level (4/5), an increase in estimated glomerular filtration ratio (4/5), and a decrease in plasma brain natriuretic peptide level (4/5), which did not reach statistical significance due to the limited number of cases (Table 2). Furthermore, there was no unexpected rehospitalization due to the deterioration of heart failure and no adverse events, such as urinary tract infection, during the mean follow-up period of 12 months (ranging from 2 to 20 months) after the initiation of a SGLT-2 inhibitor. Unfortunately, we did not assess hemodynamic status including pulmonary arterial pressure and resistance by invasive methods, such as cardiac catheterization or indwelling central venous pressure monitoring.

The phenotype of Fontan circulatory failure is not well understood. Actually, in our case series, 3 patients had tolerable central venous pressure, and 3 patients had high cardiac index. Therefore, pathophysiologic interactions between the cardiovascular system and advanced noncardiovascular end-organ dysfunction are supposed to play major roles in Fontan circulatory failure [7, 8]. Fontan circulatory failure cannot be explained by the contemporary concept of heart failure according to ventricular ejection fraction, that is, heart failure as a result of a reduced or preserved ejection fraction [9]. The application of conventional guidelines for chronic heart failure should be carefully considered in patients with the Fontan circulatory failure. Some drugs that may be beneficial for some aspects of the Fontan circulation may be difficult to use because of adverse effects for another aspect of the Fontan circulation. In addition, targets for drug treatment in patients after the Fontan procedure may vary over time and between individual patients [9]. The benefits of SGLT-2 inhibitors include natriuresis and glucose-induced osmotic diuretics, which leads to a reduction in intraglomerular pressure and an increase in glomerular filtration ratio [6]. These beneficial effects on the kidney result in improvements in

Table 1: Summary of baseline characteristics in five patients after Fontan procedure who were treated with a SGLT-2 inhibitor.

Case	Sex	Age	Primary diagnosis	Prior procedures	Age at Fontan (years) Type of Fontan	Comorbidities	BMI (kg/m^2)	CI (L.min^{-1}.m^{-2})	CVP (mmHg)	EF (%)	Valve regurg.	Peak VO_2 (%)	Times of unexpected hospitalization and reasons
1	Male	45	AVSD, MGA, PA, IVCD, left isomerism	AP shunt, TCPS, PMI	22 ECC	Heart failure PAf Chylothorax/ ascites FALD	21.0	4.87 High CI	20	53	Mod AR Mod AVVR	—	19 (0.82/year) Heart failure PAf
2	Male	36	AVSD, MGA, PS, right isomerism	AP shunt	13 ECC	Heart failure Hypertension Obesity Diabetes CKD CNS hemorrhage	31.3	2.55 Low CI	11	53	Mild AVVR	58	10 (0.45/year) Heart failure Thrombosis Infection
3	Male	35	DORV, hypoplastic LV	PAB, BCPS	11 ECC	Heart failure Obesity DM CKD FALD	37.9	5.02 High CI	18	54	Mild AVVR	52	2 (0.08/year) Heart failure
4	Male	21	HLHS	Norwood, BCPS	1 ECC	Heart failure PLE PB	16.5	5.09 High CI	11	53	Mod AVVR	—	29 (1.52/year) Heart failure PLE/PB
5	Male	24	AVSD, MGA, PA, right isomerism	AP shunt, BCPS	2 ECC	DM CKD	24.0	2.32 Low CI	12	41	Mod AVVR	71	1 (0.04/year) Heart failure

Times of admission means unexpected admission due to not scheduled examination or treatment but cardiovascular symptoms. AP shunt: aortopulmonary shunt; AVSD: atrioventricular septal defect; BMI: body mass index; CI: cardiac index; CKD: chronic kidney disease; CNS: central nervous system; CVP: central venous pressure; DM: diabetes mellitus; DORV: double outlet right ventricle; ECC: extracardiac conduit; EF: ejection fraction; FALD: Fontan-associated liver disease; HLHS: hypoplastic left ventricle; IVCD: inferior vena cava defect; LV: left ventricle; MGA: malposition of the great arteries; PA: pulmonary atresia; PAB: pulmonary arterial banding; PAf: paroxysmal atrial fibrillation; PB: plastic bronchitis; PLE: protein-losing enteropathy; PMI: pacemaker implantation; PS: pulmonary stenosis; TCPS: total cavopulmonary shunt; Valve regurg.: valve regurgitation.

Table 2: Changes in clinical data before and after administration of a SGLT-2 inhibitor.

Case	SGLT-2 inhibitor	Duration of SGLT-2 inhibitor administration (months)	Data acquisition timing	Weight (kg)	HR (min^{-1})	SO_2 (%)	Mean BP (mmHg)	HbA1C (%)	Ht (%)	Platelet ($\times 10^9/L$)	Albumin (g/dL)	Total bilirubin (mg/dL)	AST (IU/dL)	γGTP (IU/dL)	Na (mmol/L)	Creatinine (mg/dL)	eGFR ($mL/min/1.73m^2$)	BNP (pg/mL)
1	Dapagliflozin 5 mg	3	Before	55	85	83	86	5.6	43	0.93	3.3	4.6	50	155	140	1.02	64	193
			After	53	87	91	87	—	44	0.78	3.1	3.9	45	139	141	1.28	50	277
2	Empagliflozin 10 mg	20	Before	80	114	91	93	7.3	52	3.15	2.9	1.5	26	32	138	1.21	56	231
			After	85	83	92	90	7.7	56	3.30	3.4	0.5	48	51	139	1.12	60	7
3	Dapagliflozin 5 mg	12	Before	116	91	85	86	6.5	41	1.57	2.8	1.0	41	78	140	0.84	72	52
			After	106	83	89	85	6.3	53	1.18	3.8	2.7	45	138	140	0.97	140	57
4	Dapagliflozin 5 mg	2	Before	34	92	81	93	3.2	35	2.35	1.8	0.1	16	17	137	0.60	113	43
			After	33	94	79	94	—	32	2.97	2.0	0.1	17	17	132	0.74	137	38
5	Dapagliflozin 5 mg	14	Before	69	103	88	84	7.8	60	1.64	2.9	1.7	55	108	125	1.52	72	101
			After	66	75	92	81	6.6	62	1.57	4.4	2.6	39	62	141	1.07	125	12
P value				0.345	0.224	0.138	0.224	—	0.224	0.892	0.079	0.715	0.892	0.224	0.465	0.685	0.500	0.345

P value < 0.05 means statistical significance when clinical data were compared before and after administration of a sodium glucose cotransporter-2 inhibitor using the Wilcoxon signed rank test. AST: aspartate aminotransferase; BNP: brain natriuretic peptide; BP: blood pressure; γGTP: gamma-glutamyl transpeptidase; HbA1C: haemoglobin A1C; HR: heart rate; Ht: haematocrit; eGFR: estimated glomerular filtration ratio; SGLT-2 inhibitor: sodium glucose cotransporter-2 inhibitor; SO_2: systemic oxygen saturation.

ventricular filling, ventricular wall stress, and myocardial energetics [10]. From this perspective, we believe that a SGLT-2 inhibitor has the potential to elicit maximum diuretic function in the Fontan circulation. Our case series supports the postulation that SGLT-2 inhibitors can reduce rehospitalization rate of patients, although the pharmacological impacts of these drugs on heart failure are still in the black box.

In conclusions, SGLT-2 inhibitors were tolerable without acute adverse effects in adults who undergone the Fontan procedure, although the exact changes in urinary output were unknown in all patients. Large prospective studies are needed to assess the efficacy and safety of SGLT-2 inhibitors in this population.

References

[1] J. J. V. McMurray, S. D. Solomon, S. E. Inzucchi et al., "Dapagliflozin in patients with heart failure and reduced ejection fraction," *The New England Journal of Medicine*, vol. 381, no. 21, pp. 1995–2008, 2019.

[2] M. Packer, S. D. Anker, J. Butler et al., "Cardiovascular and renal outcomes with empagliflozin in heart failure," *The New England Journal of Medicine*, vol. 383, no. 15, pp. 1413–1424, 2020.

[3] F. Zannad, J. P. Ferreira, S. J. Pocock et al., "SGLT2 inhibitors in patients with heart failure with reduced ejection fraction: a meta-analysis of the EMPEROR-reduced and DAPA-HF trials," *The Lancet*, vol. 396, no. 10254, pp. 819–829, 2020.

[4] Y. Lytvyn, P. Bjornstad, J. A. Udell, J. A. Lovshin, and D. Z. I. Cherney, "Sodium glucose cotransporter-2 inhibition in heart failure: potential mechanisms, clinical applications, and summary of clinical trials," *Circulation*, vol. 136, no. 17, pp. 1643–1658, 2017.

[5] O. Vardeny, "The sweet spot: heart failure prevention with SGLT2 inhibitors," *The American Journal of Medicine*, vol. 133, no. 2, pp. 182–185, 2020.

[6] H. J. L. Heerspink, B. V. Stefánsson, R. Correa-Rotter et al., "Dapagliflozin in patients with chronic kidney disease," *The New England Journal of Medicine*, vol. 383, no. 15, pp. 1436–1446, 2020.

[7] H. Ohuchi, "Where is the "optimal" Fontan hemodynamics?," *Korean Circulation Journal*, vol. 47, no. 6, pp. 842–857, 2017.

[8] T. A. McDonagh, M. Metra, M. Adamo et al., "2021 ESC guidelines for the diagnosis and treatment of acute and chronic heart failure," *European Heart Journal*, vol. 42, no. 36, pp. 3599–3726, 2021.

[9] N. J. Oldenburger, A. Mank, J. Etnel, J. J. Takkenberg, and W. A. Helbing, "Drug therapy in the prevention of failure of the Fontan circulation: a systematic review," *Cardiology in the Young*, vol. 26, no. 5, pp. 842–850, 2016.

[10] S. Verma and J. J. V. McMurray, "The serendipitous story of SGLT2 inhibitors in heart failure," *Circulation*, vol. 139, no. 22, pp. 2537–2541, 2019.

Pericardial Tamponade following Asymptomatic SARS-CoV-2 Infection: A Diagnostic Journey

Christian Birner, Matthias Gasche, Rainer Voisard, and Christian Neumann

Joint Medical Service (Germany), Department of Internal Medicine, Military Hospital Ulm, 89081 Oberer Eselsberg 40 Ulm, Germany

Correspondence should be addressed to Christian Birner; christian1birner@bundeswehr.org

Academic Editor: Yuli Huang

Background. Pericardial tamponade is a known life-threatening condition rarely reported in COVID-19 but has not been reported following asymptomatic SARS-CoV-2 infection. Its pathomechanism is still elusive. *Case Summary.* We report the case of a 66-year-old man with progressive shortness of breath and leg swelling due to new-onset heart failure and pericardial tamponade following asymptomatic SARS-CoV-2 infection. Ultrasound-guided placement of a pericardial drainage led to significant improvement of symptoms and revealed an exudative effusion. Throughout the diagnostic process, we were confronted with a systemic inflammatory syndrome suspicion of an induced autoimmune condition. After steroid pulse therapy and oral anticoagulation for subclavian vein thrombosis, the patient was discharged and followed in our outpatient clinic. *Discussion.* Patients with asymptomatic SARS-CoV-2 infection are at risk for developing life-threatening complications. Induced autoimmune conditions could be a potential explanation for late-onset pericardial tamponade in this population. A multimodal imaging approach is crucial in the diagnosis and characterization of cardiac inflammation. An interdisciplinary approach is essential. Awareness of uncommon cardiac complications following a SARS-CoV-2 infection is crucial for the initial assessment and the appropriate treatment of these patients.

1. Introduction

Pericardial tamponade is a known life-threatening condition rarely reported in COVID-19 but has not been reported following asymptomatic SARS-CoV-2 infection. We report the case of a 66-year-old man with myopericarditis, pericardial tamponade, and polyserositis within five weeks after asymptomatic infection with SARS-CoV-2. Throughout the diagnostic process, we were confronted with a systemic inflammatory syndrome suspicious of an induced autoimmune condition. This report highlights a dedicated diagnostic workup by multimodal cross-sectional imaging studies. Induced autoimmune conditions could be a potential explanation for late-onset pericardial tamponade in this population.

2. Case Presentation

A 66-year-old man without any known comorbidities or allergies presented to our emergency department with ten-day progressive shortness of breath without chest pain, abdominal distension, decreased effort tolerance, and 12 kg weight gain within the last ten days. The first assessment showed an afebrile patient (36.5°C) with sinus tachycardia (108 bpm), hypertension (153/110 mmHg), respiratory rate 15/min, SpO2 87% on room air, signs of low voltage in ECG (Figures 1(a) and 1(b)), anasarca, ascites, pleura effusion, and a massive pericardial effusion on ultrasound evaluation.

39 days prior, the unvaccinated patient was tested positive for SARS-CoV-2 (by RT-PCR) as part of a health care

workers' screening. Prior to the infection, the patient was healthy and fit, doing cycling regularly. During the infection, the patient remained asymptomatic. On admission, the patient was tested negative for influenza, respiratory syncytial virus, and SARS-CoV-2 by RT-PCR. SARS-CoV-2-IgG was positive. Laboratory assessment (Table 1) showed leucocytosis with absolute lymphopenia, elevated C-reactive protein, and IL-6 indicating an inflammatory process. Furthermore, biomarkers of myocardial damage were elevated while NT-pro-BNP was within normal limits. We suspected concomitant shock physiology as serum lactate was elevated (3.3 mmol/l).

A CT-thorax scan showed bilateral lower lobe collapse consolidations, large bilateral pleural effusion, pericardial effusion, and ground-glass opacification in the left upper lobe. Dedicated echocardiography (supplemental files, video 1) revealed reduced left and right ventricular function, collapse of the left and right atrium, and a massive circumferential pericardial effusion (48.9 mm apical) suggesting echocardiographic tamponade (Figure 2). We suspected new-onset heart failure and echocardiographic pericardial tamponade. The patient was admitted to our medical intensive care unit for noninvasive ventilation and high-flow nasal cannula oxygen therapy for one day.

Due to pericardial tamponade, a step-by-step approach was initiated with pericardiocentesis first for symptomatic therapy and assessing the most common etiologies of pericardial effusion. An ultrasound-guided pericardial drainage was placed, and 850 ml of serosanguinous fluid was removed. Fluid analysis tested negative by RT-PCR for SARS-CoV-2, revealing high-level LDH and protein indicating an exudative process; microbiology (including mycobacterial and fungal culture) remained negative as well as serology for cardiotropic pathogens. Interferon-y (QuantiFERON) testing was positive. After pericardiocentesis, symptoms improved. Cytologic evaluation of the pericardial fluid was suspicious for high malignant lymphoma. Further flow cytometry and immunophenotyping excluded a monoclonal cell population as well as PET-CT showed no pathologic extracardiac FDG uptake, which could have indicated a highly proliferative tumor mass or active tuberculosis. Pleurocentesis was performed for diagnostic purpose and symptomatic treatment. The exudative fluid showed no evidence of malignancy or infection but indicating polyserositis. After removal of at least 1850 ml in total over 9 days, echocardiography showed minimal residual effusion and the drainage was removed. Left ventricular function recovered, but the right ventricular global function was still impaired. Echocardiography revealed hypertrophy of the free right ventricular wall. Cross-sectional studies (Figure 3) confirmed myocardial inflammation indicating myocarditis with diffuse biventricular fibrosis. Cardiac catheterization excluded occlusive coronary artery disease.

A duplex and compression sonography of the upper extremities was performed due to new-onset pain in both arms. It confirmed thrombosis of the left subclavian vein and symmetrical thrombophlebitis of the cephalic vein. An extensive vasculitis and collagenosis screening revealed elevated ANA titer (1 : 100) with high positivity for Ro52, borderline positivity for nRNP/Sm, negative anti-ds-DNA, anti-Sm-antibodies, and normal complement C3/C4. Direct Coombs test (anti-Fy(b)) was positive without evidence of hemolysis. An antiphospholipid syndrome evaluation revealed a slight elevated anti-cardiolipin-IgM titer. Serology for hepatitis A, B, C, and E and HIV was negative. Urine analysis and sediment showed no evidence of concomitant nephropathy. Past medical history was negative for joint pain, skin rash or mucosal lesions, alopecia, and neuropsychiatric abnormalities. Although ACR/EULAR criteria for SLE were negative, 100 mg oral prednisolone was administered for seven days in the set of acute myopericarditis and suspected autoimmune etiology. Within the next three weeks, the patient recovered slowly with loss of about 15 kg along with diuretics and guideline-directed medical heart failure therapy. Left and right ventricular function improved. The elevated liver enzymes had normalized along the improvement of cardiac function suggesting congestive hepatopathy. The patient was discharged after 23 days and followed in our outpatient clinic.

Two weeks later, the patient reported an improvement of his physical performance without any complaints. The laboratory assessment revealed a rise in the ANA titer up to 1 : 320 with persisting high positivity for Ro52 and a positive RT-PCR for SARS-CoV-2 in a nasopharyngeal swab with a cycle threshold of 35.5 indicating low viral shedding. Echocardiography showed a persisting moderate reduced right ventricular function and a pericardial effusion of 8 mm around the right ventricle. A rheumatologic examination was intended but is still pending due to patient's concerns. At a six-month telephone follow-up, the patient was asymptomatic and again at his prior exercise capacity but refused any further medical consultation.

3. Discussion

We report the case of a healthy 66-year-old male patient with myopericarditis, pericardial tamponade, and polyserositis within five weeks after asymptomatic infection with SARS-CoV-2.

A negative SARS-CoV-2 PCR and a positive IgG titer at admission indicated a postinfection condition on the background of a positive RT-PCR 39 days prior. At follow-up two weeks after discharge, SARS-CoV-2 PCR was positive with a cycle threshold of 35.5. Repositive tests by RT-PCR are very common in recovered COVID-19 patients. The reason is still unclear, but false RT-PCR results, intermittent virus shedding, viral reactivation, or reinfection with another SARS-CoV-2 strain are currently being discussed [1]. In our institution, sequencing was not routine at this point of time; furthermore, genetic sequencing of the first positive swab was not available and the high cycle threshold on the follow-up PCR indicated no infectivity.

Hypertension is not a characteristic feature of tamponade but is not uncommon in subacute pericardial tamponade [2, 3]. Symptoms, diagnostic findings, and point-of-care echocardiography indicated cardiac tamponade in our patient.

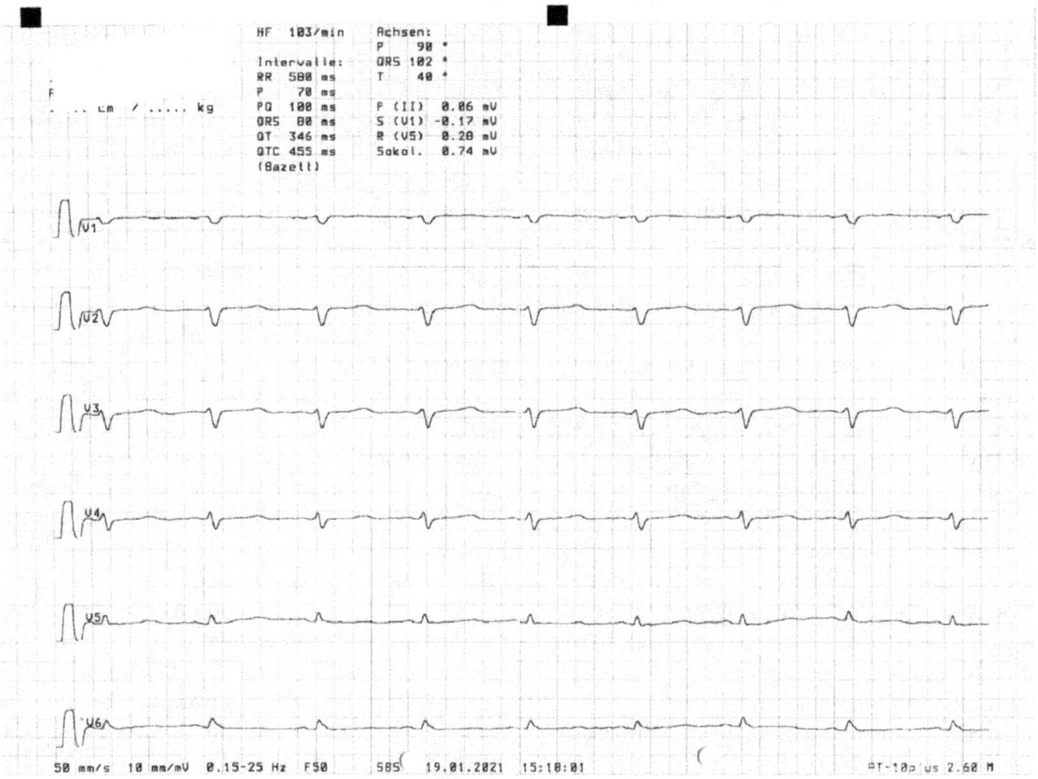

(a)

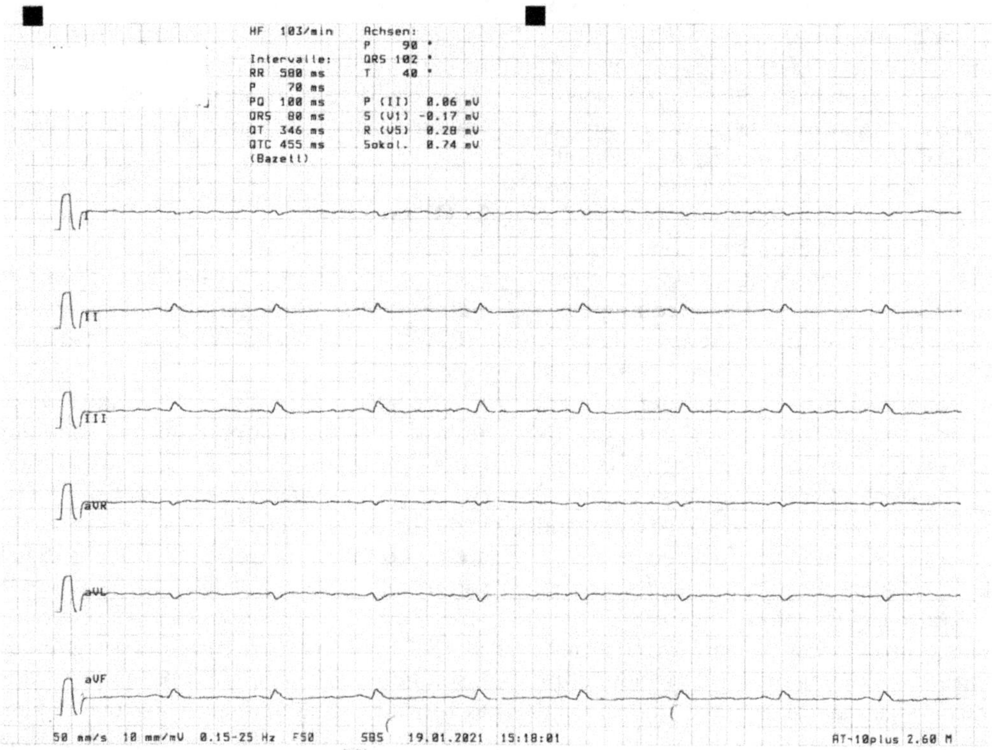

(b)

FIGURE 1: (a, b) Electrocardiogram (50 mm/s) showing low-voltage morphology, tachycardic sinus rhythm (103 bpm), and repolarization abnormalities.

Table 1: Laboratory assessment at admission and follow-up.

	Reference range	Admission	Follow-up
Hemoglobin	13.5–18.0 g/dl	13.5	10.1
Leucocytes	4.0–9.0/nl	12.5	5.9
Lymphocytes	1.1–4.0/nl	0.38	0.77
Platelet count	150–450/nl	195	260
Serum-creatinine	0.55–1.10 mg/dl	0.68	0.47
Serum-urea	16.6–48.5 mg/dl	82.6	27.8
CRP	<0.5 mg/dl	9	1
Interleukin-6	<7 pg/ml	115	—
PCT	mg/dl	0.35	—
NT-pro-BNP	<879 pg/ml	159	762
hsTropT	<0.014 ng/ml	0.026	0.037
LDH	135–225 U/l	483	221
D-dimer	<0.70 mg/l FEU	10.54	1.52
ESR (1 h)	<21 mm/h		56
GOT	<50 U/l	280	14
GPT	<50 U/l	391	12
Bilirubin	<1.20 mg/dl	2.63	0.74
ANA (IFT)	<1 : 100	1 : 100	1 : 320
ANCA (IFT)	<1 : 10	Negative	Negative
Ro52		High positivity	High positivity
nRNP/Sm		Borderline positivity	Negative
SARS-CoV-2 RT-PCR		Negative	Positive
SARS-CoV-2 ct		—	35.5
SARS-CoV-2-IgG		Positive	—
Adenovirus (ELISA)		IgG/IgM negative	—
HHV-6 (IFT)		IgG positive, IgM negative	—
CMV (CMIA)		IgG/IgM negative	—
Parvovirus B19 (CLIA)		IgG/IgM negative	—

We used a step-by-step approach for excluding the most common etiologies for pericardial effusion, which are cancer (10-25%), pericarditis and infectious causes (15-30%), and connective tissue diseases (5-15%), while tuberculosis is the dominant etiology in developing countries (>60%). Nevertheless, up to 50% still remain idiopathic [4].

Initial cytology findings of the pericardial fluid were suspicious for aggressive lymphoma. Atrial and right heart involvement in our cross-sectional studies may be suggestive for cardiac lymphoma as malignant pericardial effusions can result in tamponade, but primary lymphoma of the heart is rare. Common imaging features in these cases are ill-defined infiltrative masses, tumor extension along the epicardial surfaces, and pericardial thickening [5]. Saab et al. examined 419 pericardial effusion specimens obtained from 364 patients. Only 15% of the specimens were positive for malignancy. The most common primary malignancies were breast and lung cancers, and only 3 of 51 patients had a hematologic malignancy. The sensitivity of cytology for diagnosing malignancy was 92.1%, and false-negative rate was 14.7% [6]. In our case, PET-CT showed no evidence for malignancy and cardiac MRI findings were conclusive for diffuse myocarditis. Immunophenotypisation of the pericardial fluid and an unremarkable follow-up at six months finally excluded this rare diagnosis.

An active extrapulmonary tuberculosis was discussed, but neither microscopy nor culture or PET-CT could confirm this hypothesis. On the other hand, the professional background (volunteer in a nursing home) and the positive QuantiFERON test are still suggestive and should prompt further diagnostic workup if disease progress is suspected, but the uneventful time course argued against an active disease process.

There was no evidence for any common infectious myocarditis, but SARS-CoV-2 infection remained a potential cause.

Cardiac involvement is a salient feature in COVID-19 and is associated with a worse outcome. Pericardial tamponade is a known but rarely reported complication of myopericarditis in COVID-19. Its underlying pathomechanism is still elusive [7]. Farina et al. reported a case of cardiac tamponade 23 days after a positive SARS-CoV-2 nasopharyngeal swab in early 2020. The serohemorrhagic pericardial

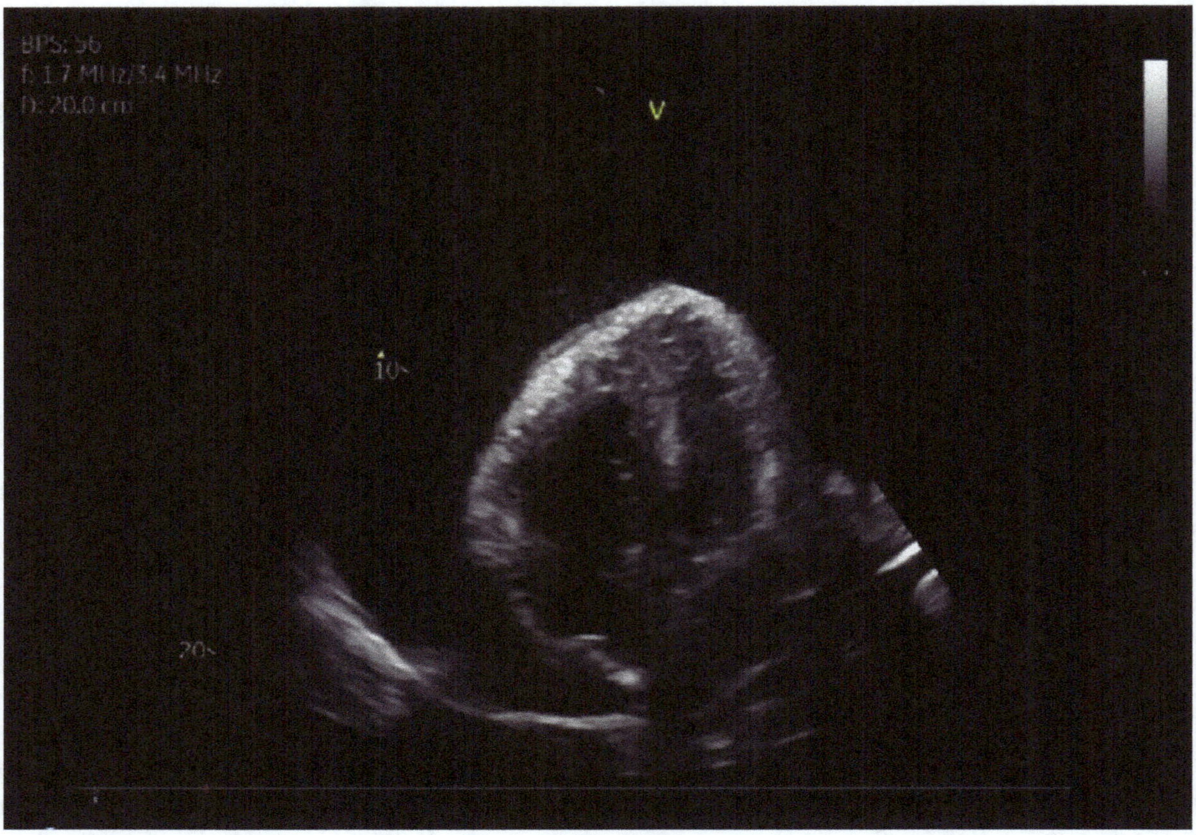

(a)

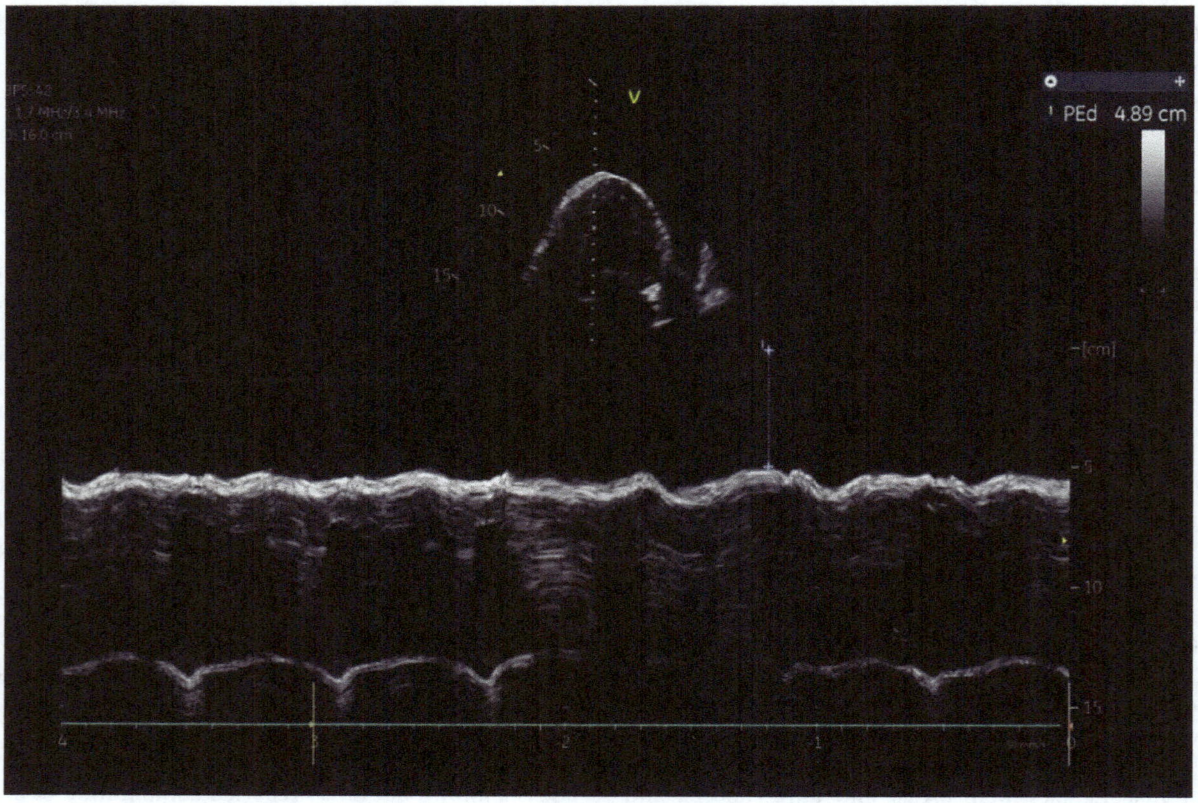

(b)

FIGURE 2: Continued.

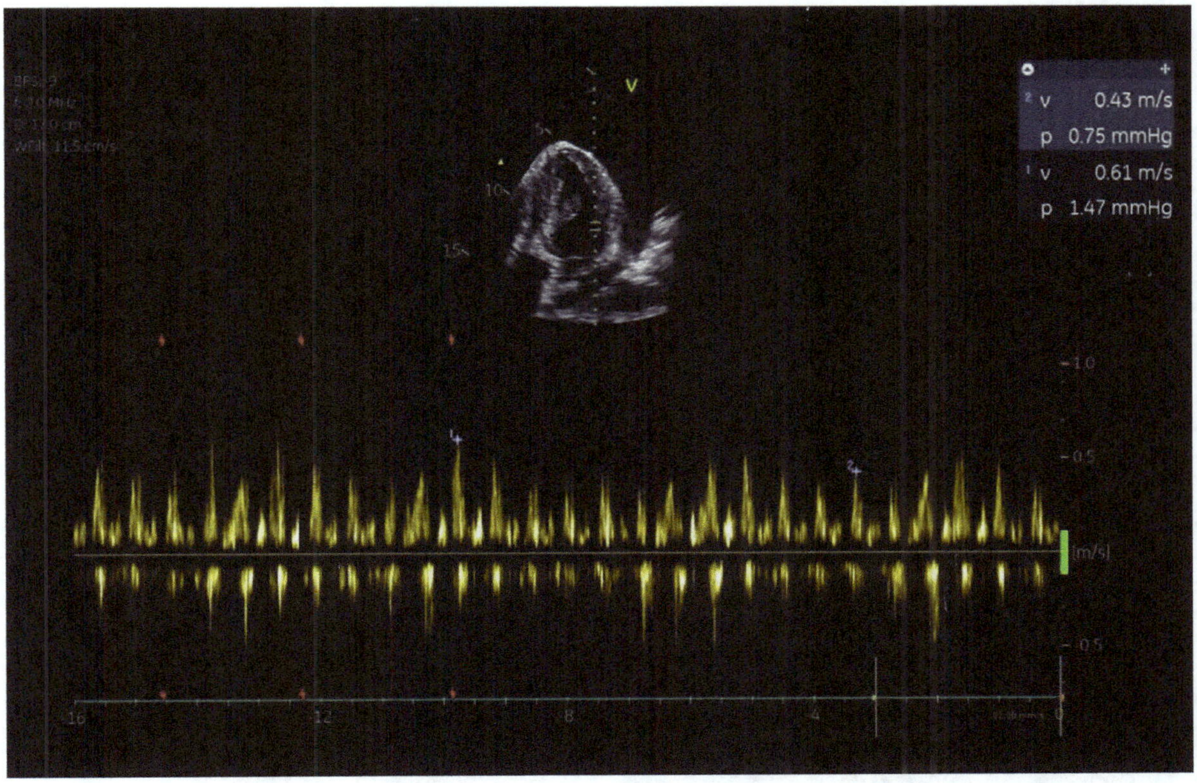

(c)

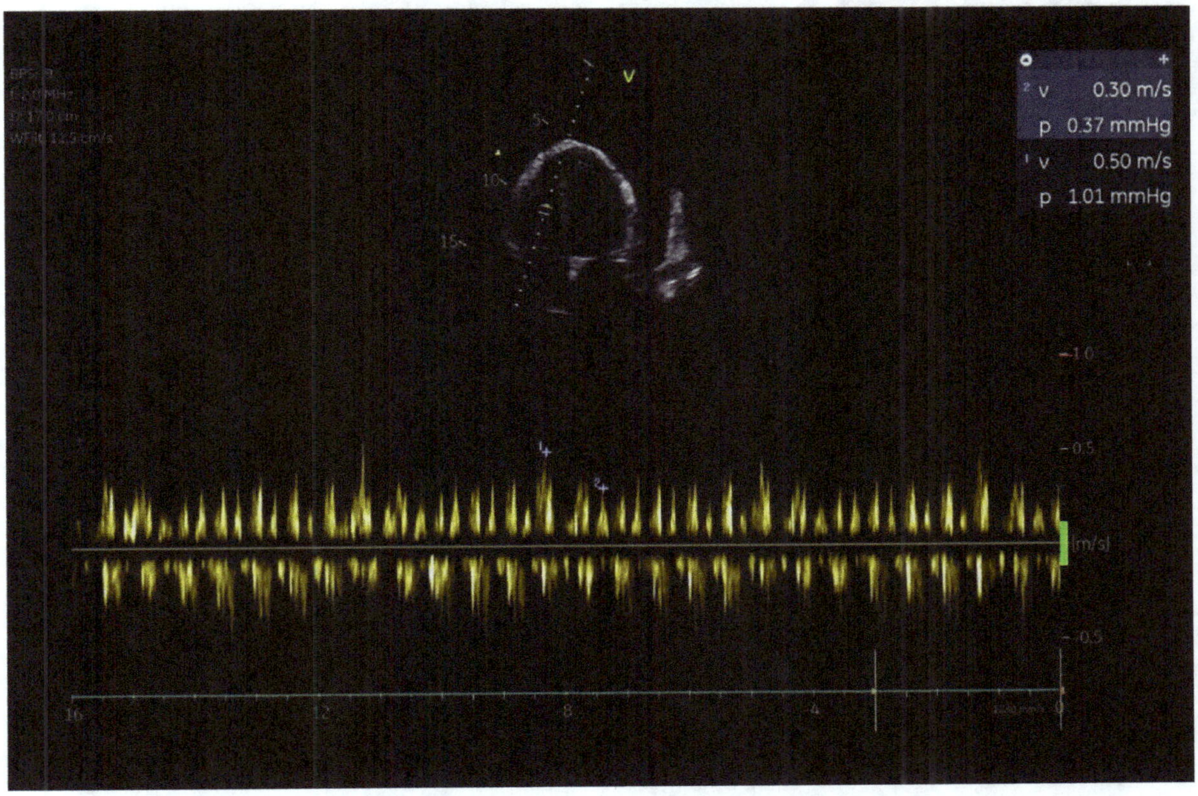

(d)

FIGURE 2: Initial transthoracic echocardiography indicating pericardial tamponade. (a) Apical 4-chamber view with large circumferential pericardial effusion. (b) Apical 4-chamber view (M-mode) with 4.89 mm pericardial effusion end diastolic. (c) Mitral inflow respiratory variation > 25% and (d) tricuspid inflow respiratory variation > 40% by PW-Doppler indicating tamponade morphology; scale and velocity settings are not optimal due to intensive care unit bedside echocardiography.

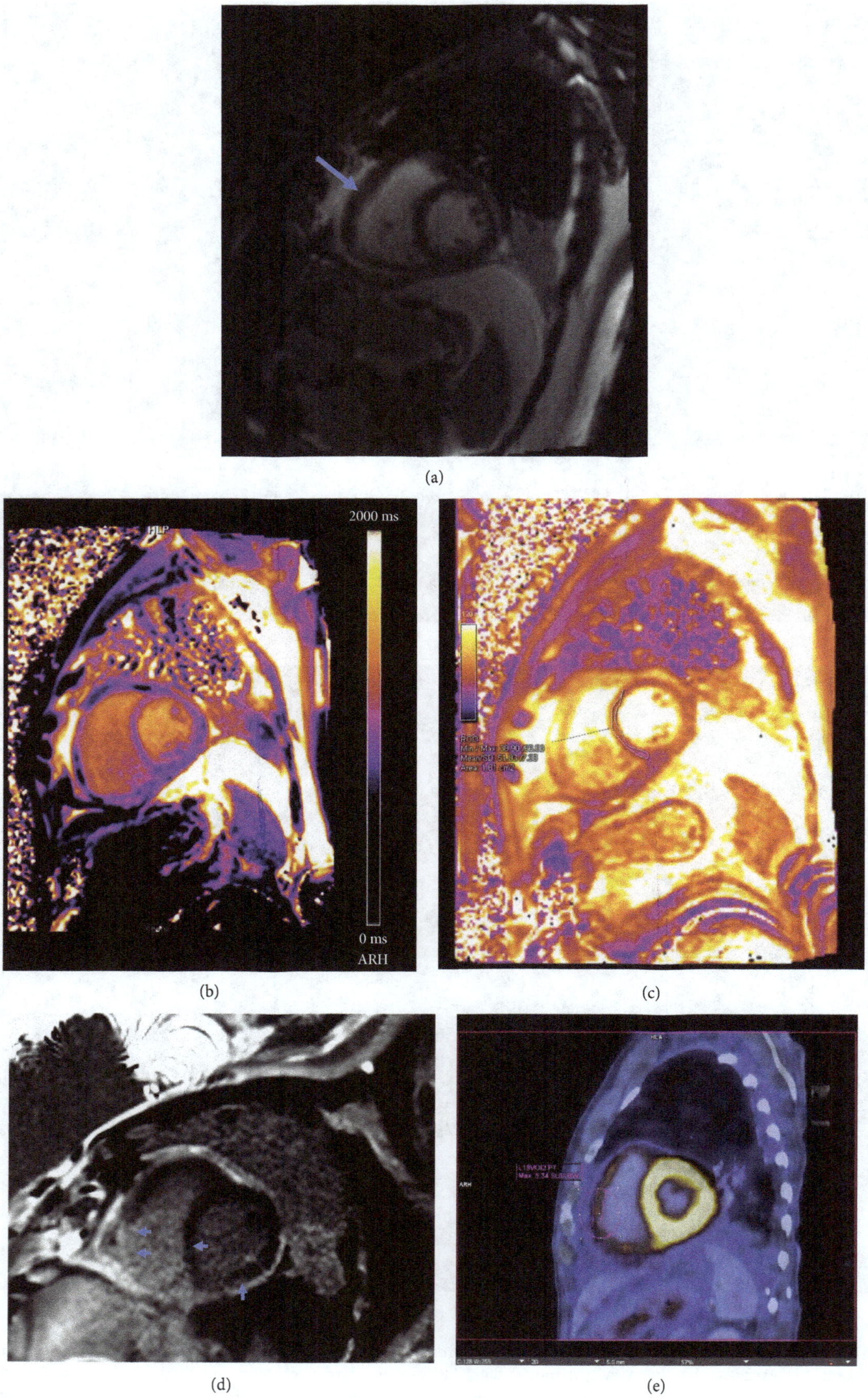

Figure 3: Continued.

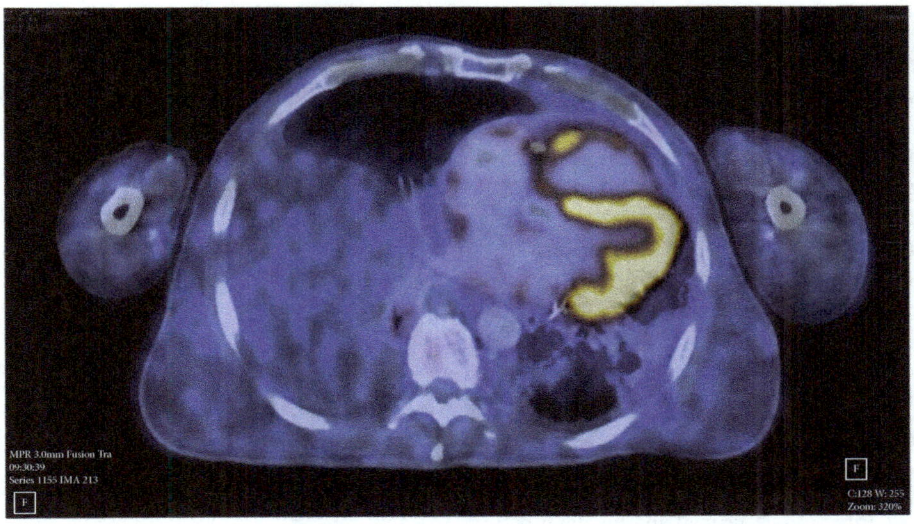

(f)

FIGURE 3: Cross-sectional studies confirmed myocardial inflammation. (a–d) Cardiac magnetic resonance imaging showing right ventricular hypertrophy (a, SSFP cine, ∗), increased T1 relaxation time (septal: 1062 ms, LV posterior wall: 1118 ms) and ECV of 33% (b, T1 map), increased T2 relaxation time to 52 ms septal and 60 ms in LV posterior wall (c, T2 map) and right ventricular, diffuse septal and left ventricular posterior wall late gadolinium enhancement (c, PSIR LGE, arrows) indicating myocarditis and diffuse biventricular fibrosis. (e, f) Positron emission tomography with computed tomography showing FDG uptake in the right ventricular myocardium (SUVmax 5.3), left ventricular uptake was within normal limits.

fluid was tested positive for SARS-CoV-2 by RT-PCR while the second nasopharyngeal swab was negative. They suspected pericardial persistence and a possible direct virus involvement [8]. Furthermore, Garcia-Cruz et al. reported another case of cardiac tamponade with hemorrhagic pericardial effusion secondary to COVID-19. For the first time, they documented changes compatible with acute pericarditis in a pericardial tissue sample with the presence of viral particles in a blood vessel and the interstitium by electron microscopy [9].

To our knowledge, there are only two cases in literature reporting asymptomatic SARS-CoV-2 infection with pericardial tamponade [10, 11]. One had no proven echocardiographic tamponade [10]; the other had upper respiratory tract infection symptoms and was thus not asymptomatic [11]. None of them revealed autoimmune laboratory abnormalities; both were drained about 700 ml bloody pericardial fluid.

However, in contrast to both cases, our patient revealed noticeable increased autoimmune laboratory abnormalities. Berger and Volc proposed a model for viral-induced autoimmunity by type I interferon production and reported an increased frequency of lupus anticoagulant, ANA, anti-erythrocyte antibodies, SSA/Ro, and anti-cardiolipin antibodies in patients with COVID-19 [12]. Thus, the question arose if these laboratory findings are unspecific parainfectious findings, directly associated with COVID-19 or initial signs of an autoimmune disease, in particular systemic lupus erythematosus (SLE).

There are two reported cases of COVID-19 associated tamponade with elevated ANA titer; one was diagnosed with SLE with possible antiphospholipid syndrome [13], and the other one had no signs of myocarditis and showed full recovery in a four-week follow-up [14]. Both presented with symptoms of upper respiratory tract infection. Our patient's demographics, symptoms, and diagnostic findings were not meeting the ACR/EULAR criteria for SLE but matched the Systemic Lupus International Collaborating Clinics (SLICC) classification criteria 2012, supporting the diagnosis of SLE with primary lupus myocarditis and possible antiphospholipid syndrome.

A multicentric lupus myocarditis case series reported myocarditis as the first manifestation of SLE in 58.6% of patients and endomyocardial biopsy (EMB) was low yield in the diagnostic process [15]. In our case, we refrained from EMB due to patient's concerns, fast clinical recovery, and diffuse septal LGE and thus low probability for positive histology. On the other hand, subclavian vein thrombosis and cephalic vein thrombophlebitis may reflect a hypercoagulatory state in the context of COVID-19. As Shah et al. suggested, it would be worthwhile to closely follow those patients with positive autoantibodies [16], because reports of COVID-19 mimicking or precipitating rheumatic musculoskeletal diseases points towards a possibility of persisting intermediate to long-term immune dysregulation.

We are aware that despite the extensive workup, the origin of myopericarditis in our case remains unclear particularly due to the lacking histologic evidence. Regardless of this, a direct or indirect association with SARS-CoV-2 still remained a possible candidate in our diagnostic journey as other differential diagnoses were ruled out and disease progression occurred in the context of a recent asymptomatic infection. Further studies are needed to show whether asymptomatic SARS-CoV-2-infected patients are at risk for potential life-threatening sequelae.

4. Conclusion

The key feature of this case was the diagnostic process in a subacute to late-onset myopericarditis following an asymptomatic SARS-CoV-2 infection and the differentiation between directly linked infectious organ damage, malignancy, and a triggered autoimmune condition. These patients need close follow-up, and an interdisciplinary approach is essential. Awareness of cardiac complications following a SARS-CoV-2 infection is crucial in the diagnostic and therapeutic approach. Due to millions of patients infected in the COVID-19 pandemic, this diagnostic dilemma will be challenging in the future.

Additional Points

Learning Points. (1) Awareness of cardiac complications following a SARS-CoV-2 infection is crucial in the diagnostic and therapeutic approach. (2) Pericardial tamponade is a rare initial presentation in patients with COVID-19 but should be considered as a potential cause of shock. (3) A multimodal imaging approach is crucial in the diagnosis and characterization of cardiac inflammation. (4) Post viral-induced autoimmune phenomena may play a role in late onset pericardial effusions. (5) Echocardiography is a mainstay in rapid bedside diagnosis of pericardial tamponade.

Consent

The authors confirm that written consent for submission and publication of this case report including images and associated text has been obtained from the patient in line with COPE guidance.

Acknowledgments

We thank Dr. Thomas Mayer for his assistance in the care of our patient and reviewing of images and the manuscript. Cardiac imaging was used with kind approval of the Department of Radiology and the Department of Nuclear Medicine (Military Hospital Ulm).

References

[1] T. L. Dao, T. van Hoang, and P. Gautret, "Recurrence of SARS-CoV-2 viral RNA in recovered COVID-19 patients: a narrative review," *European Journal of Clinical Microbiology & Infectious Diseases*, vol. 40, no. 1, pp. 13–25, 2021.

[2] E. Argulian, E. Herzog, D. G. Halpern, and F. H. Messerli, "Paradoxical hypertension with cardiac tamponade," *The American Journal of Cardiology*, vol. 110, no. 7, pp. 1066–1069, 2012.

[3] J. Brown, D. MacKinnon, A. King, and E. Vanderbush, "Elevated arterial blood pressure in cardiac tamponade," *The New England Journal of Medicine*, vol. 327, no. 7, pp. 463–466, 1992.

[4] M. Imazio and Y. Adler, "Management of pericardial effusion," *European Heart Journal*, vol. 34, no. 16, pp. 1186–1197, 2013.

[5] J. Jeudy, J. Kirsch, F. Tavora et al., "From the radiologic pathology archives: cardiac lymphoma: radiologic-pathologic correlation," *Radiographics*, vol. 32, no. 5, pp. 1369–1380, 2012.

[6] J. Saab, R. S. Hoda, N. Narula et al., "Diagnostic yield of cytopathology in evaluating pericardial effusions: clinicopathologic analysis of 419 specimens," *Cancer Cytopathology*, vol. 125, no. 2, pp. 128–137, 2017.

[7] A. Khatri and F. Wallach, "Coronavirus disease 2019 (Covid-19) presenting as purulent fulminant myopericarditis and cardiac tamponade: a case report and literature review," *Heart & Lung*, vol. 49, no. 6, pp. 858–863, 2020.

[8] A. Farina, G. Uccello, M. Spreafico, G. Bassanelli, and S. Savonitto, "SARS-CoV-2 detection in the pericardial fluid of a patient with cardiac tamponade," *European Journal of Internal Medicine*, vol. 76, pp. 100-101, 2020.

[9] E. García-Cruz, D. Manzur-Sandoval, E. A. Lazcano-Díaz, E. Soria-Castro, and S. Jiménez-Becerra, "Cardiac tamponade in a patient with myocardial infarction and COVID-19: electron microscopy," *JACC Case Rep*, vol. 2, no. 12, pp. 2021–2023, 2020.

[10] B. Amoozgar, V. Kaushal, U. Mubashar, S. Sen, S. Yousaf, and M. Yotsuya, "Symptomatic pericardial effusion in the setting of asymptomatic COVID-19 infection: a case report," *Medicine (Baltimore)*, vol. 99, no. 37, article e22093, 2020.

[11] A. Heidari, S. E. Hashemi, M. Parsa Mahjoob, and A. N. Jadbabaei, "Hemorrhagic pericardial effusion leading to cardiac tamponade, as presenting feature of COVID-19 in a young man: a case report," *Acta Biomed*, vol. 91, no. 4, article e2020146, 2020.

[12] J. Berger and S. Volc, "Autoantibodies in Covid-19 - a model for viral induced autoimmunity," *Journal of the European Academy of Dermatology and Venereology*, vol. 35, no. 9, pp. e571–e573, 2021.

[13] E. Mantovani Cardoso, J. Hundal, D. Feterman, and J. Magaldi, "Concomitant new diagnosis of systemic lupus erythematosus and COVID-19 with possible antiphospholipid syndrome. Just a coincidence? A case report and review of intertwining pathophysiology," *Clinical Rheumatology*, vol. 39, no. 9, pp. 2811–2815, 2020.

[14] K. Fox, J. A. Prokup, K. Butson, and K. Jordan, "Acute effusive pericarditis: a late complication of COVID-19," *Cureus*, vol. 12, no. 7, article e9074, 2020.

[15] G. Thomas, F. Cohen Aubart, L. Chiche et al., "Lupus myocarditis: initial presentation and longterm outcomes in a multicentric series of 29 patients," *The Journal of Rheumatology*, vol. 44, no. 1, pp. 24–32, 2017.

[16] S. Shah, D. Danda, C. Kavadichanda, S. Das, M. B. Adarsh, and V. S. Negi, "Autoimmune and rheumatic musculoskeletal diseases as a consequence of SARS-CoV-2 infection and its treatment," *Rheumatology International*, vol. 40, no. 10, pp. 1539–1554, 2020.

12

Saved by the VAC: Minimally Invasive Removal of a Surely Fatal Right Heart Thrombus in a Patient with Advanced Heart Failure

James Keeton,[1] Pedro Engel Gonzalez,[2] Julie Cox,[3] Robert M. Morlend,[2] Alpesh A. Amin,[2] Pradeep P. A. Mammen,[2] Lynn C. Huffman,[2] and Faris G. Araj[2]

[1]*University of Texas Health Science Center, San Antonio, Texas, USA*
[2]*University of Texas Southwestern Medical Center, Dallas, Texas, USA*
[3]*Baylor Scott and White Health, Dallas, Texas, USA*

Correspondence should be addressed to Faris G. Araj; faris.araj@utsouthwestern.edu

Academic Editor: Hajime Kataoka

Intracardiac thrombi are associated with an increased morbidity and mortality due to their unpredictability and embolic potential. Right heart thrombus is infrequently encountered in clinical practice outside the scenario of acute pulmonary embolism with hemodynamic compromise, and even more uncommon is the presence of a massive right heart thrombus. Embolic potential is high, and historically, management has revolved around open surgical removal or systemic thrombolysis. We hereby present a case of a massive right heart thrombus in a high surgical risk patient, which was successfully removed using a percutaneous aspiration device.

1. Introduction

A right heart thrombus (RHT) in transit is an increasingly recognized medical emergency despite its low prevalence because it is associated with a very high mortality, especially if associated with hemodynamic instability, shock, or cardiac arrest [1, 2]. The optimal therapeutic approach is unclear given the absence of randomized control studies. However, the accepted treatment modalities include anticoagulation with systemic thrombolysis or surgical thrombectomy [2, 3]. An emerging treatment option is via catheter-based therapies, but there is still a paucity of data in this area. Critically ill patients are often at high risk of bleeding complications from thrombolytics and can have a forbiddingly high surgical risk. We hereby present a case to illustrate the complexity of treating a critically ill patient who presented with a massive RHT in transit.

2. Case Presentation

A 61-year-old male with a history of inotrope-dependent end-stage nonischemic cardiomyopathy with a severely depressed left ventricular ejection fraction and an implantable cardioverter defibrillator (ICD) presented with bilateral lower extremity edema and seven-pound weight gain. He had no history of atrial fibrillation or venous thrombosis. This was his second hospitalization for acute on chronic decompensated systolic heart failure in a matter of a few months. His examination was notable for a heart rate of 100 bpm, a BP of 85/66 mmHg, and an oxygen saturation of 100% breathing ambient air. He was in no apparent respiratory distress. He had jugular venous distention and a third heart sound, clear lung fields, and bilateral lower extremity pitting edema. He was continued on his inotrope, and treatment with intravenous diuretic therapy was initiated. A transthoracic echocardiogram (TTE) was performed mainly to assess his right ventricular (RV) function since he was being considered for a possible orthotopic heart transplant or left ventricular assist device implant. In addition to severely depressed RV systolic function, he was found to have a new large highly mobile echo density in the right atrium intermittently prolapsing through the tricuspid valve into the right ventricle (Figure 1, Movie 1). The patient had no evidence of infectious signs or symptoms, serial blood cultures

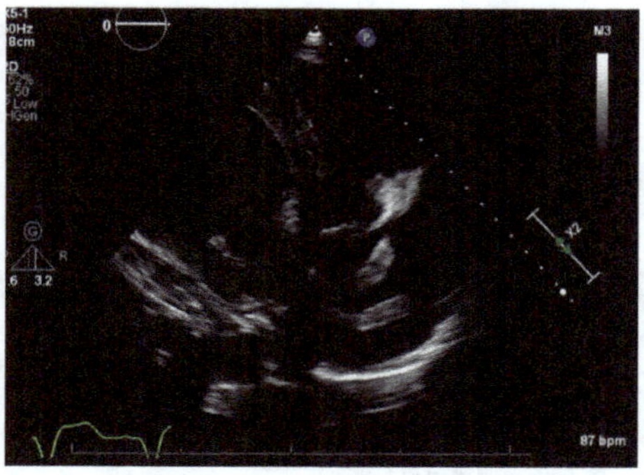

FIGURE 1: Large mobile thrombus in the right atrium prolapsing into the right ventricle.

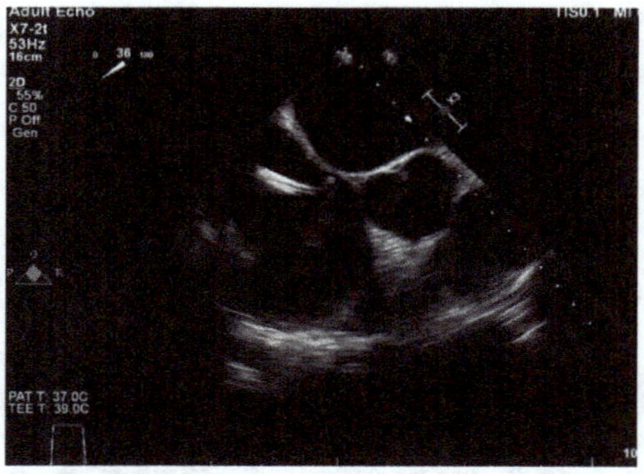

FIGURE 2: Aspiration catheter engaging the thrombus.

remained sterile, and the elongated serpiginous echocardiographic appearance was more suggestive of thrombus than a vegetation. Systemic anticoagulation with intravenous heparin was initiated, and a surgical consultation was obtained. Doppler ultrasound of the bilateral lower extremities did not demonstrate any deep venous thrombosis, and the TTE did not show that the thrombus was clearly attached to the lead. Testing for Factor V Leiden mutation was negative, as was testing for heparin-induced thrombocytopenia. Age-appropriate cancer screening (colon, prostate) was normal, and computed tomography of the head, chest, and abdomen/pelvis did not show any masses or pathologic lymph node enlargement. Additionally, a bone marrow biopsy was negative for any infiltrative or malignant process.

He was deemed to be too high risk for conventional surgical thrombectomy given his severe heart failure, and we were hesitant to administer systemic thrombolytic therapy given the high embolic and bleeding risk. Despite therapeutic systemic anticoagulation, a subsequent TTE 2 days later did not demonstrate reduction in the right atrial thrombus size. After discussions with the cardiothoracic surgery team and the interventional radiology team, the decision was made to attempt a minimally invasive percutaneous thrombectomy using the AngioVac Aspiration System (AngioDynamics, Latham, NY).

Transesophageal echocardiography (TEE) was performed intraoperatively to confirm persistence of the right atrial thrombus prior to proceeding. Under general anesthesia, venous access was obtained via bilateral femoral veins to perform aspiration and reinfuse the blood. An AngioVac device was advanced to the right atrium in proximity to the thrombus (Figure 2, Movie 2). Subsequently, a 22 cm thrombus (Figure 3) was removed, and no residual thrombus was seen on intraoperative imaging. There were no apparent procedural complications, and the patient was continued on systemic intravenous anticoagulation afterwards. Subsequent cultures of the excised thrombus did not reveal any growth. The patient underwent successful cardiac transplantation three weeks later.

3. Discussion

The incidence of echocardiographically detected RHT in the setting of acute pulmonary embolism (PE) is low, approximating 2-4%, with the highest incidence observed in cases of acute PE with associated hemodynamic instability [1–3]. The presence of RHT in the setting of acute PE increases mortality, suggesting that detection with echocardiography may have both prognostic and therapeutic implications [1–3]. It is uncertain if the presence of a right heart thromboembolism is an independent risk factor for increased mortality, or a marker of hemodynamic dysfunction and more severe PE [3]. Without treatment, RHT in acute PE carries a 100% mortality [4, 5]. Morphologically, RHT are either elongated and serpiginous (occasionally prolapsing into the right ventricle) or either ovoid or round (typically nonmobile) [6]. Serpiginous thrombi have been associated with higher mortality, suggesting that the morphology of RHT may be a significant predictor of prognosis, although data are conflicting in this regard [3, 6].

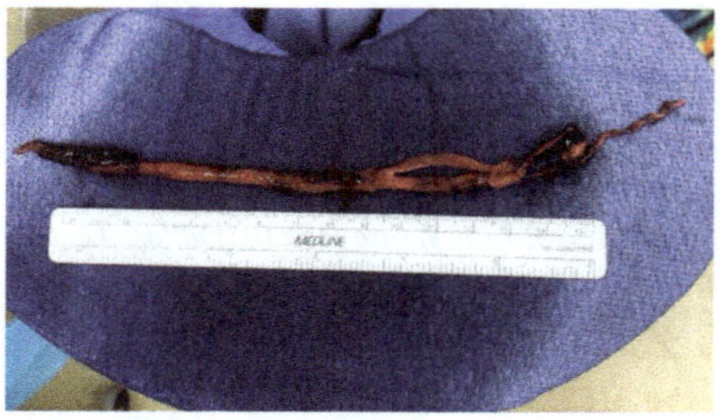

FIGURE 3: 22 cm thrombus removed by the aspiration device.

There are no randomized clinical trial data to date to provide evidence-based guidance for any specific therapeutic modality. The main treatment options for RHT includes systemic anticoagulation, thrombolytic therapy, and either surgical or percutaneous aspiration thrombectomy. Systemic anticoagulation is considered an appropriate first line therapy for hemodynamically stable patients, although it may not be entirely effective in cases of large thrombi [3, 7]. Systemic thrombolysis can be administered rapidly and dissolves clots in several locations simultaneously (heart, pulmonary, and femoral vasculature). Systemic thrombolysis has the potential to embolize clot fragments or the entire clot by disruption of the attachment site, which can be fatal [8, 9]. Furthermore, one in five patients may suffer a bleeding complication, most feared of which would be an intracranial bleed [9]. Although small retrospective observational studies suggest that thrombolysis may be superior to anticoagulation and surgical thrombectomy, the data are conflicting [8, 9]. Open surgical thrombectomy is an invasive procedure with restrictions based on surgical risk, which leads to the exclusion of otherwise eligible candidates. Apart from the high procedural mortality [7], this involves scheduling delays and cardiopulmonary bypass.

Percutaneous aspiration thrombectomy represents a novel and less invasive method to address right heart thrombi in select patients. This treatment innovation has previously been utilized for aspiration of DVTs, including thrombi associated with inferior vena cava filters, as well as vegetations, tumors, and foreign bodies [10, 11]. The AngioVac system essentially functions as a venovenous extracorporeal membrane oxygenation circuit connected to a thrombus filter and centrifugal pump. The thrombus is aspirated, passed through a filter, and trapped in a reservoir. Then, thrombus-free blood is returned to the body [11]. Based on a single-center case series, this technique is commonly successful (up to 80%) in the removal of RHT [12]. In comparison to open surgical thrombectomy, and in the appropriately selected patient, percutaneous aspiration thrombectomy is considered a relatively safer procedure with the most common complication being access site bleeding and hematoma [12, 13]. However, there are other practical limitations to consider as well, including the device's larger profile cannula preventing use in smaller veins, rigidity of the cannula creating difficulty with maneuvering, and lack of operator experience. Additionally, patients with a contraindication to anticoagulation would not be candidates for this therapy [12, 13].

In conclusion, percutaneous aspiration thrombectomy offers a minimally invasive and potentially safer alternative to systemic thrombolytics or open surgical thrombectomy. This method successfully removed a surely fatal massive right heart thrombus in our patient with advanced heart failure, allowing him the opportunity to continue to heart transplant.

Disclosure

This work has been accepted as a poster presentation at the ACC.20 World Congress of Cardiology that will take place in March 2020 in Chicago, Illinois.

Acknowledgments

The manuscript was funded through the Endowed Alfred W. Harris, M.D., Professorship in Cardiology awarded to Pradeep P.A. Mammen.

References

[1] A. Torbicki, N. Galié, A. Covezzoli et al., "Right heart thrombi in pulmonary embolism: results from the International Cooperative Pulmonary Embolism Registry," *Journal of the American College of Cardiology*, vol. 41, no. 12, pp. 2245–2251, 2003.

[2] K. M. KoćM, W. Elikowski, and N. Meneveau, "Outcome of patients with right heart thrombi: the Right Heart Thrombi European Registry," *European Respiratory Journal*, vol. 47, no. 3, pp. 869–875, 2016.

[3] N. M. Dabbouseh, J. J. Patel, and P. A. Bergl, "Role of echocardiography in managing acute pulmonary embolism," *Heart*, vol. 105, no. 23, pp. 1785–1792, 2019.

[4] P. S. Rose, N. M. Punjabi, and D. B. Pearse, "Treatment of right heart thromboemboli," *Chest*, vol. 121, no. 3, pp. 806–814, 2002.

[5] L. Lazar, R. Dave, and R. Tabibiazar, "Dilemma of right atrial thrombi, to dissolve or to extract," *Proceedings of UCLA Healthcare*, vol. 16, pp. 1–4, 2012.

[6] G. Koronik, "The European Cooperative Study on the clinical significance of right heart thrombi," *European Heart Journal*, vol. 10, no. 12, pp. 1046–1059, 1989.

[7] G. Pierre-Justin and L. A. Pierard, "Management of mobile right heart thrombi: a prospective series," *International Journal of Cardiology*, vol. 99, no. 3, pp. 381–388, 2005.

[8] M. Ruiz-Bailén, C. López-Caler, A. Castillo-Rivera et al., "Giant right atrial thrombi treated with thrombolysis," *The Canadian Journal of Cardiology*, vol. 24, no. 4, pp. 312–314, 2008.

[9] R. Agarwal, A. N. Aggarwal, and D. Gupta, "Is right heart thromboemboli another indication for thrombolysis?," *Internal Medicine Journal*, vol. 37, no. 5, pp. 333–335, 2007.

[10] C. Basman, U. Rashid, Y. J. Parmar, C. Kliger, and I. Kronzon, "The role of percutaneous vacuum-assisted thrombectomy for intracardiac and intravascular pathology," *Journal of Cardiac Surgery*, vol. 33, no. 10, pp. 666–672, 2018.

[11] F. Casazza, C. Becattini, E. Guglielmelli et al., "Prognostic significance of free-floating right heart thromboemboli in acute pulmonary Embolism," *Thrombosis and Haemostasis*, vol. 111, no. 1, pp. 53–57, 2014.

[12] M. D'Ayala, B. Worku, L. Gulkarov, A. Sista, J. Horowitz, and A. Salemi, "Factors associated with successful thrombus extraction with the AngioVac device: an institutional experience," *Annals of Vascular Surgery*, vol. 38, pp. 242–247, 2017.

[13] T. H. Enezate, A. Kumar, K. Aggarwal, S. Balla, and J. Omran, "Non-surgical extraction of right atrial mass by AngioVac aspiration device under fluoroscopic and transesophageal echocardiographic guidance," *Cardiovascular Diagnosis and Therapy*, vol. 7, no. 3, pp. 331–335, 2017.

13

A Case of Quadricuspid Aortic Valve Regurgitation: The Cardiac Clover

John S. Dayco[1] **and Shaun Cardozo**[2]

[1]*PGY-I, Internal Medicine, Department of Internal Medicine, Detroit Medical Center, USA*
[2]*Division of Cardiology, Physician, Division of Cardiology, Detroit Medical Center, Wayne State University, Wayne State University Physician Group, USA*

Correspondence should be addressed to John S. Dayco; jdayco@med.wayne.edu

Academic Editor: Francesco Nappi

A quadricuspid aortic valve is a very rare congenital heart condition that can present as aortic regurgitation in the 5th and 6th decade of life. The following case report will describe a patient who presented with symptoms of severe aortic regurgitation and was found to have a quadricuspid aortic valve on echocardiography. The case will describe the clinical manifestations in which the patient presented and the subsequent diagnosis of the quadricuspid aortic valve. The rationale for the surgical approach will also be discussed, along with the patient's clinical response.

1. Introduction

A quadricuspid aortic valve (QAV) is a very rare congenital heart condition with an incidence of only 0.008-0.033% in an autopsy series of patients and 0.013-0.043% in patients undergoing transthoracic echocardiography (TTE) [1]. The pathogenesis is usually due to an abnormal fusion of the aorticopulmonary septum during embryogenesis, which leads to an aortic valve with an extra 4th cusp [2]. The complications manifested by QAVs are mainly aortic regurgitation, and a QAV is often incidentally discovered during an echocardiogram [3]. Aortic stenosis can also be observed along with regurgitation; however, aortic stenosis by itself is a rare presentation of a QAV. These complications usually arise during the 5th to 6th decade of life, as is observed in the following patient. This case report will highlight the nonspecific manifestation of a QAV, the classification with the Hurwitz and Roberts model, and the rationale for surgical intervention.

2. Case

Our patient is a 62-year-old female with a past medical history of heart failure with preserved ejection fraction (55-60% visually estimated ejection fraction) New York Heart Associate (NYHA) Class III, hypertension, and hyperlipidemia who was seen in clinic for worsening dyspnea on exertion. Her vital signs were stable, and on exam, she had a grade III/VI diastolic murmur along the left upper sternal border that increased with expiration. The EKG was normal sinus rhythm. ATTE was performed, which showed moderate to severe aortic regurgitation. In order to delineate the pathology and severity of the regurgitation, a transesophageal echocardiogram (TEE) was performed and showed an aortic valve morphology suspicious for a quadricuspid aortic valve (Figure 1). The valve demonstrated doming and four areas of commissural fusion were noted (Figure 2). The aortic root was mildly enlarged at 4.51 cm (Figure 3). There

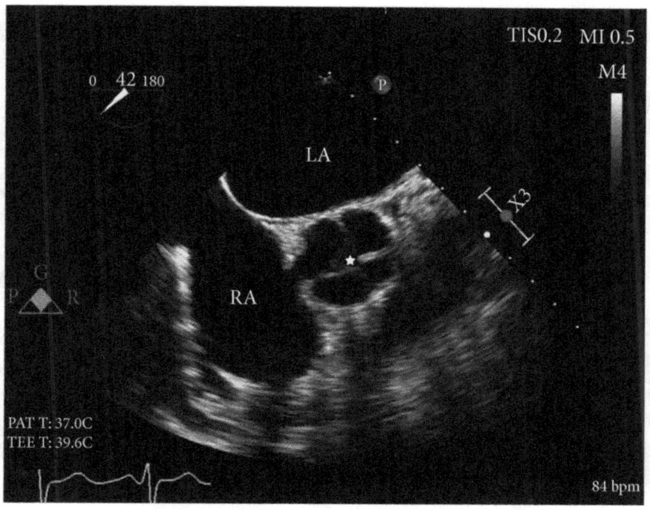

FIGURE 1: Mid epigastric short axis view. The closed aortic valve is demonstrating the characteristic X pattern as seen in QAVs in a TEE. The incomplete closure is marked with a star, leading to significant aortic regurgitation.

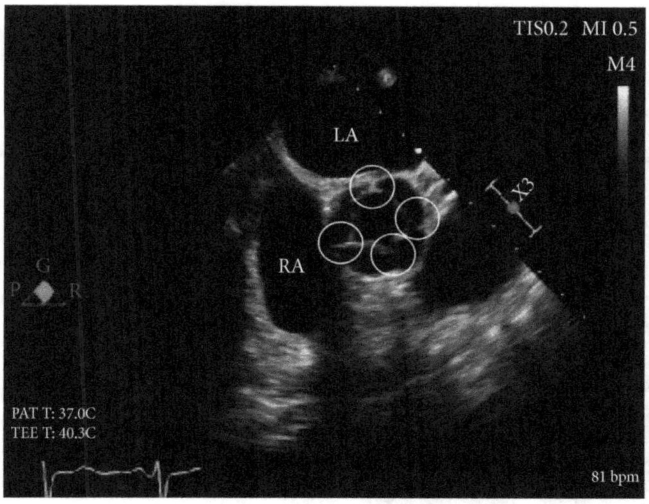

FIGURE 2: Mid Epigastric Short Axis View. During systole, 4 areas of commissural cusps fusion are noted (circled), suggesting aortic stenosis.

was holodiastolic flow reversal noted at the proximal descending aorta which helped to support severe regurgitation (Figures 4 and 5). The presence of a systolic aortic cusp doming also suggested a superimposed aortic stenosis (Figure 3). A coronary angiogram showed no significant coronary artery stenosis, and subsequently, the patient then underwent an aortic valve replacement (AVR) with a 21 mm Edwards Magna Ease bovine pericardial bioprosthetic valve. During the surgery, the presence of the quadricuspid aortic valve was confirmed on gross pathology. Immediately, postoperatively, the patient developed ventricular tachycardia and atrial fibrillation. She was then transferred to the surgical intensive care unit to receive an amiodarone drip for two days, which has resolved her atrial fibrillation and ventricular tachycardia. A repeat EKG showed normal sinus rhythm. She was then discharged with oral metoprolol. The patient underwent an uncomplicated recovery process, and her dyspnea on exertion has improved tremendously after a course of cardiac rehabilitation. A repeat TEE revealed a left ventricular end diastolic diameter of 4.7 cm, which is an improvement from 4.96 cm before the AVR, indicating a reduction in aortic regurgitation.

3. Discussion

This patient initially presented for dyspnea on exertion, along with a loud diastolic murmur in the left upper sternal border. While this kind of presentation is concerning for aortic regurgitation, the suspicion for a QAV did not arise until the patient received a TEE, which showed the characteristic "X" pattern of the aortic valve, as opposed to the normal "Y" (aka *Mercedes-Benz* pattern) of a normal tricuspid aortic valve (Figure 1). Aortic regurgitation is the most common

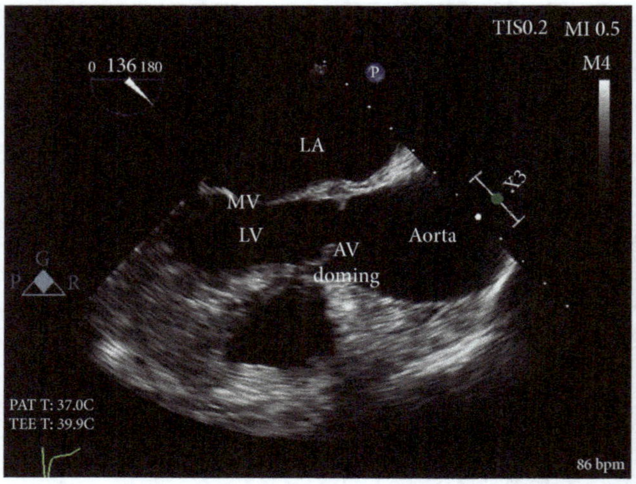

Figure 3: Mid epigastric long axis view. In Figure 3, aortic valve doming is seen during midsystole, suggesting asymmetry and restriction. In Figure 4, taken with doppler ultrasonography during middiastole, a "mosaic pattern" (star) is evident in the left ventricular area, suggesting aortic regurgitant flow.

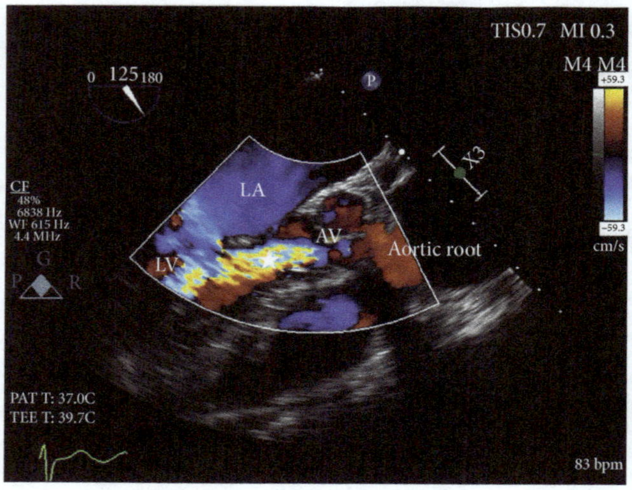

Figure 4: Mid epigastric long axis view. In Figure 3, aortic valve doming is seen during midsystole, suggesting asymmetry and restriction. In Figure 4, taken with doppler ultrasonography during middiastole, a "mosaic pattern" (star) is evident in the left ventricular area, suggesting aortic regurgitant flow.

complication of a QAV, and the finding of a holodiastolic flow reversal in the descending aorta supported this (Figure 5). Aortic stenosis could also be observed, such as when commissural fusion occurs (Figure 2). In Figure 4, the doppler image showed the characteristic "mosaic pattern," as seen during the reversal of flow through the insufficient aortic valve in diastole. For the purpose of visualization and ease of access, cardiac echocardiography remains to be the imaging standard for a QAV. With the recent advent of more advanced imaging modalities, studies such as cardiac MRIs are proving to be particularly useful in the diagnosis of QAV. The gold standard in the classification of QAVs

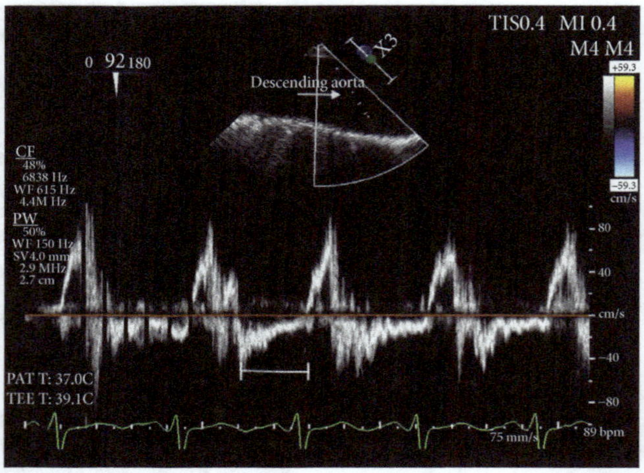

Figure 5: Descending aorta long axis view. In this image, a holosystolic aortic regurgitation is shown by the waveform labeled "I."

remains to be the Hurwitz-Robinson classification [2], which classifies QAVs into 7 different subtypes, depending on the cusp morphology (Table 1).

Types A, B, and C comprise the vast majority of cases at >80% [2]. Our patient, as seen in the images obtained in the TEE (Figure 1), has 3 identical cusps and 1 smaller cusp, classifying it as Type B.

The decision to perform a surgical aortic valve replacement on the patient was made on the basis of worsening dyspnea on exertion, with the QAV producing aortic regurgitation. By this time, the patient had progressed to New York Heart Associate Class III, exhibiting symptoms with mild exertion, such as going to the bathroom. Based on the ACC/AHA guidelines, AVR is indicated for symptomatic patients with severe AR regardless of LV systolic function. For such patients, immediate surgical intervention is indicated to greatly improve the patient's quality of life, as well as to prevent long-term sequela, such as left ventricular cavity dilation from the volume overload due to constant aortic regurgitation. In addition, a serious complication may also arise in which one of the supernumerary cusps may develop bacterial seeding, leading to infective endocarditis [4]. This usually occurs at the extra cusp, such as the one smaller cusp in Type B cases like our patient. Some authors recommend antibiotic prophylaxis unconditionally for any dental procedures [5]. However, per current ACC/AHA guidelines, antibiotics prophylaxis is only indicated for symptomatic patients with active infection [6]. The treatment of choice is surgical aortic valve replacement (SAVR) [7]. The surgical approach includes tricuspidization, bicuspidization, or a complete aortic valve replacement. These choices depend on factors such as the quality of the native aortic valve, the presence of calcification and stenosis, and surgeon capabilities. Our patient received a 21 mm Edwards Magna Ease bovine pericardial bioprosthetic valve, with a noncomplicated post-op recovery period. The SAVR procedure proved to be very effective for the

Table 1: Hurtwitz-Robinson classification of quadricuspid aortic valve.

Type	Description	Morphology
Type A	(4) Identical cusps	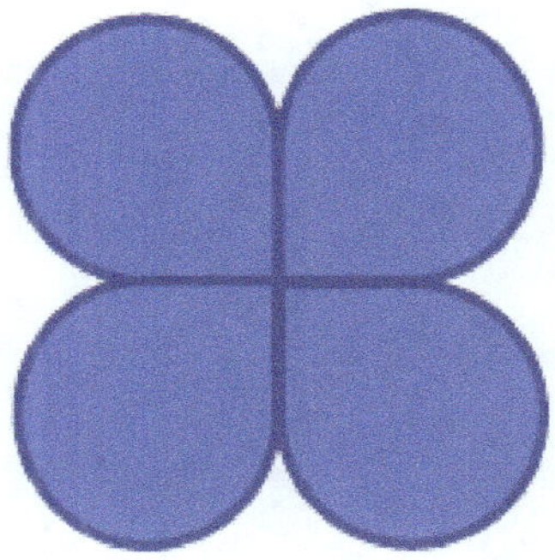
Type B	(3) Identical and (1) smaller cusp	
Type C	(2) Identical and (2) smaller cusps	
Type D	(1) Large, (2) intermediate, and (1) small cusp	
Type E	(3) Identical and (1) larger cusp	

Table 1: Continued.

Type	Description	Morphology
		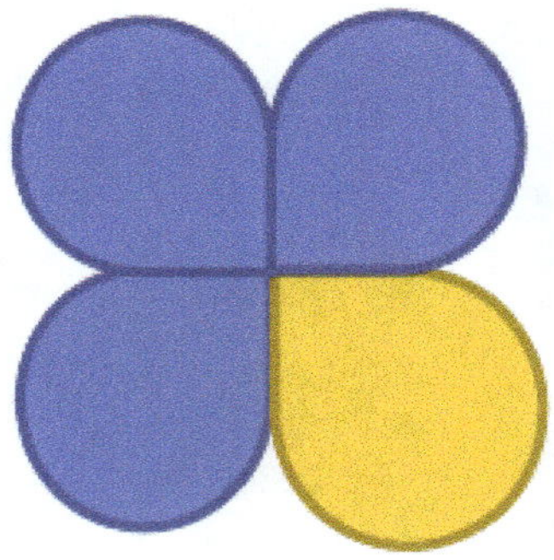
Type F	(2) Larger identical and (2) smaller nonidentical cusps	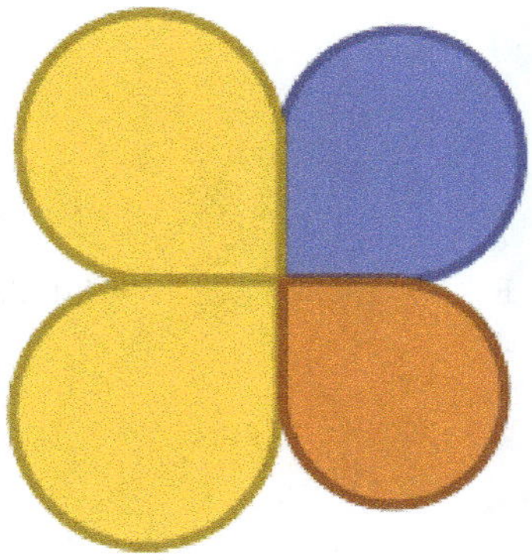
Type G	(4) Nonidentical cusps	

patient, as a repeat TTE showed a significant improvement in the aortic regurgitation. More importantly, the shortness of breath and dyspnea on exertion has tremendously improved. The patient will require constant monitoring, such as a yearly TTE, due to the lower durability of bioprosthetic aortic valves as compared to a mechanical valve or native valve tricuspidization.

References

[1] B. J. Feldman, B. K. Khandheria, C. A. Warnes, J. B. Seward, C. L. Taylor, and A. J. Tajik, "Incidence, description and functional assessment of isolated quadricuspid aortic valves," *The American Journal of Cardiology*, vol. 65, no. 13, pp. 937-938, 1990.

[2] L. E. Hurwitz and W. C. Roberts, "Quadricuspid semilunar valve," *The American Journal of Cardiology*, vol. 31, no. 5, pp. 623–626, 1973.

[3] M. Y. Tsang, M. M. Abudiab, N. M. Ammash et al., "Quadricuspid aortic valve: characteristics, associated structural cardiovascular abnormalities, and clinical outcomes," *Circulation*, vol. 133, no. 3, pp. 312–319, 2016.

[4] N. Takeda, E. Ohtaki, H. Kasegawa, T. Tobaru, and T. Sumiyoshi, "Infective endocarditis associated with quadricuspid aortic valve," *Japanese Heart Journal*, vol. 44, no. 3, pp. 441–445, 2003.

[5] Y. Kawanishi, H. Tanaka, K. Nakagiri, T. Yamashita, K. Okada, and Y. Okita, "Congenital quadricuspid aortic valve associated with severe regurgitation," *Asian Cardiovascular & Thoracic Annals*, vol. 16, no. 5, pp. e40–e41, 2008.

[6] R. A. Nishimura, B. A. Carabello, D. P. Faxon et al., "ACC/AHA 2008 Guideline update on valvular heart disease: focused update on infective endocarditis: a report of the American College of Cardiology/American Heart Association Task Force on Practice Guidelines endorsed by the Society of Cardiovascular Anesthesiologists, Society for Cardiovascular Angiography and Interventions," vol. 118, Tech. Rep. 8, .

14

The First Case of Native Mitral Valve Endocarditis due to *Micrococcus luteus* and Review of the Literature

Alisha Khan, Thu Thu Aung, and Debanik Chaudhuri

State University of New York Upstate University Hospital, USA

Correspondence should be addressed to Alisha Khan; khanali@upstate.edu

Academic Editor: Expedito E. Ribeiro

Gram-positive cocci species, notably *Staphylococcus*, *Streptococcus*, and *Enterococcus* account for 80 to 90% of infective endocarditis cases. HACEK microorganisms (*Haemophilus* spp., *Aggregatibacter actinomycetemcomitans*, *Cardiobacterium hominis*, *Eikenella corrodens*, and *Kingella kingae*) account for approximately 3% of cases and *Candida* species account for 1-2% of cases. *Micrococcus luteus* is a rare cause of endocarditis. To our knowledge, only 17 cases of prosthetic valve endocarditis have been described due to *M. luteus* and a single case of native aortic valve endocarditis has been described. The following case is the only documented case of native mitral valve endocarditis. A review of the literature pertaining to Micrococcus endocarditis was performed to further characterize the entity.

1. Case Presentation

A 67-year-old gentleman presented to our hospital with complaints of dyspnea and orthopnea. His past medical history included diabetes, hypertension, three cerebrovascular accidents, peripheral vascular disease status post right below knee amputation (BKA), and moderate-to-severe mitral valve insufficiency. He was admitted with acute on chronic diastolic heart failure and was started on a bumetanide infusion. Of note, the patient's BKA was three months prior to admission and was complicated by bacteremia and sepsis.

On admission, his vital signs were stable and within normal limits. He was intermittently noted to be tachypneic with his respiratory rate reaching 26 breaths per minute. Physical examination was remarkable for jugular venous distention, grade 4/6 systolic murmur best heard at the mitral position, decreased lung breath sounds at the bases, and trace pedal edema. Complete blood count and comprehensive metabolic panel laboratory values were within normal limits. Pro b-type natriuretic peptide level was elevated at 5309 pg/mL. Two sets of blood cultures showed no growth at 5 days. Chest radiograph revealed large bilateral pleural effusions. Transthoracic echocardiogram revealed prolapse of the anterior mitral leaflet with moderate-to-severe mitral regurgitation, hyperdynamic left ventricular (LV) systolic function with an ejection fraction between 65 and 70%, no evidence of vegetation, and an estimated pulmonary artery systolic pressure of 71 mmHg with moderate-to-severe tricuspid regurgitation. Preoperative left heart catheterization showed 80-90% stenosis of the diagonal artery and elevated left ventricular diastolic pressure. Snapshot hemodynamic recordings of the aortic pressure revealed 109/70 mmHg (mean 86 mmHg), whereas the left ventricle measured 110/11 mmHg (mean 27 mmHg).

The patient was diuresed over several days with partial relief of his respiratory symptoms. Cardiac catheterization showed occlusion of one of the diagonal branches that was not amenable to endovascular intervention. The cardiothoracic surgery team evaluated the patient for replacement of his mitral valve. He was brought to the operating room where he underwent cardiopulmonary bypass and had his native mitral valve replaced with a 29-Medtronic Mosaic porcine bioprosthetic valve. Upon visual inspection, the native mitral valve was found to have fibrinopurulent exudate on the anterior and posterior leaflets. Surgical tissue cultures of the excised mitral valve grew *Micrococcus luteus*. Surgical pathology of the excised valve showed acute endocarditis with focal necrosis. Antibiotic susceptibility testing revealed that the

Micrococcus luteus was sensitive to vancomycin, clindamycin, erythromycin, and penicillin. Replacement of his mitral valve and concurrent diuresis resulted in significant symptomatic and echocardiographic findings. Transthoracic echocardiogram performed approximately one week following valve replacement showed resolution of the mitral and tricuspid regurgitation as well as normalization of the pulmonary artery systolic pressure, indicating that the initial derangements noted on the echocardiogram were likely dynamic changes resulting from the mitral regurgitation. Ejection fraction at this time was noted to be 60-65%.

The patient was initially treated with empiric antibiotics including vancomycin, gentamicin, and rifampin. However, the patient developed acute kidney injury due to acute tubular necrosis from vancomycin and gentamicin and was subsequently transitioned to rifampin 300 mg by mouth every 12 hours and daptomycin 8 mg/kg intravenously every 48 hours at 100 mL/hour over 30 minutes to complete his treatment course for a total of six weeks of antibiotics. The patient was subsequently discharged to cardiac rehabilitation while receiving a total of six weeks of intravenous antibiotics to treat for endocarditis from the date of his mitral valve replacement.

Since treatment for his infective endocarditis, the patient's bioprosthetic valve appeared to have been functioning well for several months. However, approximately nine months after replacement, he was diagnosed with end-stage renal disease. Due to the associated fluid overload, his most recent echocardiogram shows that he has recurrent moderate mitral valve regurgitation; however, the prosthetic valve is well seated and does not rock. He is currently undergoing preparation for hemodialysis.

2. Discussion

Micrococcus species are Gram-positive, catalase-positive, oxidase-positive, nonmotile, and nonspore-forming cocci that comprise oropharyngeal and skin flora and rarely cause disease [1]. In fact, *M. luteus* used to be considered a nonpathogenic saprophyte or pure contaminant.

Micrococcus species, along with coagulase negative-staphylococci, viridans group streptococci, *Propionibacterium acnes*, *Corynebacterium* spp., and *Bacillus* spp., are the microorganisms the College of American Pathologists considers to be the most common blood culture contaminants when isolated from one out of two or three blood sets [2, 3]. However, in rare circumstances, *Micrococcus* spp. may be the causative organism for infectious diseases such as endocarditis. The first documented disease due to the organism was septic shock in 1978, when it was simultaneously recovered from a patient's blood cultures and gallbladder isolate [4]. In our case, the patient's diagnosis of infective endocarditis was confirmed by histology of the surgical specimen and the presence of new valvular regurgitation, according to the Modified Duke Infective Endocarditis Criteria.

The five species in the *Micrococcus* genus include *M. luteus*, *M. lylae*, *M. antarcticus*, *M. endophyticus*, and *M. flavus*. *Micrococcus luteus* is an obligate aerobe and has one of the smallest genomes of free-living actinobacteria sequenced to date, comprised of a single circular chromosome of 2,501,097 base pairs encoding 2,403 proteins [5].

M. luteus is a rare cause of endocarditis. Although low in virulence and usually sensitive to penicillin, it may colonize the surface of heart valves in immunosuppressed patients [1]. It has now been proposed as the pathogenic organism responsible for bacteremia, ventriculitis, peritonitis, pneumonia, endophthalmitis, keratolysis, and septic arthritis in isolated case reports [6].

In November 2018, a case of bacteremia due to *Micrococcus luteus* was described in an immunocompromised patient with a central venous catheter [7]. In December 2018, *M. luteus* was found to be the cause of a brain abscess in an immunocompromised patient with systemic lupus erythematosus who was being treated with immunosuppressive therapy for lupus nephritis [8]. Our patient's uncontrolled diabetes mellitus, with an HbA1c level of 7.4% on admission appears to have been his only known predisposing factor for immunosuppression, which would make him more susceptible to infection with a low virulence organism such as *M. luteus*.

In a review of the literature published by Miltiadous and Elisaf in 2011, only 17 cases of native valve endocarditis secondary to *M. luteus* had been reported and all involved prosthetic valves. A single case of native aortic valve endocarditis due to *M. luteus* has been described in an immunosuppressed patient [9]. To our knowledge, there are no case reports describing isolated native mitral valve endocarditis due to *M. luteus*.

We suspect that our patient became bacteremic with *M. luteus* during his BKA surgery three months prior to admission. Interestingly, in the case of native aortic valve endocarditis described by Miltiadous and Elisaf, the authors presumed that orthopedic surgery (total knee replacement) three weeks prior to admission was the source of bacteremia [9]. This supports the theory that in order for low virulence organisms such as *M. luteus* to become pathogenic and cause serious and invasive infections such as endocarditis, a significant bacterial load is required.

Due to the rarity of this microorganism as a cause for infective endocarditis, the optimal therapeutic regimen remains undefined. Of note, in the case of native aortic valve endocarditis secondary to *M. luteus* mentioned above, a treatment regimen consisting of vancomycin, gentamicin, and rifampicin for four weeks was *not* successful and the patient ultimately required aortic valve replacement [9]. Our patient who was treated with rifampin and daptomycin in addition to mitral valve replacement appears to have been successfully treated thus far.

Consent

Written informed consent was obtained from the patient for publication of this case report.

References

[1] U. N. Durst, E. Bruder, L. Egloff, J. Wust, J. Schneider, and H. O. Hirzel, "Micrococcus luteus: a rare pathogen of valve prosthesis endocarditis," *Zeitschrift fur Kardiologie*, vol. 80, no. 4, pp. 294–298, 1991.

[2] S. Dargere, H. Cormier, and R. Verdon, "Contaminants in blood cultures: importance, implications, interpretation and prevention," *Clinical Microbiology and Infection*, vol. 24, no. 9, pp. 964–969, 2018.

[3] K. Alcorn, F. Meier, and R. Schifman, *Blood Culture Contamination. Q-Tracks 2013 Monitor Instructions*, College of American Pathologists, Northfield, IL, 2013.

[4] D. Albertson, G. A. Natsios, and R. Gleckman, "Septic shock with Micrococcus luteus," *Archives of Internal Medicine*, vol. 133, no. 3, pp. 487-488, 1978.

[5] M. Young, V. Artsatbanov, H. R. Beller et al., "Genome sequence of the Fleming strain of Micrococcus luteus, a simple free-living actinobacterium," *Journal of bacteriology*, vol. 192, no. 3, pp. 841–860, 2010.

[6] C. von Eiff, N. Kuhn, M. Herrmann, S. Weber, and G. Peters, "Micrococcus luteus as a cause of recurrent bacteremia," *The Pediatric Infectious Disease Journal*, vol. 15, no. 8, pp. 711–713, 1996.

[7] J. M. M. Guerra, M. M. Asenjo, and C. R. Martín, "Bacteriemia por Micrococcus luteus en un paciente inmunodeprimido," *Medicina Clínica*, vol. 152, no. 11, pp. 469-470, 2019.

[8] F. Erbasan, "Brain abscess caused by Micrococcus luteus in a patient with systemic lupus erythematosus: case-based review," *Rheumatology International*, vol. 38, no. 12, pp. 2323–2328, 2018.

[9] G. Miltiadous and M. Elisaf, "Native valve endocarditis due to Micrococcus luteus: a case report and review of the literature," *Journal of Medical Case Reports*, vol. 5, no. 1, article 1611, p. 251, 2011.

15

Proximal Left Main Coronary Artery Aneurysm Presenting as ST-Elevation Myocardial Infarction Treated by Stenting

Vijay Chander Vinod, Zuhair Eltayeb Yousif, Najat Omer Salim, and Talib Majwal

Mediclinic City Hospital, Dubai, UAE

Correspondence should be addressed to Vijay Chander Vinod; vijay.chander@mediclinic.ae

Academic Editor: Manabu Shirotani

Coronary artery aneurysm (CAA) is a rare cardiac anomaly with a reported incidence of 0.3-4.9% of patients who undergo coronary angiography. The term is used when the coronary artery diameter exceeds more than 50% or 1.5 times the reference diameter. It can be congenital or acquired. The commonest acquired cause in an adult is atherosclerosis and in a child is Kawasaki's disease. The commonest culprit vessel is the Right Coronary Artery (RCA), followed by Left Circumflex (LCx) and Left Anterior Descending (LAD). Left main coronary aneurysms are extremely rare in clinical practice. Coronary angiography is the gold standard procedure, both for diagnosis and treatment. We report a 49-year-old male who presented with anterior wall ST-Elevation Myocardial Infarction (STEMI). The initial angiography showed LAD stent thrombosis, but when the second angiography was done, there was spontaneous recanalization of the LAD. Coronary angiography was performed at our hospital, which revealed a long left main coronary artery aneurysm measuring 9.8 mm—maximum diameter. This was treated with a size 5×24 mm Begraft coronary stent.

1. Introduction

Coronary artery aneurysm (CAA) is a rare cardiac anomaly with a reported incidence of 0.3-4.9% of patients who undergo coronary angiography. The term is used when the coronary artery diameter exceeds more than 50% or 1.5 times the reference diameter [1, 2].

It can be congenital or acquired. The commonest acquired cause in an adult is atherosclerosis and in a child is Kawasaki's disease. The commonest culprit vessel is the Right Coronary Artery (RCA), followed by Left Circumflex (LCx) and Left Anterior Descending (LAD). Left main coronary aneurysms are extremely rare in clinical practice. It is usually diagnosed incidentally either during a coronary angiogram or intravascular ultrasound or during postmortem. Coronary angiography is the gold standard procedure, both for diagnosis and treatment.

2. Study Setting

This case has been reported at the Emergency Department (ED) of Mediclinic City Hospital (MCH) situated in Dubai Health Care City (DHCC), Dubai, United Arab Emirates. MCH is a 230 bedded multidisciplinary tertiary care hospital and a Level 1 Cardiac Centre in the region. We see around 45,000 patients per year in our ED, of which 2400 patients present with cardiac symptoms. On average, the Cardiac Catheterization Lab carries out 300 coronary angioplasty procedures per year.

3. Case Presentation

A 49-year-old male was referred to our Emergency Department (ED) from a local hospital where he presented with a 10-hour history of central chest pain, radiating to the left

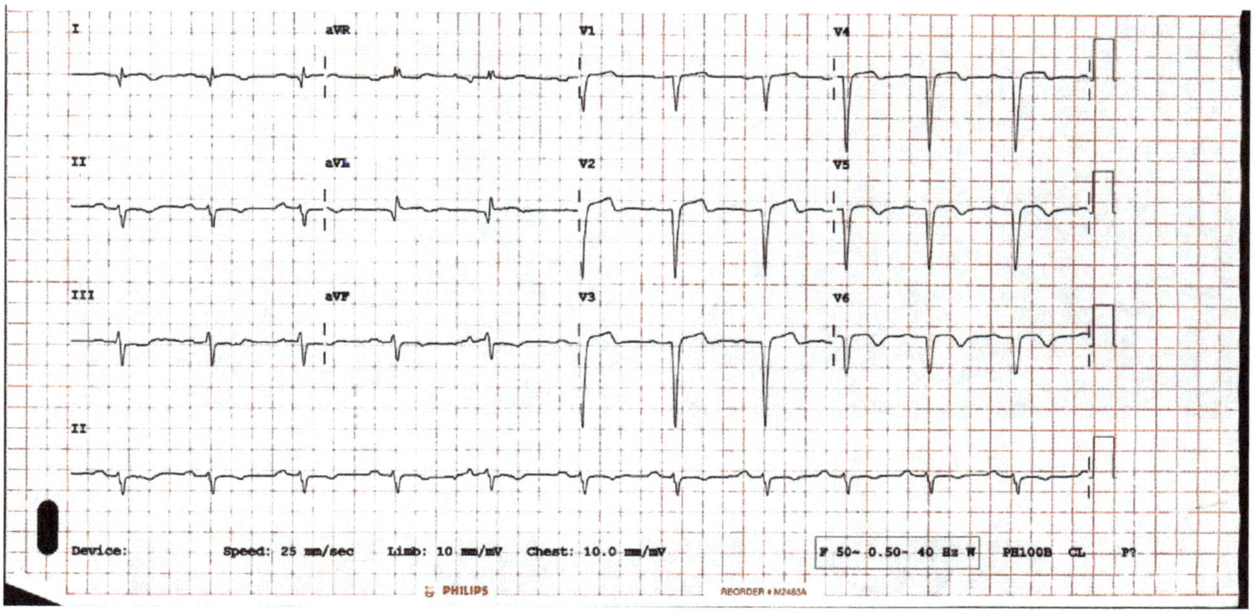

FIGURE 1: ECG at presentation.

arm and upper back. There was no history of shortness of breath, palpitations, or exertional symptoms; no history of headache, dizziness, or syncope; and no history of fever or respiratory symptoms. He has documented coronary artery disease with previous percutaneous coronary intervention to Left Anterior Descending and Ramus arteries. Other cardiovascular risk factors include hypertension, dyslipidemia, smoking, and first-degree family history of premature coronary artery disease.

Electrocardiogram (ECG) showed ST-segment elevation and T wave inversion in Leads I, aVL, and V1-V6. ST-segment depression in II, III, and aVF confirms acute STEMI (Figure 1).

Urgent coronary angiography was performed which revealed long left main aneurysm with thrombus, stent thrombosis of LAD, patent Ramus, ectatic RCA, and severe left main ectasia (Figure 2).

At the local hospital, he had been advised to have urgent Coronary Artery Bypass Grafting (CABG). Hence, the patient came to Mediclinic City Hospital for a second opinion regarding surgical versus medical management. On admission to our hospital, the patient's pain scale was 1/10. Vitals were stable. ECG still showed the same changes as in the local hospital. Examination of the cardiovascular and respiratory systems was normal. Abdomen examination was unremarkable. Full blood count (FBC), C-reactive protein (CRP), urea and electrolytes, prothrombin time (PT), and international normalized ratio (INR) were all within normal limits. Troponin I was 0.668 ng/ml (<0.034), and creatine kinase (MB fraction) was 16.6 ng/ml (0.00-5.10). Echocardiography showed impaired left ventricular (LV) function with an ejection fraction (EF) of 35-40%. The septum and apex were akinetic. There was hypokinesia of the anterior and inferior walls. Dilated LV and LV apical clot were noted. The patient was admitted to the Intensive Care Unit (ICU) and was maintained on antiplatelet and anticoagulant therapy.

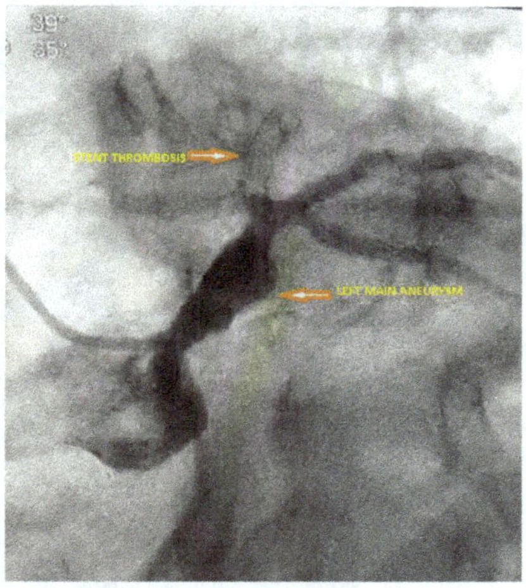

FIGURE 2: Initial coronary angiogram showing left main coronary aneurysm and stent thrombosis.

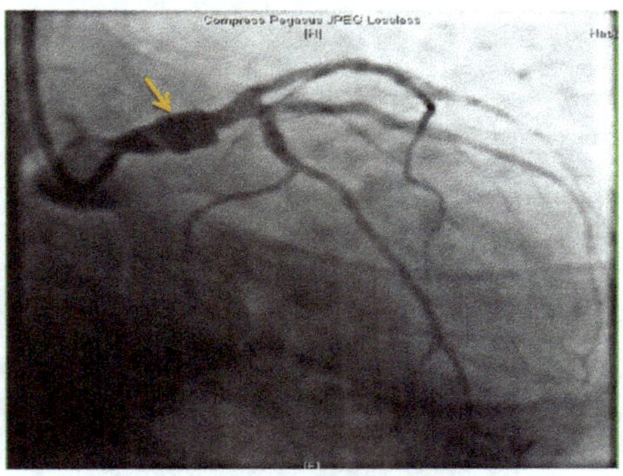

FIGURE 3: AP caudal view showing left main coronary artery aneurysm.

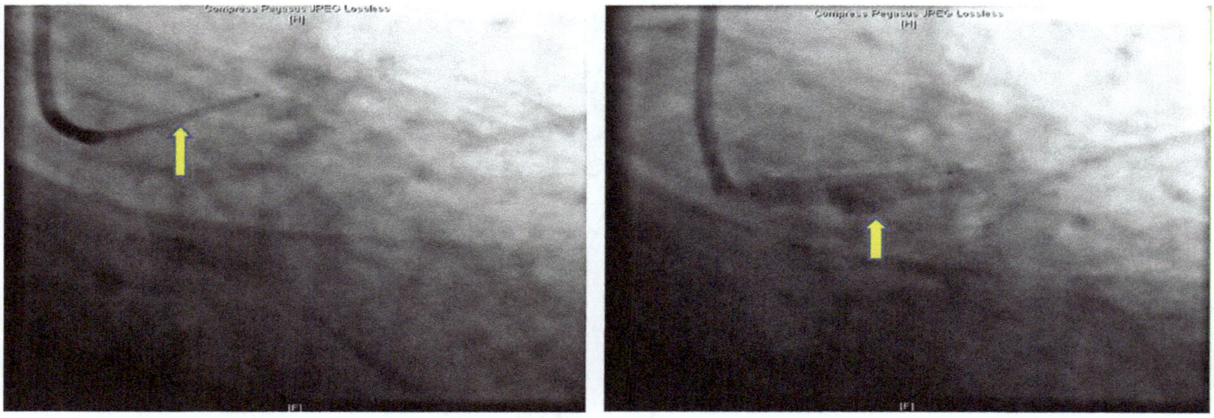

FIGURE 4: Positioning and deploying the stent in the left main coronary artery.

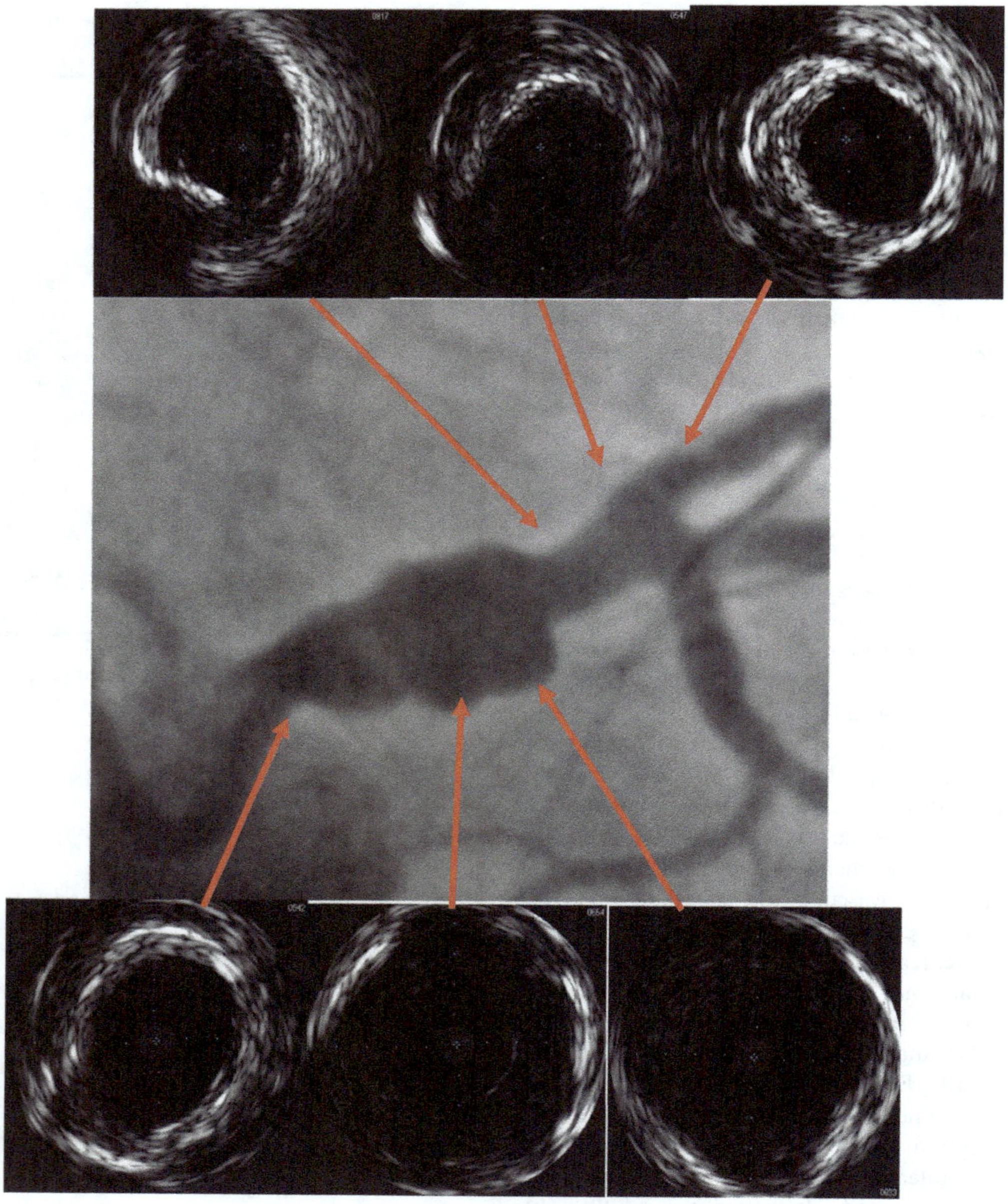

FIGURE 5: Baseline IVUS shows the aneurysm diameter and length. Healthy ostial and distal end of the left main coronary artery. Maximum diameter at aneurysm 10.6 mm, healthy segment 5.2 mm.

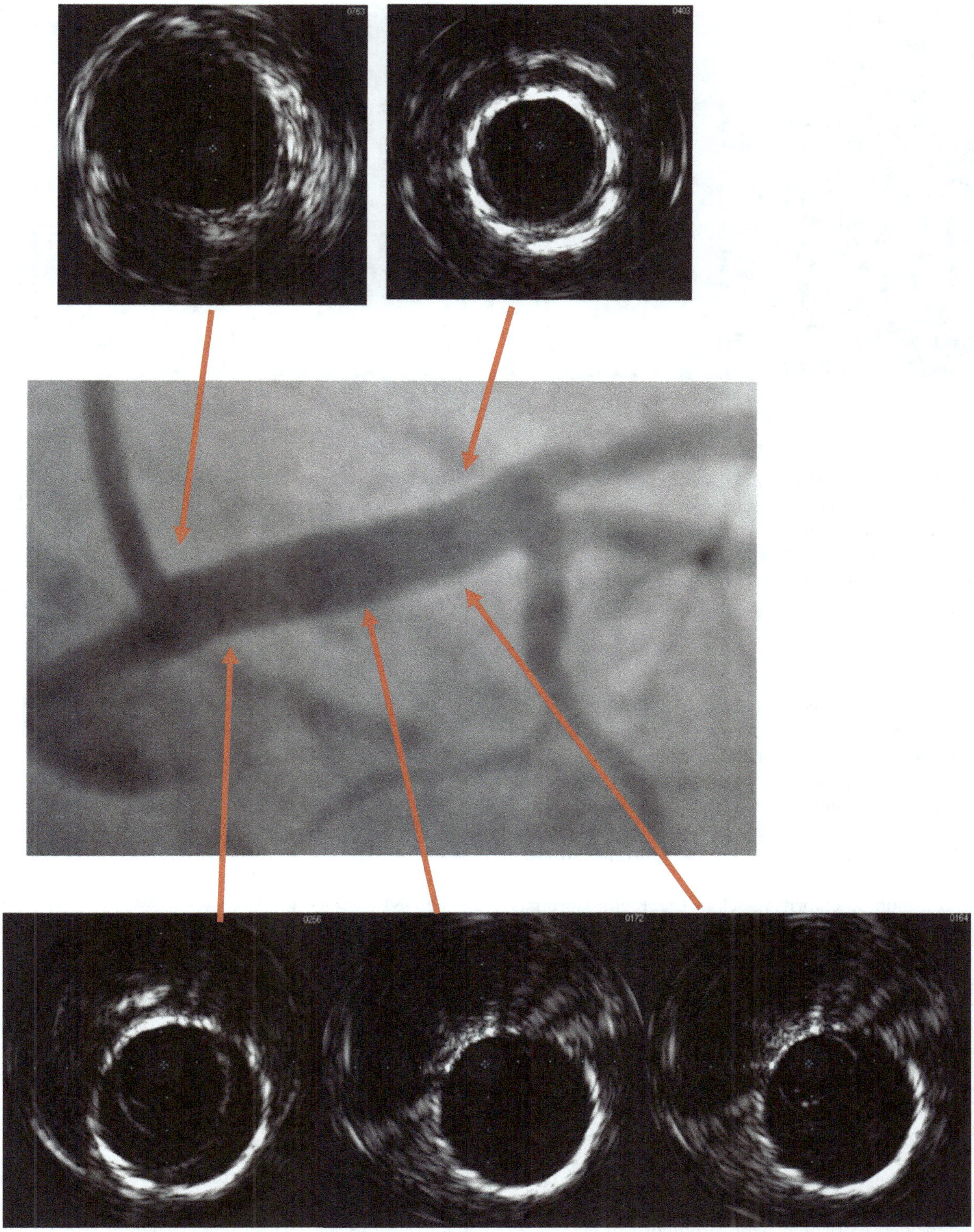

FIGURE 6: Final IVUS result with single-layer covered stent with diameter of 5 mm and complete exclusion of the aneurysm.

The revascularization strategy was discussed amongst the multidisciplinary team. It was a one-stage procedure, as the initial angiography showed LAD stent thrombosis, but when the second angiography was done, there was spontaneous recanalization of the LAD. A decision was made to go ahead with PCI, because if surgical revascularization was performed, there would be a risk of thrombus formation in the LMCA with distal embolization to the LAD/LCx resulting in STEMI, thus increasing the morbidity and mortality of the patient. Coronary angiography was performed at our hospital, which revealed a long left main coronary artery aneurysm measuring 9.8 mm—maximum diameter. This was treated with a size 5 × 24 mm Begraft coronary stent, and there was spontaneous recanalization of the LAD (Figures 3 and 4).

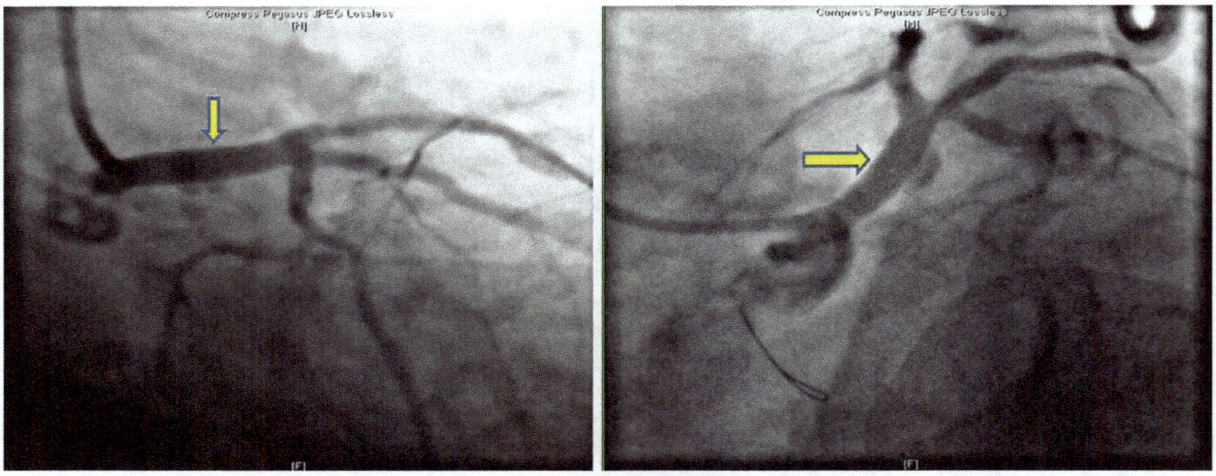

FIGURE 7: AP caudal and spider view showing post left main aneurysm stenting.

Intravascular ultrasound (IVUS) was done (Figures 5 and 6) which confirmed excellent results (Figure 7).

The patient was discharged 2 days after the procedure. He remained stable on further follow-up. Six-week control angiography was not done, and the plan is to do 1-year angiography and IVUS imaging.

4. Discussion

Coronary artery aneurysms (CAA) are rare in clinical practice. Left main coronary artery aneurysms (LMCAA) are extremely rare, with a reported incidence of 0.1% [3].

It can be congenital or acquired. The commonest acquired cause in an adult is atherosclerosis and in a child is Kawasaki's disease. The other causes could be connective tissue disorders like Ehlers-Danlos syndrome, Marfan syndrome, and scleroderma [4].

The commonest culprit vessel is the Right Coronary Artery (RCA), followed by Left Circumflex (LCx) and Left Anterior Descending (LAD). It is usually diagnosed incidentally either during a coronary angiogram or intravascular ultrasound or during postmortem. Coronary angiography is the gold standard procedure, both for diagnosis and treatment. Noninvasive imaging modalities such as CT coronary angiogram and MR coronary angiogram when done electively can increase the chances of detection in asymptomatic patients [5].

Various studies have reported an increased incidence of CAA after coronary angioplasty with drug-eluting stents (DES), which can range from 0.2 to 10.5%. There is an increased incidence of latent stent thrombosis in DES when compared to bare metal stents (BMS), and this is associated with increased risk of CAA [6, 7, 8]. There are case reports and literature to suggest that the chances of coronary artery aneurysms, in-stent thrombosis, and restenosis with drug-eluting stents are increasing. The preferred treatment of choice in such patients who develop coronary artery aneurysms is single-layer covered stent [9, 10, 11, 12].

The selection of coronary stents is very important, and the diameter of the coronary artery aneurysm plays an important role with regard to postprocedure complications like restenosis and in-stent thrombosis. Diameters less than 3 mm are at higher risk of restenosis, and those more than 4.5 mm have a low risk of restenosis [13]. Our patient's coronary artery aneurysm was 5 mm and has a low risk of restenosis. Moreover, the patient was started on dual antiplatelet therapy and advised to continue for life.

When it comes to treatment modality of choice, there is no statistical significance in the survival rates of patients treated either medically or surgically, between patients who had CAA and patients who had obstructive CAD but did not have CAA [1, 14].

There is still a great amount of controversy about whether to treat CAA medically or surgically. The decision is usually based on individual patient criteria like CAA with proximal stenosis or emboli from the thrombus, patient's overall clinical condition and coexisting CV risk factors, and of course the expertise of the treating physician. Surgical management is usually recommended in symptomatic patients who demonstrate thrombus within the CAA which embolised to the distal coronary segment causing myocardial ischemia. However, in our case, the LMCAA was successfully treated with stenting rather than surgical management. We deployed the new generation single-layered covered stent (polytetrafluoroethylene), which has got better safety profile, higher efficacy, and reduced risk of restenosis and in-stent thrombosis when compared to the old generation double-layered stents [15, 16].

Since these cases are extremely rare, there is no standard guideline or protocol to treat LMCAA when they present to the ED with acute myocardial infarction. Hence, this poses a diagnostic challenge to the treating clinician.

5. Conclusion

Coronary artery aneurysms (CAA) are rare and left main CAA is extremely rare in clinical practice. The patient we presented had left main coronary artery aneurysm (maximum diameter 9.8 mm) with a thrombus that embolised the distal coronary segment causing acute myocardial infarction. He was treated percutaneously with the deployment of 5×24 mm Begraft-Bentley coronary stent, with excellent angiographic and clinical outcome.

Consent

Written informed consent could not be obtained from the patient for publication as the patient could not be contacted. The entire case report has been sufficiently anonymized as per the ICMJE guidelines. Consent waiver has been issued by Mediclinic Research and Ethics Committee, and a copy of the waiver is available for review by the editor-in-chief of this journal on request.

References

[1] P. S. Swaye, L. D. Fisher, P. Litwin et al., "Aneurysmal coronary artery disease," *Circulation*, vol. 67, no. 1, pp. 134–138, 1983.

[2] K. Y. Wang, C. T. Ting, M. St John Sutton, and Y. T. Chen, "Coronary artery aneurysms: a 25-patient study," *Catheterization and Cardiovascular Interventions*, vol. 48, no. 1, pp. 31–38, 1999.

[3] O. Topaz, G. DiSciascio, M. J. Cowley et al., "Angiographic features of left main coronary artery aneurysms," *The American Journal of Cardiology*, vol. 67, no. 13, pp. 1139–1142, 1991.

[4] J. E. Everett and H. M. Burkhart, "Coronary artery aneurysm: case report," *Journal of Cardiothoracic Surgery*, vol. 3, no. 1, 2008.

[5] H. Doustkami, N. Maleki, and Z. Tavosi, "Left main coronary artery aneurysm," *The Journal of Tehran Heart Center*, vol. 11, no. 1, pp. 41–45, 2016.

[6] E. Stabile, E. Escolar, G. Weigold et al., "Marked malapposition and aneurysm formation after sirolimus-eluting coronary stent implantation," *Circulation*, vol. 110, no. 5, pp. e47–e48, 2004.

[7] E. Abergel and A. Roguin, "Coronary aneurysm occurring late after drug-eluting stent implantation," *ISRN Cardiology*, vol. 2011, Article ID 367512, 3 pages, 2011.

[8] X. Zhong, H. Li, C. Li et al., "Clinical outcomes and risk factors of coronary artery aneurysms after successful percutaneous coronary intervention and drug-eluting stent implantation for chronic total occlusions," *IJC Heart & Vessels*, vol. 4, pp. 108–115, 2014.

[9] S. Bajaj, R. Parikh, A. Hamdan, and M. Bikkina, "Covered-stent treatment of coronary aneurysm after drug-eluting stent placement: case report and literature review," *Texas Heart Institute Journal*, vol. 37, no. 4, pp. 449–454, 2010.

[10] P. Patil, A. Sethi, and U. Kaul, "Stent thrombosis with an aneurysm 7 years after a drug eluting stent implantation," *Indian Heart Journal*, vol. 66, no. 2, pp. 216–219, 2014.

[11] S. E. Lee, S. H. John, J. H. Lim, and J. Y. Rhew, "Very late stent thrombosis associated with multiple stent fractures and peri-stent aneurysm formation after sirolimus-eluting stent implantation," *Circulation Journal*, vol. 72, no. 7, pp. 1201–1204, 2008.

[12] J. P. Levisay, R. M. Roth, and R. A. Schatz, "Coronary artery aneurysm formation after drug-eluting stent implantation," *Cardiovascular Revascularization Medicine*, vol. 9, no. 4, pp. 284–287, 2008.

[13] A. Colombo, G. Stankovic, and J. W. Moses, "Selection of coronary stents," *Journal of the American College of Cardiology*, vol. 40, no. 6, pp. 1021–1033, 2002.

[14] F. C. Robinson, "Aneurysms of the coronary arteries," *American Heart Journal*, vol. 109, no. 1, pp. 129–135, 1985.

[15] S. Kufner, N. Schacher, M. Ferenc et al., "Outcome after new generation single-layer polytetrafluoroethylene-covered stent implantation for the treatment of coronary artery perforation," *Catheterization and Cardiovascular Interventions*, vol. 93, no. 5, pp. 912–920, 2018.

[16] S. Neupane and K. Dass, "Use of polytetrafluoroethylene (PTFE)-covered stent in treatment of RCA aneurysm," *Heart Asia*, vol. 6, no. 1, p. 144, 2014.

16

The Insidious Cardiac Tumor: A Primary Left Atrium Intimal Cardiac Sarcoma in a Young Patient

Chika-Nwosuh Ogechukwu, Nnaoma Christopher, Sossou Christoph, Okundaye Etinosasere, and Bustillo Jose

Department of Medicine, Newark Beth Israel Medical Center, Robert Wood Johnson Barnabas Health, Newark, NJ, USA

Correspondence should be addressed to Chika-Nwosuh Ogechukwu; ochikanwosuh@gmail.com

Academic Editor: Assad Movahed

This case presentation discusses a rare cardiac malignancy initially thought to be a benign tumor. A 36-year-old presented with syncope, dyspnea, Computed Tomography Pulmonary angiography study obtained was negative for pulmonary emboli but revealed a left atrial mass. A transesophageal echocardiogram (TEE) confirmed a mass with multiple lobes and a broad base attached to the septum, encroaching into the right atrium, aortic root wall, base of the anterior mitral leaflet flowing to the mitral orifice in diastole also obstructing the right pulmonary vein. Despite a quick diagnosis and plan to begin treatment, the patient rapidly declined owing to the extent and aggressive nature of this cardiac malignancy. This case reports the insidious nature of these tumors as well as how challenging and life threatening they are at the time of their clinical manifestation.

1. Introduction

Primary cardiac sarcomas are rare clinical entities and pose challenges in their management, given their aggressive nature and high recurrence rate [1]. Over 75% of primary cardiac tumors are benign, the remaining 25% are malignant [1]. Of the 25% of malignant cardiac tumors, 75% are sarcomas [2]. Up until 2006, fewer than 20 cases had been reported about cardiac sarcomas [1]. Intimal sarcoma also tends to present in the right atrium, albeit rare, they can be seen in the left atrium [3]. The diagnosis relies mainly on image modalities such as echocardiography, computed tomography, coronary angiography, and magnetic resonance imaging. Without tissue sampling, they could easily be mistaken for myxoma or a clot which could delay management [4]. Immediate diagnosis is essential to avoid cardiac complications such as arrhythmias, ischemia due to obstruction of coronary arteries, heart failure, sudden cardiac death, metastasis, or delay in management [5]. Treatment involves resection, chemotherapy, and radiation, with the median survival of six months [6]. Surgical resection remains the most common treatment for most cardiac tumors and involves the complex cardiac reconstruction especially in malignant cases [4].

2. Case

A 36-year-old male with no past medical history presented to the hospital with two syncopal episodes, worsening palpitations, and progressive dyspnea on exertion (NYHA class II-III). He reported no prodromal symptoms, immediately regained consciousness after a few seconds without any post-ictal signs. First syncopal episode occurred 2 weeks earlier while in a passenger seat; he sought no medical attention at the time. The second episode was during a coughing fit the evening of his presentation. Both episodes were said to be witnessed without any seizure activity. Six months prior to the onset of the syncopal episodes, he began experiencing dyspnea with mild exertion which progressed, limiting his functional activities. He reported a 40 lbs weight loss over six months which he had attributed to his intent to lose

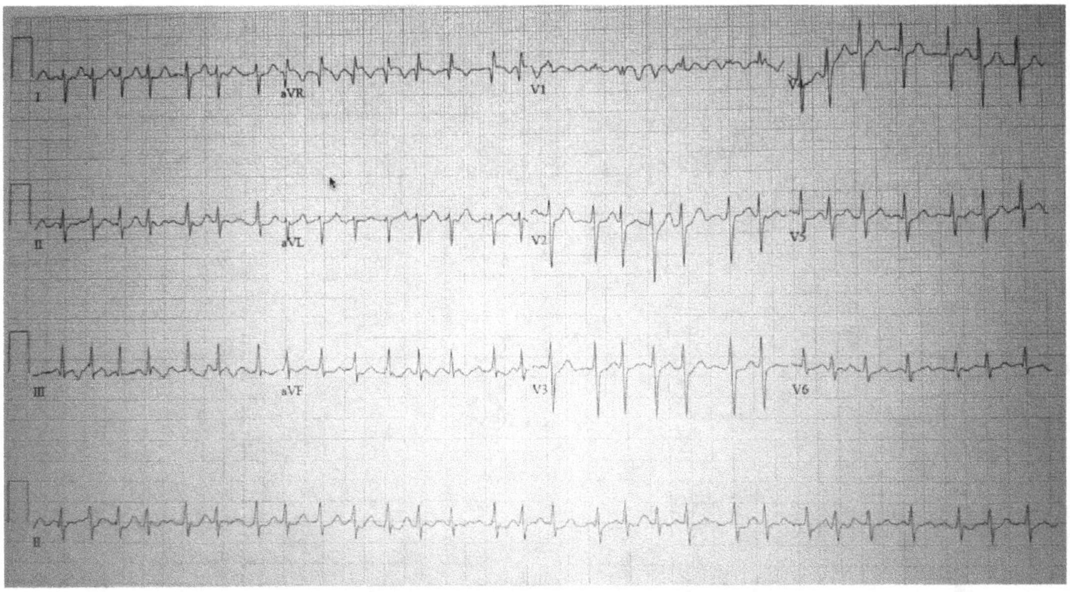

Figure 1: EKG on presentation demonstrating atrial fibrillation with rapid ventricular response.

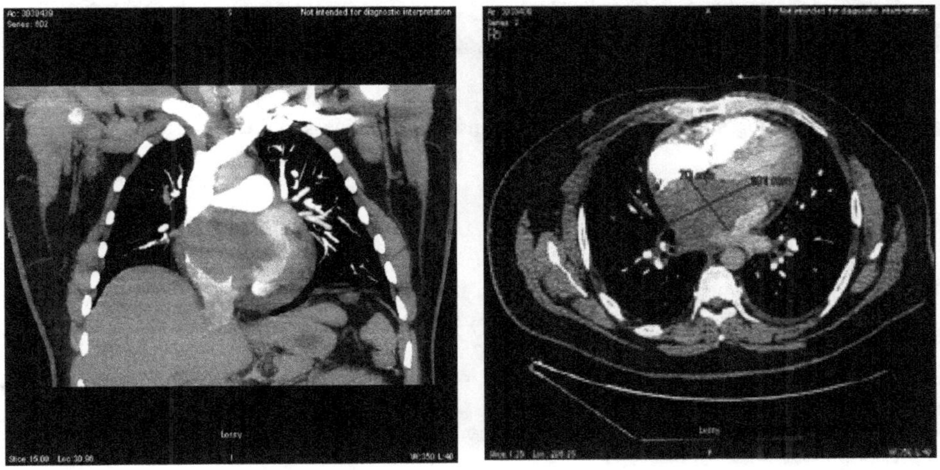

(a) (b)

Figure 2: Computed tomography of the chest demonstrating the mass in the left atrium.

weight (BMI 38). He also admitted to night sweats but denied chest discomfort, increased abdominal girth, or leg swelling.

Physical examination revealed BP 123/78 mmHg, HR 120-150 bpm which was irregularly irregular, RR 26 breaths per minute, hypoxic at 88% on room air with improvement in Bipap, and laying in Trendelenburg position, negative orthostatic. There was a presence of bibasilar crackles in the lung field, no jugular venous distention or peripheral edema noted, cardiovascular examination was limited due to body habitus and rapid irregular heart rate, and the rest of the exam was unremarkable except for morbid obesity. Electrocardiogram (EKG) showed supraventricular tachycardia and subsequently atrial fibrillation (Figure 1); there was no old EKG to compare. He was started on Cardizem drip at 5 mg/hour and titrated up to maintain a goal heart rate of 80-110 bpm. Chest radiography remarkable for bilateral pleural effusion is worse on the left than the right.

A Computed Tomography Pulmonary angiography study was negative for pulmonary emboli but revealed a left atrial mass (Figure 2). A transthoracic echocardiogram (TTE) showed an 8-9 cm atrial mass attached to the interatrial septum (Video 1). Given significant outflow obstruction, the patient was taken to the operating room (OR) for possible resection. Transesophageal echocardiogram (Figure 3) in the OR demonstrated similar mass with multiple lobes and a broad base attached to the septum, encroaching into the right atrium, aortic root wall, base of the anterior mitral leaflet flowing to the mitral orifice in diastole also obstructing the right pulmonary vein seen in. A biopsy and partial resection were performed with no much change in size; the patient was not a candidate for complete resection due to the extensive cardiac involvement.

Pathology (Figure 4) revealed intimal sarcoma evidenced by markers positive for MDM2, CDK4 gene, and KIT and

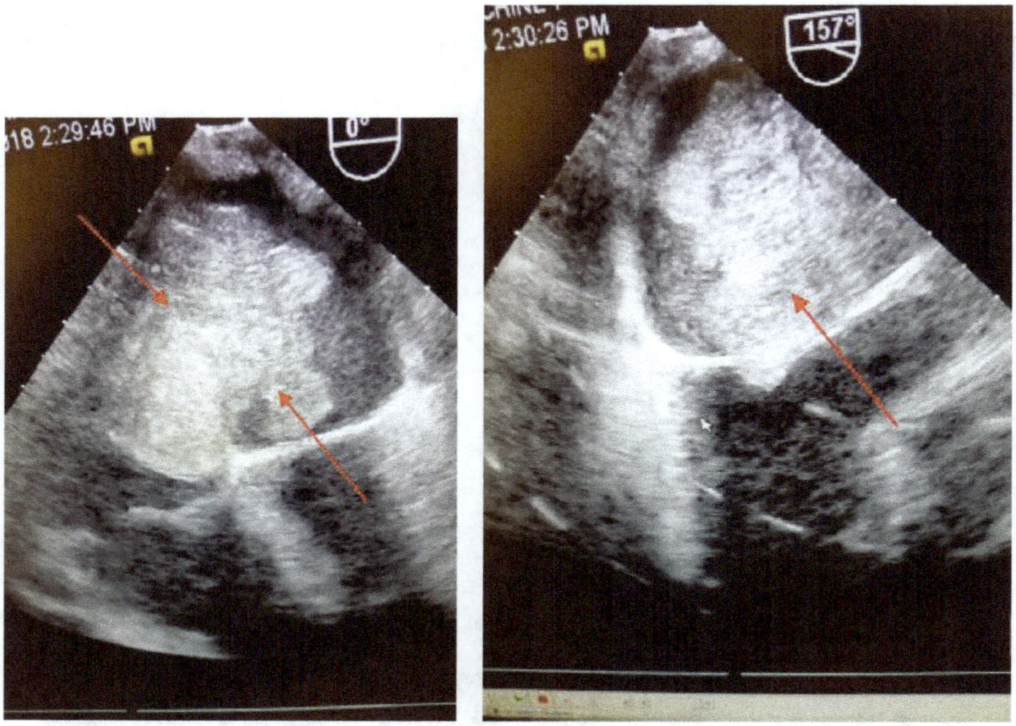

(a) (b)

FIGURE 3: Transesophageal echocardiogram (intraoperative) demonstrating the mass in the left atrium invading the interatrial septum.

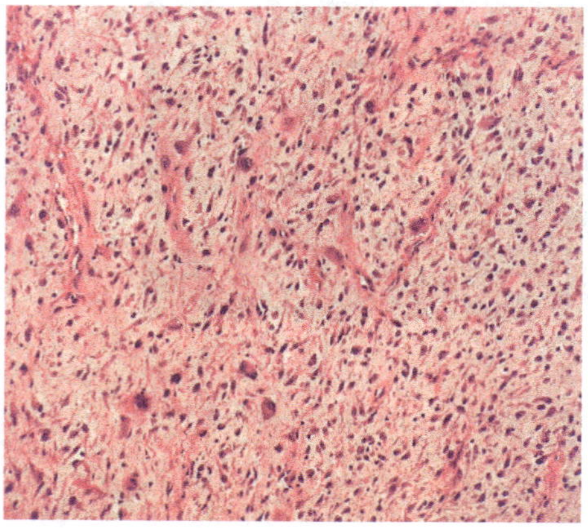

FIGURE 4: This histopathology illustrates multiple pleomorphic cells (tumor cells) from the partial resection of the left intimal sarcoma.

PDGFRA amplification. The patient was rate and rhythm controlled with Cardizem and digoxin. An oncologist was consulted with a plan of treatment with doxorubicin and olaratumab. However, the patient against medical advice wanted to delay treatment for few days. He unfortunately expired from pulseless electrical activity arrest during the same hospital admission after 3 weeks of hospitalization.

3. Discussion

Cardiac sarcomas are quite rare, with the male predisposition being 2.5 : 1 [3], and usually occurs in the 3rd and 4th decade of life [3]. It typically occurs in the right atrium and rarely in the left [1]. They often infiltrate into the septum and other structures of the heart resulting in significant outflow obstruction, thus, are very aggressive [3].

In majority of cases, cardiac tumors can be silent; however, when symptoms occur, they are determined based mainly on the size and anatomical location of the tumor [4]. They classically present with signs of congestive heart failure depending on the obstructing atrium. Right heart outflow obstruction can present with jugular venous distention, lower extremities swelling, and ascites mimicking symptoms of right sided heart failure. Involvement of the left side of the heart typically presents with dyspnea due to pulmonary congestion, syncope, and cardiogenic shock from lack of forward flow. Most times, these sarcomas can be confused with benign conditions such as myxoma which are more common tumors of the left atrium [6].

Image studies such as TTE and transesophageal echocardiography, computed tomography, coronary angiography, and magnetic resonance imaging are used for diagnosis and guiding surgical intervention [4]; however, specific diagnosis is made by tissue biopsy and histopathology.

Surgical resection is possible in about 33% of these cases; however, they have a tendency to recur, while others are deemed nonresectable [3]. The standard of treatment involves resection with chemotherapy and radiation. A study by Bakaeen et al. showed a median survival of 24 months in 27 patients after surgical resection and also better outcome with multimodality treatment [6]. In recent studies, neoadjuvant chemotherapy followed by radical resection has been deemed safe and effective in primary sarcoma on the right heart [7]. This mode of treatment enhances resection and can be translated to improvement in survival [7]. Our patient rapidly deteriorated given a significant poor prognosis due to the extent of the mass coupled with his delayed presentation in seeking medical attention. The delay in medical attention, initiation of chemotherapy, the aggressive nature, and the nonresectable mass all compounded to his rapid decline. Early surgical resection with chemotherapy and or radiotherapy may help improve survival in these patients.

4. Conclusion

Given the rarity of these cardiac malignancy, very little studies have been conducted regarding the management of these rare tumors especially in nonsurgical candidates; hence, this calls for a meta-analysis on the outcome of surgical candidates and nonsurgical candidates who are treated with chemotherapy and or radiotherapy. This case also calls to question the differences between the left and right atria sarcoma in terms of their presentation, management, and prognosis.

Authors' Contributions

All authors contributed significantly to this manuscript.

References

[1] M. Talukder, L. Joyce, R. Marks, and K. Kaplan, "Primary cardiac synovial sarcoma," *Interactive CardioVascular and Thoracic Surgery*, vol. 11, no. 4, pp. 490–492, 2010.

[2] B. Ramlawi, M. J. Leja, W. K. Abu Saleh et al., "Surgical treatment of primary cardiac sarcomas: review of a single-institution experience," *The Annals of Thoracic Surgery*, vol. 101, no. 2, pp. 698–702, 2016.

[3] M. Hosseinzadeh Maleki, M. Aboobakri Makouei, F. Hatami, and R. Zeinabadi Noghabi, "Primary cardiac synovial sarcoma: a case report," *The Journal of Tehran Heart Center*, vol. 12, no. 1, pp. 32–34, 2006.

[4] B. Yanagawa, A. Mazine, E. Y. Chan et al., "Surgery for tumors of the heart," *Seminars in Thoracic and Cardiovascular Surgery*, vol. 30, no. 4, pp. 385–397, 2018.

[5] C. DeZorzi and K. I. Harris, "Secret sarcoma: a cardiac mass disguised as influenza," *Case Reports in Cardiology*, vol. 2018, Article ID 8628365, 3 pages, 2018.

[6] F. G. Bakaeen, D. E. Jaroszewski, D. C. Rice et al., "Outcomes after surgical resection of cardiac sarcoma in the multimodality treatment era," *The Journal of Thoracic and Cardiovascular Surgery*, vol. 137, no. 6, pp. 1454–1460, 2009.

[7] W. K. Abu Saleh, B. Ramlawi, O. M. Shapira et al., "Improved outcomes with the evolution of a neoadjuvant chemotherapy approach to right heart sarcoma," *The Annals of Thoracic Surgery*, vol. 104, no. 1, pp. 90–96, 2017.

17

Post-Myocardial Infarction Ventricular Septal Defect Successfully Treated with Impella as Bridge to Cardiac Transplantation

Lauren Giudicatti,[1] Benjamin Silbert,[2] Xiao-Fang Xu,[1] Anthony Putrino,[1] Felicity Lee,[2] Amit Shah,[2] Robert Larbalestier,[3] Karim Slimani,[3] Andrew Laycock,[4] and Kaitlyn Lam[2]

[1]*Department of Cardiology, Fiona Stanley Hospital, Perth, Australia*
[2]*Advanced Heart Failure and Cardiac Transplantation Unit, Fiona Stanley Hospital, Perth, Australia*
[3]*Department of Cardiothoracic Surgery, Fiona Stanley Hospital, Perth, Australia*
[4]*PathWest, Fiona Stanley Hospital, Perth, Australia*

Correspondence should be addressed to Lauren Giudicatti; lgiudicatti@gmail.com

Academic Editor: Muhammad Zia-Ul-Haq

A 63-year-old female presented late with anterior ST-elevation myocardial infarction and cardiogenic shock. This was complicated by acute ventricular septal defect with large left-to-right shunt. An Impella CP was inserted on day seven with rapid haemodynamic improvement. This facilitated bridge to cardiac transplant on day twelve post-MI.

1. History of Presentation

A 63-year-old female presented following several days of central chest pain and dyspnoea. Past medical history was remarkable for mild intermittent asthma, ex-smoking status, and overweight body habitus (82 kg, body mass index 27). 12-lead electrocardiogram showed anterior ST-segment elevation myocardial infarction (MI). The patient underwent urgent coronary angiography. The left anterior descending artery (LAD) was occluded with ostial thrombus. Revascularisation of the LAD was performed with Xience Sierra 3.5 × 33 mm drug-eluting stent. Slow flow improved following intracoronary eptifibatide. A 50 cc intra-aortic balloon pump (IABP) was inserted for persistent hypotension at full augmentation. Intravenous heparin and eptifibatide infusions were continued. The patient returned to the coronary care unit for routine post-MI management.

2. Differential Diagnosis and Investigations

Transthoracic echocardiogram (TTE) on day two demonstrated 1.3 cm ventricular septal defect (VSD) at the basal anteroseptum with a large eccentric shunt from left ventricle (LV) to right ventricular (RV) outflow tract (Figure 1). The LV ejection fraction was 40% with akinesis of the interventricular septum (IVS) and LV apex on mechanical and inotropic support. On day five, trial of IABP removal failed due to rapid deterioration into cardiogenic shock and multiorgan failure, requiring prompt reinsertion. Right heart catheterisation was performed on day six. A significant step-up in oxygen saturation was demonstrated between RV (74%) and pulmonary artery (88%), and calculated shunt fraction (Qp : Qs) was 3.4, consistent with a haemodynamically significant shunt. Pulmonary capillary wedge pressure and transpulmonary gradient were elevated at 21 mmHg and 15 mmHg, respectively.

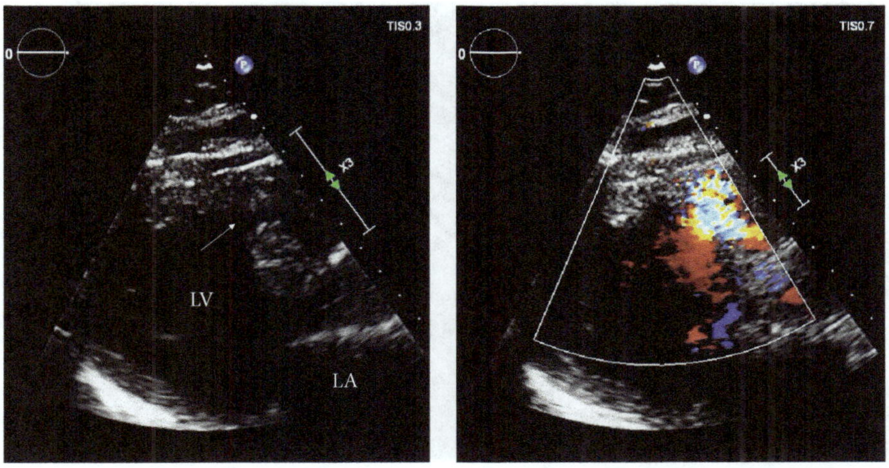

(a) (b)

Figure 1: Transthoracic echocardiogram, parasternal long axis view, demonstrating a 1.3 cm muscular VSD in the basal anteroseptum ((a), arrow) with left-to-right shunting on colour Doppler (b).

3. Management

The patient developed refractory cardiogenic shock despite IABP support and escalating inotrope and vasodilator therapy. Following heart team meeting, a decision was made to insert a percutaneous microaxial flow pump (Impella) as a bridge to either VSD repair at approximately six weeks post-MI, with or without left ventricular assist device (LVAD), or urgent cardiac transplantation. Urgent insertion of an Impella CP was performed on day seven post-MI via surgical cut down to the left axillary artery. The higher power Impella 5 or Impella 5.5 was not available at the time of insertion. The patient experienced rapid haemodynamic improvement within minutes and complete wean of inotropic/IABP support within hours which was sustained over the following days. Transesophageal echocardiogram (TEE) and continuous SvO2 monitoring were used to guide manipulation of Impella flow and shunt fraction, to good effect (Table 1). Figure 2 demonstrates persistent left-to-right shunt on TEE following Impella insertion.

The patient had no contraindications to cardiac transplant and was urgently listed. A suitable donor became available on day five post-Impella insertion (12 days post-MI). Total donor ischemia time was 100 minutes. Immunologic matching profile was favourable. Macroscopic and microscopic examinations of the explanted heart are shown in Figure 3. The patient was extubated on day five.

Table 1: Haemodynamics and biochemistry pre versus post-Impella insertion demonstrating rapid improvement without increase in right-to-left shunting or right heart pressures.

Variable	Baseline (on IABP)	<6-hours post-Impella	24-hours post-Impella
CVP	20	10	12
PCWP	21	23	23
PASP	45	49	42
CI	3.3	2.8	3.5
SvO2	43	84	76
Lactate	1.1	1.1	0.8
Creatinine	172	200	99

IABP: intra-aortic balloon pump; CVP: central venous pressure; PCWP: pulmonary capillary wedge pressure; PASP: pulmonary artery systolic pressure: CI: cardiac index; SvO2: oxygen saturation in venous blood.

4. Follow-Up

The patient experienced a postoperative stroke requiring inpatient rehabilitation and was discharged home on day 47 with residual right foot drop.

5. Discussion

Acute ischaemic VSD is a rare but catastrophic mechanical complication of acute MI [1, 2]. Post-MI VSDs are typically diagnosed between 3 and 7 days postinfarct, although it can occur as early as 24 hours [3]. Contemporary management of MI with early revascularisation has led to a reduction in prevalence to less than 1% [2, 3]. Despite this, untreated mortality remains over 90% at 30 days [2, 3]. With intervention, mortality is reduced to approximately 65% at 30 days [4].

Timing of repair for post-MI VSD remains a major challenge. Data from the Society of Thoracic Surgeons National Database ($n = 2876$) demonstrated a reduction in mortality from 54% to 18% with early (<7 days) versus delayed (7 days or later) surgical repair, respectively [5]. The durability of early surgical is largely hindered by friable peri-infarct tissue which may cause incomplete closure and residual shunting in up to 20% of patients [3]. Transcatheter repair provides a less invasive alternative where surgical repair is contraindicated, although it is also limited by defect location and peri-infarct tissue quality [3]. Where suitable, it may be used either as a bridge to haemodynamic stability and definitive surgical repair, or as a definitive therapy in itself [4].

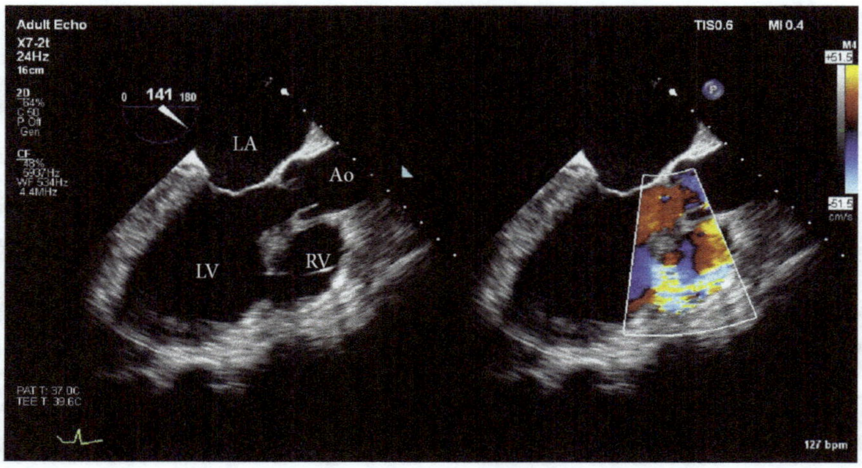

FIGURE 2: Transesophageal echocardiogram, midesophageal 3-chamber view taken whilst on Impella support, showing large VSD with left-to-right shunting on colour Doppler.

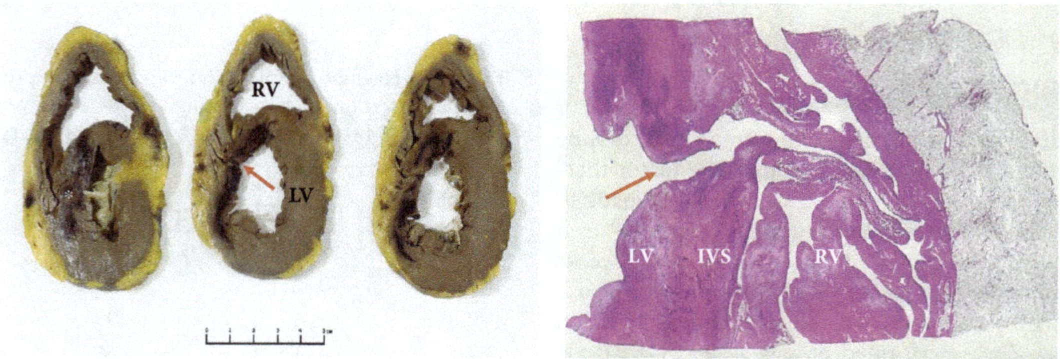

(a) (b)

FIGURE 3: Explanted heart showing. (a) Cross-section through the basal (left) to apical (right) left ventricle (LV) demonstrating haemorrhagic infarct involving the interventricular septum (IVS) and anterior LV (asterisk). A defect is evident through the infarcted region of the IVS (arrow). (b) At low power, a full thickness defect is evident through the region of infarction (arrow), allowing communication from LV to RV, via a tortuous path.

Temporary mechanical circulatory support (MCS) is increasingly utilised in patients with cardiogenic shock post-MI VSD to reduce left-to-right shunting and augment cardiac output [6]. This allows time for the scar to consolidate and improves likelihood of durable repair. The optimal timing and method of MCS remain contentious [6]. Thiele and colleagues describe the use of IABP in 23 patients as a bridge to early or delayed surgical repair [4, 7]. Peri-operative mortality remained high at 83% and 57%, respectively, and later studies have failed to show any significant mortality benefit [4, 7]. Peripheral veno-arterial extracorporeal membrane oxygenation (VA-ECMO) provides more complete circulatory support compared to IABP, with more favourable outcomes when used as a bridge to reparative surgery [8]. Limitations include a high risk of complications, insufficient LV unloading, and worsening of left-to-right shunting [6, 8]. Finally, LVAD has been used with success in isolated VSD cases as a longer term MCS option, both at the time of surgical repair and following absence of postoperative myocardial recovery [6].

In recent years, the Impella intracardiac microaxial pump (Abiomed Danvers, Massachusetts) has gained popularity as a less invasive and more durable alternative to traditional MCS strategies following acute MI [9]. The Impella offers superior reduction in wedge pressure and minimisation of left-to-right shunting compared to IABP, with conceivable benefit for patients with VSD, although it remains off-label for this indication [4, 6, 9]. The Impella CP provides a maximum output of approximately 3.7 L/minute [9]. In patients with VSD, excessive pump power and flow may result in right to left shunting and subsequent hypoxia, and careful manipulation with a goal of maintaining saturations above 92% is therefore required. In our case, after several days of minimal improvement on IABP, we observed a dramatic haemodynamic response and rapid reversal of end organ damage following Impella CP insertion. This reflects the superior augmentation of cardiac output provided by the Impella. Isolated case reports have previously shown similar success with Impella in post-MI VSD [10]. Patanè and colleagues have described the use of the Impella Recovery as a bridge to transplantation in a post-MI VSD unsuitable for surgical repair [10]. The importance of timely implantation of Impella before irreversible haemodynamic deterioration is again emphasised in our case.

6. Conclusion

Post-MI VSD is an important and life-threatening complication of acute MI. Conventional MCS options including IABP and VA-ECMO can help achieve temporary haemodynamic stability where delayed surgical intervention is preferable, but may be limited by incomplete LV unloading and high risk of complications. We have demonstrated that the Impella is an effective alternative bridge to transplantation in patients with VSD and refractory cardiogenic shock. Future experience with this device in acute post-MI VSD will help form treatment pathways.

7. Learning Objectives

(1) To use a multidisciplinary and haemodynamic-based approach to determine optimal timing of intervention in patients with acute post-MI VSD and refractory cardiogenic shock.

(2) To understand the role of mechanical circulatory support in providing a bridge to definitive therapy in the setting of acute post-MI VSD.

Abbreviations

MI: Myocardial infarction
LAD: Left anterior descending artery
IABP: Intra-aortic balloon pump
TTE: Transthoracic echocardiogram
VSD: Ventricular septal defect
LV: Left ventricle
RV: Right ventricle
IVS: Interventricular septum
LVAD: Left ventricular assist device
TEE: Transesophageal echocardiogram
MCS: Mechanical circulatory support
VA-ECMO: Veno-arterial extracorporeal membrane oxygenation.

References

[1] B. Crenshaw, C. Granger, Y. Birnbaum et al., "Risk factors, angiographic patterns, and outcomes in patients with ventricular septal defect complicating acute myocardial infarction," *Circulation*, vol. 101, no. 1, pp. 27–32, 2000.

[2] M. Shahreyar, O. Akinseye, M. Nayyar, U. Ashraf, and U. N. Ibebuogu, "Post-myocardial infarction ventricular septal defect: a comprehensive review," *Cardiovascular Revascularization Medicine*, vol. 21, no. 11, pp. 1444–1449, 2020.

[3] S. Omar, G. Morgan, H. Panchal et al., "Management of post-myocardial infarction ventricular septal defects: a critical assessment," *Journal of Interventional Cardiology*, vol. 31, no. 6, pp. 939–948, 2018.

[4] A. Cinq-Mars, P. Voisine, F. Dagenais et al., "Risk factors of mortality after surgical correction of ventricular septal defect following myocardial infarction: retrospective analysis and review of the literature," *International Journal of Cardiology*, vol. 206, pp. 27–36, 2016.

[5] G. Arnaoutakis, Y. Zhao, T. George, C. Sciortino, P. McCarthy, and J. Conte, "Surgical repair of ventricular septal defect after myocardial infarction: outcomes from the Society of Thoracic Surgeons National Database," *The Annals of Thoracic Surgery*, vol. 94, no. 2, pp. 436–444, 2012.

[6] D. HlaváÊek, M. Pokorný, P. Ivák, I. Netuka, and O. Szárszoi, "Implantation of durable left ventricular assist device in patient with postmyocardial infarction ventricular septal defect," *Journal of Cardiac Surgery*, vol. 36, no. 10, pp. 3944–3947, 2021.

[7] H. Thiele, B. Lauer, R. Hambrecht et al., "Short- and long-term hemodynamic effects of intra-aortic balloon support in ventricular septal defect complicating acute myocardial infarction," *The American Journal of Cardiology*, vol. 92, no. 4, pp. 450–454, 2003.

[8] P. Artemiou, I. Gasparovic, B. Bezak, V. Hudec, I. Glonek, and M. Hulman, "Preoperative extracorporeal membrane oxygenation for postinfarction ventricular septal defect: case series of three patients with a literature review," *Journal of Cardiac Surgery*, vol. 35, no. 12, pp. 3626–3630, 2020.

[9] D. Ouweneel, E. Eriksen, K. Sjauw et al., "Percutaneous mechanical circulatory support versus intra-aortic balloon pump in cardiogenic shock after acute myocardial infarction," *Journal of the American College of Cardiology*, vol. 69, no. 3, pp. 278–287, 2017.

[10] F. Patanè, P. Centofanti, E. Zingarelli, F. Sansone, and M. La Torre, "Potential role of the Impella Recover left ventricular assist device in the management of postinfarct ventricular septal defect," *The Journal of Thoracic and Cardiovascular Surgery*, vol. 137, no. 5, pp. 1288-1289, 2009.

18

Esmolol Use in Dual Axis Defibrillation Resistant Ventricular Fibrillation

Ankit Agrawal,[1] Maria Cardinale,[2,3] Douglas Frenia,[4] Tarun Dalia,[5] and Chirag Shah[6]

[1]*Division of Internal Medicine Rutgers Robert Wood, Johnson Medical School/Saint Peter's University Hospital, New Jersey, USA*
[2]*Division of Pharmacy, Saint Peter's University Hospital, New Jersey, USA*
[3]*Ernest Mario School of Pharmacy, Rutgers University, New Jersey, USA*
[4]*Division of Pulmonary and Critical Care Medicine, Rutgers Robert Wood Johnson Medical School/Saint Peter's University Hospital, New Jersey, USA*
[5]*Division of Internal Medicine, University of Kansas Medical Center, Kansas, USA*
[6]*Division of Cardiovascular Sciences Rutgers, Robert Wood Johnson Medical School/Saint Peter's University Hospital, New Jersey, USA*

Correspondence should be addressed to Ankit Agrawal; drankit.agrawal91@gmail.com

Academic Editor: Filippo M. Sarullo

Cardiac arrest in an event of acute myocardial infarction most commonly results in life-threatening ventricular tachycardia or ventricular fibrillation (VF). Patients who remain in VF despite optimal epinephrine, amiodarone, and three or more attempts at 200 joules of biphasic current defibrillation are known to be in an electrical storm. Here, we describe a case of defibrillation refractory VF responding to intravenous esmolol resulting in a successful return of spontaneous circulation. *Learning objective.* This case reinforces the growing body of evidence supporting esmolol as a novel treatment approach for refractory VF before the cessation of resuscitative efforts.

1. Introduction

Sudden cardiac death in cases of acute myocardial infarction commonly results from ventricular tachyarrhythmias such as ventricular tachycardia (VT) or ventricular fibrillation (VF). The development of these malignant arrhythmias may depict ongoing cardiac ischemia. About 18% of in-hospital cardiac arrest (IHCA) present with VF or VT as the initial rhythm [1]. Cardiopulmonary resuscitation (CPR) with guideline-recommended medications like epinephrine and amiodarone and appropriate defibrillation for shockable rhythms remain the cornerstone of advanced cardiac life support (ACLS) [2]. VF is considered refractory if return of spontaneous circulation (ROSC) is not achieved despite at least 10 minutes of high-quality CPR, three defibrillation attempts, 3 mg of epinephrine, and 300 mg of amiodarone [3]. Small observational studies of patients with recurrent VF suggest that beta-blockade may improve long-term survival after cardiac arrest. However, limited data exists supporting the use of intra-arrest beta-blockade. Here, we present a case of defibrillation-refractory VF responding to intravenous intra-arrest esmolol.

2. Literature Search

Literature review was done using PubMed and ovid MEDLINE. Keywords like "esmolol", "refractory ventricular fibrillation", "double sequential defibrillation", and "electrical storm" were searched.

3. Case

A 52 years old Caucasian male with a history of hypertension presented to the emergency department with severe pressure-like left-sided chest pain of 1-hour duration which radiated to the ipsilateral arm. He was administered 0.4 mg of sublingual nitroglycerin which improved the pain significantly. Vital signs showed a blood pressure of 100/72 mmHg,

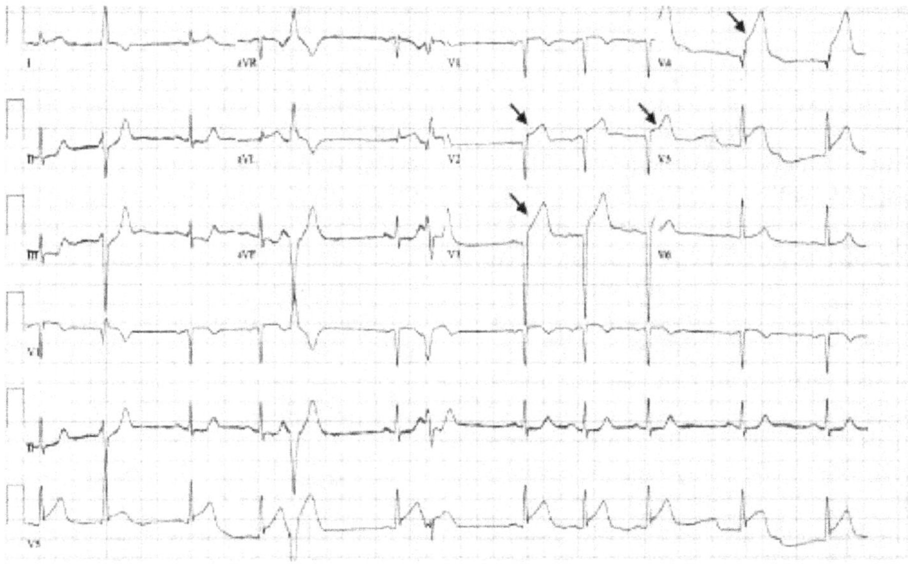

FIGURE 1: 12-lead EKG showing ST segment elevation (black arrows) in leads V2, V3, V4, and V5 suggestive of ST-segment elevation myocardial infarction.

heart rate of 71/min, respiratory rate of 19/min with a saturation of 96% on room air, and a temperature of 97.8 F. His cardiopulmonary examination was within normal limits. An electrocardiogram was obtained which reflected a new ST segment elevation in leads V2-V5 (Figure 1). The cardiac catheterization laboratory was activated, and the patient was given loading doses of aspirin 325 mg, ticagrelor 180 mg, and atorvastatin 80 mg. Meanwhile, laboratory investigation was significant for troponin-I of more than 80.00 ng/mL. While in the emergency room, the patient started complaining of palpitations and he lost consciousness. Upon examination, there was no palpable pulse and the cardiac monitor showed ventricular fibrillation. A code blue was called and cardiopulmonary resuscitation was initiated. Immediate successful intubation was performed. In total, the patient received 9 rounds of 1 mg intravenous (IV) epinephrine every 3-5 minutes, 300 mg IV amiodarone bolus, 1 gram of 10% calcium chloride, 2 doses of 50 mEq sodium bicarbonate, and 5 biphasic defibrillator shocks of 200 joules (J) each. The cardiac monitor still showed VF.

Considering it as a resuscitation failure, double sequential defibrillation was performed and he received 4 additional shocks of 400 J each. Despite this, the patient was still in an electrical storm and at this moment intravenous esmolol 500 mcg/kg (35 mg) IV bolus was administered. The patient subsequently experienced an immediate return of spontaneous circulation. The total resuscitation time was 50 minutes. The therapeutic hypothermia protocol was initiated, and the patient was urgently transferred to the cardiac catheterization laboratory. A loading dose of tirofiban IV 25 mcg/kg and bivalirudin IV 0.75 mg/kg was administered, and a tirofiban maintenance infusion was continued for 12 hours. Emergent catheterization revealed a 100% occlusion of the left anterior descending artery (LAD) (Video 1) with subsequent placement of two drug-eluting stents (DES) in the LAD (Video 2).

The patient was then promptly transferred to the coronary care unit. Therapeutic hypothermia was stopped after 24 hours and meanwhile echocardiography revealed an ejection fraction of 30% with anterior and apical wall akinesis confirming a diagnosis of ischemic cardiomyopathy. The patient was successfully extubated after 4 days, and his neurological function was at his baseline. His hospital stay was complicated by an isolated episode of atrial fibrillation with rapid ventricular response and aspiration pneumonia. The former responded to beta-blockade for rate control. Aspiration pneumonia was treated with 7 days of intravenous ceftriaxone and metronidazole as per the sensitivity results of sputum culture which grew *Haemophilus influenzae*. The patient was discharged from the hospital on day 12 on aspirin 81 mg once daily, ticagrelor 90 mg two times a day, metoprolol succinate extended-release tablet 150 mg once a day, lisinopril 5 mg once a day, and a life vest. He was followed up within a week at our cardiac rehabilitation clinic where he was found to be asymptomatic and compliant with medications.

4. Discussion

The optimal management of VF that is unresponsive to multiple defibrillation attempts is unknown. Several novel interventions have been described in the literature. One such intervention is double sequence defibrillation (DSD). DSD was first described by Hoch and colleagues in 1994 in a case series of five patients in whom DSD was successful in achieving ROSC in VF that was refractory to standard defibrillation [4]. Since then, several case reports demonstrate the potential usefulness of DSD in resuscitation attempts for refractory VF [5]. Extracorporeal cardiopulmonary resuscitation using extracorporeal membrane oxygenation (ECMO) can also be considered in institutions with immediate access to ECMO, as some studies have demonstrated positive results in these patients [6]. Although these strategies show promise, survival rates for refractory VF remain exceptionally poor, and low-quality evidence precludes the widespread adaptation of these strategies into routine ACLS management.

In the present case, DSD was ineffective in terminating the VF arrhythmia, and ECMO was not readily available, so esmolol was administered, with subsequent ROSC. The rationale for esmolol was based on the understanding that beta-adrenergic myocardial hyperstimulation is known to lower the threshold for refractory VF and broaden the ischemic insult in patients with an electrical storm. Electrical storm is defined as the occurrence of three or more episodes of ventricular tachyarrhythmias in 24 hours [7]. Apart from the acute phase of myocardial infarction, an electrical storm can also manifest in the setting of any structural heart disease or genetic arrhythmia syndromes [7]. Activation of the sympathetic nervous system plays a major role in the propagation of electrical storm, and beta-blocking agents are recommended to decrease the incidence of sudden cardiac death [7].

In the setting of cardiac arrest, beta-adrenergic hyperstimulation may be exaggerated as a result of frequent administration of epinephrine in accordance with ACLS guidelines. Esmolol is an intravenous cardioselective beta-1 adrenergic antagonist that is often used in supraventricular tachycardia but also carries an off-label use in the management of electrical storm. In one study of 49 patients with electrical storm and recent myocardial infarction, sympathetic blockade using either beta-blocker agents or left stellate ganglionic blockade was associated with improved survival compared to standard antiarrhythmic therapies [8].

The data supporting the use of beta-blocking therapies during cardiac arrest is very weak. Lee et al. conducted a single-center retrospective prepost study in which sustained ROSC was more common for patients who received esmolol for refractory VF compared to those who did not (p value of 0.007) [3]. Esmolol-treated patients were also more likely to be discharged from the hospital with a favorable neurologic outcome (50% vs. 10.5%) [3]. In another retrospective study of 90 cardiac arrest patients with refractory VF performed by Driver et al., patients that received esmolol were more likely to achieve temporary or sustained ROSC, survive to ICU admission, and survive to hospital discharge with good neurological outcomes as compared to those who did not get esmolol [9]. Although these are small, retrospective studies, they demonstrate a potential role for esmolol in refractory VF.

Few case reports describe the successful use of esmolol in refractory VF. Boehm et al. reported a case of refractory VF successfully treated with DSD and esmolol [10]. In this case, DSD was administered at the 15th minute, followed by a bolus of 80 mg of esmolol IV push (approximately 1000 mcg/kg) followed by a continuous infusion. A second DSD was administered, followed by ROSC after 21 minutes of CPR [10]. More recently, Hwang and colleagues described a similar case, in which ROSC was achieved virtually immediately after esmolol was administered [11]. In this case, a dose of 500 mcg of IV esmolol was given, significantly less than the usual bolus dose administered in other tachyarrhythmias of 500 mcg/kg [11]. Like the previous cases, our patient was refractory to both standard defibrillation and DSD. He received five standard defibrillations and four additional DSD in addition to standard ACLS management, with no ROSC. After 45 minutes of CPR, esmolol 500 mcg/kg (35 mg) IV bolus was administered, and the patient achieved ROSC within minutes. In addition, the patient had an excellent neurologic outcome with no apparent sequelae of anoxic brain injury. This case is unique because CPR was performed for a prolonged period of time before ROSC, and he still experienced a favorable outcome. Our patient also received repetitive attempts at DSD without success.

5. Conclusion

Refractory VF is a rare but extremely life-threatening condition for which the optimal treatment remains unknown. DSD is a stepping-stone in the management of the same, but cases of shock refractory VF may warrant consideration of the use of beta-adrenergic blockade. This case reinforces the growing body of evidence supporting esmolol as a novel treatment approach for refractory VF before the cessation of resuscitative efforts and describes the successful use of esmolol even in cases of extended CPR time. Prospective studies are needed to define the optimal use of esmolol during cardiac arrest. Until these are available, esmolol may be considered in patients with refractory VF that is unresponsive to standard management.

References

[1] A. S. Go, D. Mozaffarian, V. L. Roger et al., "Heart disease and stroke statistics—2013 update a report from the American Heart Association," *Circulation*, vol. 127, no. 1, pp. e6–e245, 2013.

[2] M. S. Link, L. C. Berkow, P. J. Kudenchuk et al., "Part 7: adult advanced cardiovascular life support. 2015 American Heart Association guidelines update for cardiopulmonary resuscitation and emergency cardiovascular care," *Circulation*, vol. 132, 18 suppl 2, pp. S444–S464, 2015.

[3] Y. H. Lee, K. J. Lee, Y. H. Min et al., "Refractory ventricular fibrillation treated with esmolol," *Resuscitation*, vol. 107, pp. 150–155, 2016.

[4] D. H. Hoch, W. P. Batsford, S. M. Greenberg et al., "Double sequential external shocks for refractory ventricular fibrillation," *Journal of the American College of Cardiology*, vol. 23, no. 5, pp. 1141–1145, 1994.

[5] K. Hajjar, I. Berbari, C. el Tawil, R. Bou Chebl, and G. Abou Dagher, "Dual defibrillation in patients with refractory ventricular fibrillation," *The American Journal of Emergency Medicine*, vol. 36, no. 8, pp. 1474–1479, 2018.

[6] F. Y. Siao, C. C. Chiu, C. W. Chiu et al., "Managing cardiac arrest with refractory ventricular fibrillation in the emergency department: conventional cardiopulmonary resuscitation versus extracorporeal cardiopulmonary resuscitation," *Resuscitation*, vol. 92, pp. 70–76, 2015.

[7] M. Eifling, M. Razavi, and A. Massumi, "The evaluation and management of electrical storm," *Texas Heart Institute Journal*, vol. 32, no. 8, pp. 111–121, 2011.

[8] K. Nademanee, R. Taylor, W. E. Bailey, D. E. Rieders, and E. M. Kosar, "Treating electrical storm: sympathetic blockade versus advanced cardiac life support-guided therapy," *Circulation*, vol. 102, no. 7, pp. 742–747, 2000.

[9] B. E. Driver, G. Debaty, D. W. Plummer, and S. W. Smith, "Use of esmolol after failure of standard cardiopulmonary resuscitation to treat patients with refractory ventricular fibrillation," *Resuscitation*, vol. 85, no. 10, pp. 1337–1341, 2014.

[10] K. M. Boehm, D. Keyes, L. M. Mader, and M. Moccia, "First report of survival in refractory ventricular fibrillation after dual-axis defibrillation and esmolol administration," *The Western Journal of Emergency Medicine*, vol. 17, no. 6, pp. 762–765, 2016.

[11] C. W. Hwang, G. Gamble, M. Marchick, and T. K. Becker, "A case of refractory ventricular fibrillation successfully treated with low-dose esmolol," *BML Case Reports*, vol. 12, no. 3, article e228208, 2019.

19

Successful Percutaneous Coronary Intervention using Intravascular Ultrasound-Guided Rewiring Technique in a Case of Spontaneous Coronary Artery Dissection Involving Left Main Bifurcation

Yohei Numasawa, Souichi Yokokura, Yasuhiro Hitomi, Shohei Imaeda, Makoto Tanaka, Ryota Tabei, and Masaki Kodaira

Department of Cardiology, Japanese Red Cross Ashikaga Hospital, Ashikaga, Japan

Correspondence should be addressed to Yohei Numasawa; numasawa@cpnet.med.keio.ac.jp

Academic Editor: Assad Movahed

We herein describe a 49-year-old woman without significant cardiovascular risk factors who was transferred to our hospital with sudden onset of chest pain. The patient was diagnosed with non-ST-elevation acute myocardial infarction, and coronary angiography revealed a dissection at the proximal site of the left anterior descending artery (LAD) extending from the left main trunk (LMT) suggestive of spontaneous coronary artery dissection (SCAD). Because coronary flow was impaired after contrast injection and the patient had chest pain with ST elevation, urgent percutaneous coronary intervention was performed. The first guide wire was initially introduced from the LMT to the distal LAD, but intravascular ultrasound (IVUS) imaging revealed that the guide wire had passed through the true lumen of the left coronary artery ostium, false lumen at the ostium of the left circumflex artery, and true lumen of the distal LAD. We then reinserted another guide wire using an IVUS-guided rewiring technique from the true lumen of the LMT to the distal LAD. Finally, a drug-eluting stent was deployed to cover the dissected segment, and final coronary angiography revealed acceptable results with a patent left circumflex artery. This case report highlights that physicians should consider SCAD among the differential diagnoses in patients presenting with acute coronary syndrome, particularly in young women. In the present case, IVUS played a pivotal role in not only detecting the arterial dissection but also correctly introducing the guide wire into the true lumen.

1. Introduction

Spontaneous coronary artery dissection (SCAD) is a relatively rare but important cause of acute coronary syndrome, especially in young women without significant cardiovascular risk factors and coronary atherosclerosis [1, 2]. In general, conservative medical therapy is recommended in clinically stable patients with SCAD because observational studies have shown favorable short-term outcomes and a high rate of spontaneous angiographic healing of the dissected segment [2–4]. In contrast, in patients with high-risk features such as ongoing ischemia with ST elevation, dissection involving the left main trunk (LMT), and hemodynamic instability, urgent revascularization strategies including percutaneous coronary intervention (PCI) or coronary artery bypass surgery should be considered for the treatment of SCAD [5–7]. However, PCI has a relatively low success rate and a high complication rate in patients with SCAD, and a previous study showed that the failure rate of PCI was 53% [8].

We herein describe a 49-year-old woman who was diagnosed with non-ST-elevation acute myocardial infarction due to SCAD involving left main bifurcation. Because the coronary blood flow of the left anterior descending artery (LAD) was impaired by an enlargement of the false lumen after contrast injection, we performed urgent PCI. The first guide wire was initially introduced from the LMT to the distal LAD, but intravascular ultrasound (IVUS) imaging revealed that the guide wire had passed through the false lumen at the ostium of the left circumflex artery (LCX). We then successfully reinserted another guide wire using an IVUS-guided rewiring technique from the true lumen of the LMT to the distal LAD. In this case, IVUS played a pivotal role in not only detecting the dissection but also introducing the guide wire into the compressed true lumen.

2. Case Presentation

A 49-year-old woman without significant cardiovascular risk factors was transferred to our hospital with a 1-hour history of sudden-onset chest pain. She had taken no medication and experienced no physical or emotional stress preceding the chest pain. On arrival, physical examination revealed stable vital signs with no abnormal findings. Electrocardiography revealed no clear findings of ischemic ST-T changes or prior Q-wave myocardial infarction, but laboratory testing showed elevated cardiac enzymes such as troponin T (0.855 ng/mL) as well as creatine phosphokinase (565 U/L) and its MB isozyme (66 U/L). Bedside transthoracic echocardiography revealed impaired contractility in the focal apical segment of the left ventricle, but there was no clear finding of basal hypercontractility or an apical ballooning sign suggestive of stress-induced cardiomyopathy. Overall, the estimated ejection fraction of the left ventricle was broadly preserved (60%). The patient was diagnosed with non-ST-elevation acute myocardial infarction. Because her condition was stable without chest pain on arrival, we initially administered conservative medical therapy including aspirin, prasugrel, nicorandil, perindopril, pitavastatin, and bisoprolol.

Three days later, we electively performed coronary angiography via the right radial artery using a 6 Fr sheath to determine the etiology of the myocardial injury. Coronary angiography showed no significant atherosclerotic stenosis in the right coronary artery and LCX, but a dissection was found from the midportion of the LMT to the proximal site of the LAD, suggestive of type 1 SCAD (Figure 1(a), Video1) [9]. Because the coronary blood flow of the LAD was impaired from thrombolysis in myocardial infarction (TIMI) flow grade III to I after contrast injection (Figure 1(b)) and the patient had chest pain with ST elevation, we decided to perform urgent PCI. The first wire (SION Blue; Asahi Intecc Co., Ltd., Nagoya, Japan) was initially introduced into the distal LAD, but IVUS imaging revealed that the guide wire had passed through the true lumen of the left coronary artery ostium, false lumen at the ostium of the LCX, and true lumen of the distal LAD (true-false-true) (Figure 2(a)). In addition, the true lumen of the proximal LAD was compressed by the false lumen (Figure 3(a)), and no significant atherosclerosis was observed within the vessel on IVUS. We then inserted the second guide wire (SION Blue; Asahi Intecc Co., Ltd.) into the LCX (Figure 2(b)), and IVUS imaging confirmed that it had been placed in the true lumen from the LMT to LCX (Figure 3(b)). Next, we inserted the third guide wire (SION Blue; Asahi Intecc Co., Ltd.) from the true lumen of the LCX to the compressed true lumen of the LAD using a double-lumen catheter (Crusade Type R; Kaneka Corporation, Tokyo, Japan) by referring to the IVUS findings of the dissected segment (Video2). We initially inserted the third guide wire into the true lumen of the obtuse marginal branch using a double-lumen catheter that was placed in the true lumen of the LCX (Figure 2(c)). We then pulled the wire back and controlled it toward the true lumen of the LAD, which was located under the first guide wire from the right anterior oblique and caudal view (Figures 1(c) and 2(d)). The IVUS-guided rewiring technique was successful, and the subsequent IVUS imaging confirmed that the third guide wire had passed entirely through the true lumen from the LMT to LAD (Figure 3(c), Video3). After the successful rewiring from the true lumen of the LMT to distal LAD, we removed the first wire (Figure 2(e)) and deployed a drug-eluting stent (Resolute Onyx, 3.5 × 30 mm; Medtronic plc, Fridley, MN, USA) from the LMT to LAD (Figures 1(d), 1(e), and 2(f)). Because the blood flow of the LCX was preserved after stenting, we did not perform rewiring of the side branch and final kissing balloon inflation. Final coronary angiography showed acceptable results and TIMI grade III flow in both the LAD and LCX (Figure 1(f)).

The postprocedural course was uneventful, and no major adverse cardiovascular events were observed. The peak levels of creatine phosphokinase and its MB isozyme were 1155 and 142 U/L, respectively. Follow-up coronary computed tomography (CT) angiography was performed 12 months after the procedure and showed acceptable results with no clear findings of in-stent restenosis or incomplete stent apposition (Figures 4(a) and 4(b)). The patients' clinical course was uneventful during an 18-month follow-up.

3. Discussion

This case report highlights that SCAD should always be included among the differential diagnoses in patients with acute coronary syndrome, particularly in young women. Furthermore, IVUS plays a pivotal role in detecting not only the presence of a dissection but also the optimal position of the guide wire in patients with SCAD.

The treatment strategy for SCAD is controversial because of the lack of randomized controlled clinical trials. Recent large-scale observational studies have suggested that conservative medical therapy is generally recommended in hemodynamically stable patients with SCAD because of the reportedly favorable short-term outcomes and high rate of spontaneous angiographic healing of the dissection [2–4]. However, urgent revascularization strategies should be considered in patients with SCAD complicated by high-risk features such as ongoing ischemia with TIMI flow grade 0 to I and/or ST-elevation findings on the electrocardiogram, dissection involving the LMT, and hemodynamic instability [5–7]. In addition, a previous study showed that a left main culprit was relatively common (13%) in patients with SCAD presenting with ST-elevation acute myocardial infarction [7]. In the present case, we decided to perform urgent PCI because the coronary flow was suddenly impaired from TIMI flow grade III to I (which was mainly due to the progression of the dissection involving the left main bifurcation after

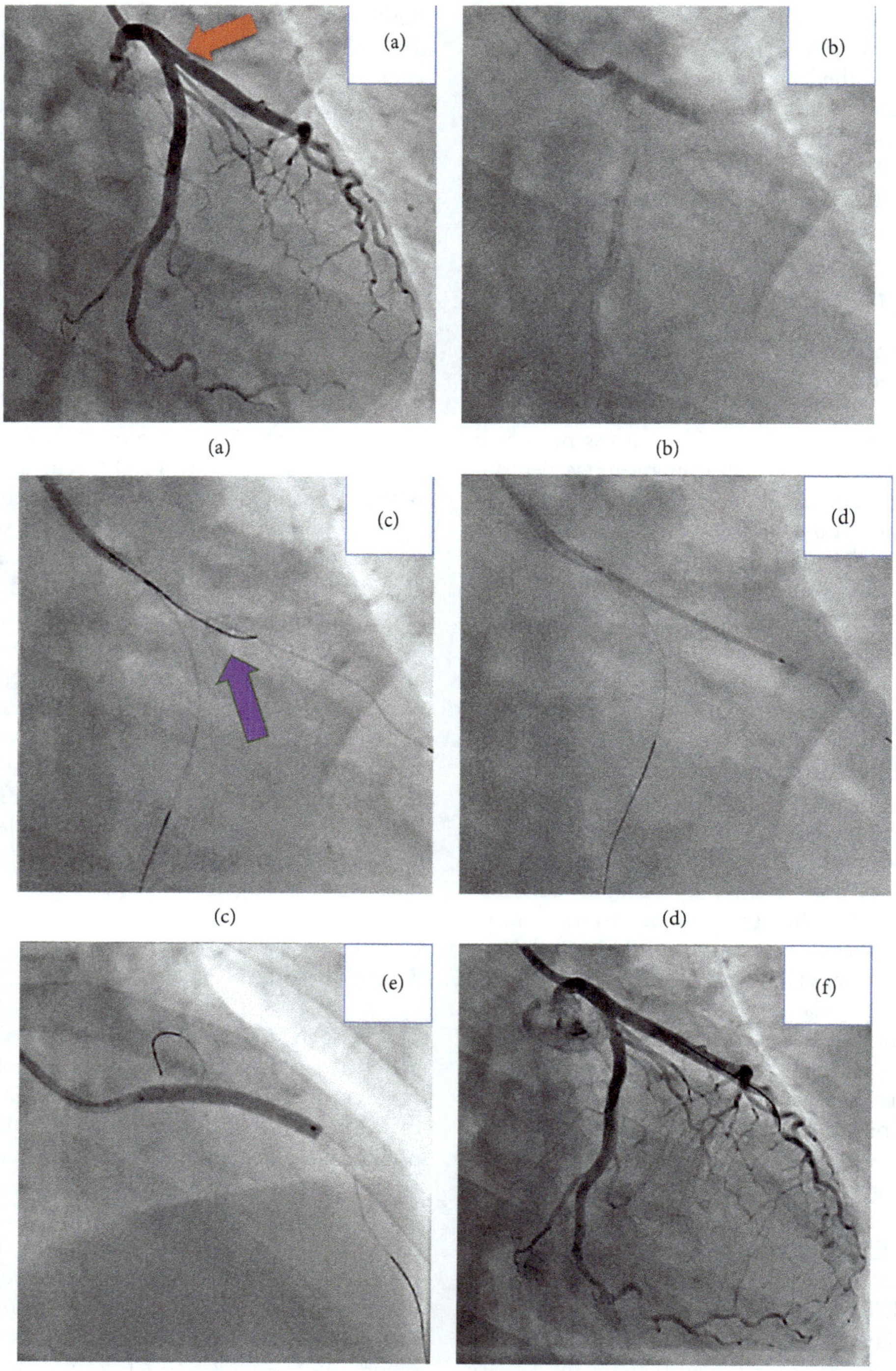

(a) (b) (c) (d) (e) (f)

Figure 1: Coronary angiography and percutaneous coronary intervention. (a) Left coronary angiography (right anterior oblique caudal view) revealed a dissection at the proximal site of the LAD extending from the LMT, suggestive of type 1 spontaneous coronary artery dissection (red arrow). (b) Coronary blood flow of the LAD was impaired after coronary angiography. (c) The IVUS-guided rewiring technique was performed, and the third guide wire (purple arrow) was inserted from the true lumen of the LCX to the true lumen of the LAD by referring to the IVUS findings of the dissected segment. (d and e) A drug-eluting stent was deployed to cover the dissected segment. (f) Final coronary angiography revealed acceptable results. LMT: left main trunk; LAD: left anterior descending artery; LCX: left circumflex artery; IVUS: intravascular ultrasound.

coronary angiography) and the patient had chest pain with ST elevation.

PCI for patients with SCAD is technically challenging mainly because of difficulties in wiring into the true lumen and the risk of extending the dissection or intramural hematoma by the catheter-based procedure [5, 6, 8]. Indeed, the reported rate of successful PCI in patients with SCAD ranges from 47% to 91% [5, 7, 8, 10]. In this case, it was difficult to

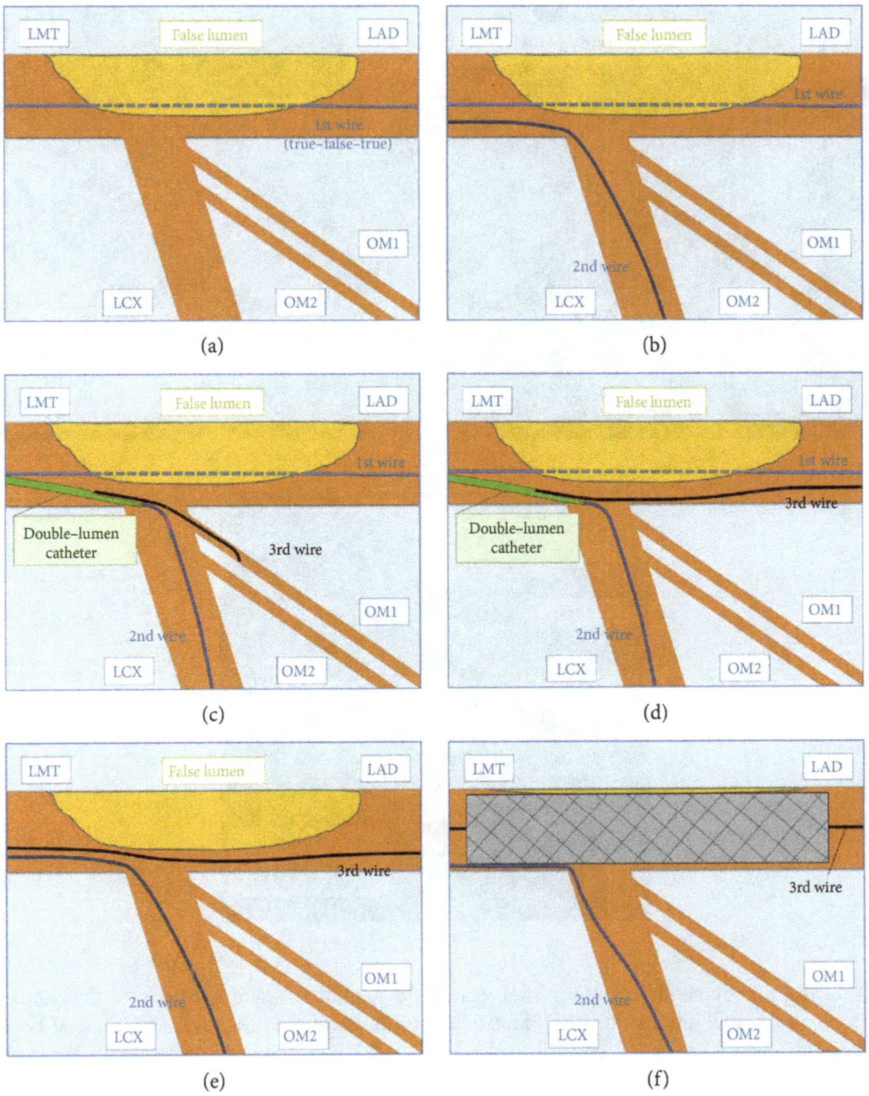

FIGURE 2: The scheme of the percutaneous coronary intervention. (a) The first guide wire passed through the false lumen from the midportion of the LMT to the proximal site of the LAD. (b) The second guide wire was inserted into the true lumen of the LCX. (c) The third guide wire was initially introduced into the true lumen of the obtuse marginal branch using a double-lumen catheter that was placed in the true lumen of the LCX. (d) We pulled the third guide wire back and controlled it toward the true lumen of the LAD, which was located under the first guide wire from the right anterior oblique and caudal view. (e) After the successful rewiring, the first guide wire was removed. (f) A drug-eluting stent was deployed from the LMT to LAD. LMT: left main trunk; LAD: left anterior descending artery; LCX: left circumflex artery; OM: obtuse marginal branch.

insert the guide wire into the true lumen of the dissected segment involving the left main bifurcation. Although the first guide wire seemed to have been successfully introduced from the LMT to LAD, IVUS imaging confirmed that the wire had passed through the true lumen of the left coronary artery ostium, false lumen at the ostium of the LCX, and true lumen of the distal LAD (true-false-true). If we had deployed a drug-eluting stent from the LMT to LAD in this situation, the LCX would have been completely occluded. Thus, we inserted the second guide wire into the true lumen of the LCX and the third guide wire into the true lumen of the LMT and LAD using an IVUS-guided rewiring technique. Although the true lumen of the LAD was compressed by the enlarged false lumen, IVUS imaging from both the true lumen of the LCX and the false lumen of the LAD clearly confirmed that the true lumen of the proximal LAD was close to the ostium of the LCX and obtuse marginal branch. Therefore, we initially inserted the third guide wire into the true lumen of the obtuse marginal branch using a double-lumen catheter that was placed in the true lumen of the LCX; we then pulled the wire back and controlled it toward the true lumen of the LAD, which was located under the first guide wire from the right anterior oblique and caudal view. Although the IVUS-guided wiring technique is commonly used in patients undergoing PCI for chronic total occlusion lesions [11], the present case suggests that it is also useful during PCI for SCAD, especially that involving left main bifurcation. During the procedure, IVUS played a pivotal role in not only detecting the dissection but also introducing the guide wire into the compressed true lumen. After the successful rewiring into the

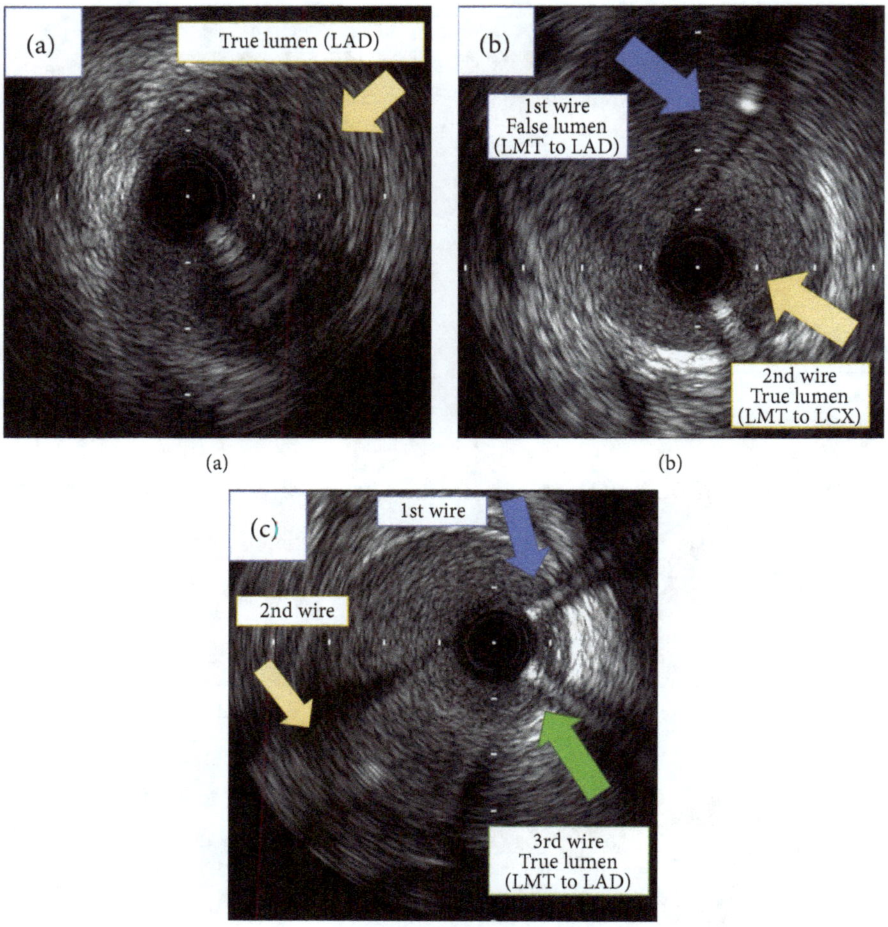

(a) (b)

(c)

FIGURE 3: IVUS findings during percutaneous coronary intervention. (a) The first guide wire passed through the false lumen from the midportion of the LMT to the proximal site of the LAD, and the true lumen of the LAD was compressed by the enlarged false lumen (orange arrow). (b) The second guide wire was inserted into the LCX, and IVUS imaging confirmed that it had been placed in the true lumen from the LMT to LCX (yellow arrow). (c) The third guide wire passed entirely through the true lumen from the LMT to LAD (green arrow). LMT: left main trunk; LAD: left anterior descending artery; LCX: left circumflex artery; IVUS: intravascular ultrasound.

true lumen, a drug-eluting stent was deployed to cover the dissected segment. Because the blood flow of the LCX was preserved after stenting and a complex procedure was considered to be associated with adverse outcomes, including extension of the dissection to the LCX, we did not perform rewiring of the side branch and final kissing balloon inflation.

Several PCI strategies have been reported in patients with SCAD, including balloon angioplasty using a cutting balloon, placement of stents, and use of bioabsorbable scaffolds [5, 6, 12]. Cutting balloon angioplasty to fenestrate the intima is one of the useful alternatives, especially in patients with SCAD characterized by a long and diffuse lesion [6, 13]. If decompression of the intramural hematoma occurs from the false lumen to the true lumen, stent implantation may be avoided in some cases [13, 14]. However, because the coronary arteries of patients with SCAD are vulnerable, cutting balloon angioplasty is associated with a risk of coronary perforation. In addition, creating a large flap after cutting balloon angioplasty, especially in the LMT, may increase the risk of fatal ischemia due to vessel occlusion. In the present case, because the dissection involved the left main bifurcation and could be covered by a single stent, we selected a direct stenting strategy using a drug-eluting stent.

In this case, because laboratory testing showed elevated cardiac enzymes on arrival and coronary angiography and IVUS imaging revealed no findings of atherosclerosis in the coronary arteries, the diagnosis of non-ST-elevation acute myocardial infarction due to SCAD was valid. However, catheter insertion and contrast injection might worsen the dissection and coronary blood flow of the LAD in such patients. Because iatrogenic catheter-induced coronary artery dissections are more common in patients with than without SCAD [15], we should have performed catheter manipulation and contrast injection more carefully. In addition, because the patient's condition was stable on admission and the culprit lesion was present in the proximal portion of the left coronary artery, coronary CT angiography prior to invasive coronary angiography might have been a noninvasive and reasonable alternative. Physicians should consider SCAD among the differential diagnoses in patients presenting with acute coronary syndrome; physicians should also be aware that both diagnostic coronary angiography and

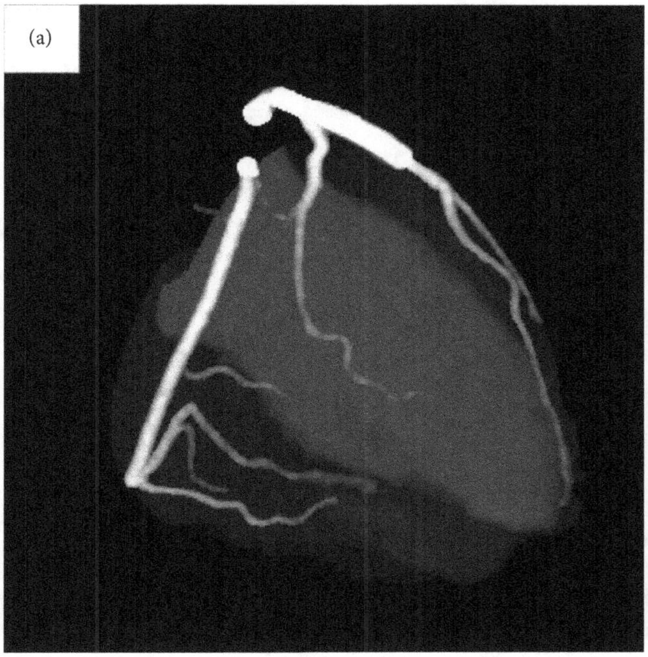

(a)

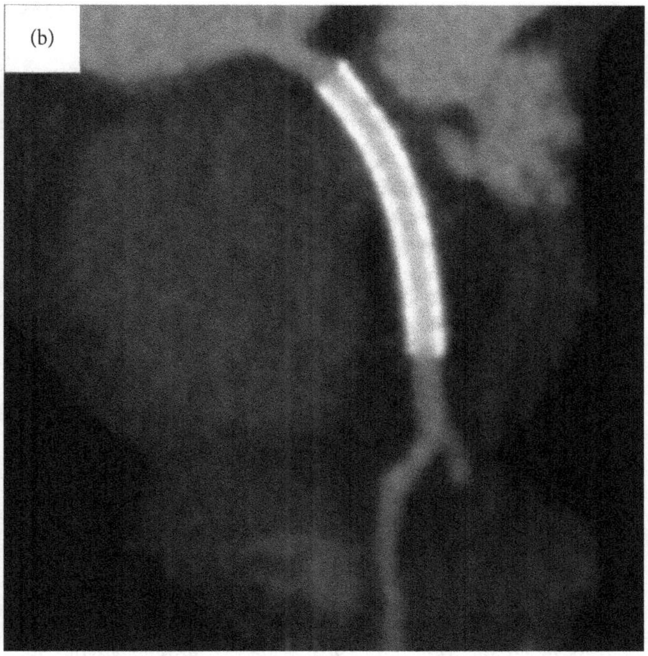

(b)

Figure 4: Coronary CT angiography performed 12 months after percutaneous coronary intervention. (a) Follow-up coronary CT angiography revealed no atherosclerotic stenosis in both the right and left coronary arteries. (b) There were no clear findings of in-stent restenosis or incomplete stent apposition. CT: computed tomography.

PCI are associated with a risk of iatrogenic catheter-induced coronary artery dissection in these patients. In this aspect, coronary CT angiography is a noninvasive and useful alternative in both the acute and chronic phases of SCAD in clinically stable patients [12, 16].

4. Conclusions

This case report suggests that IVUS is useful in not only detecting the dissection but also introducing the guide wire into the true lumen in patients with SCAD, especially that involving left main bifurcation.

Abbreviations

LMT: Left main trunk
LAD: Left anterior descending artery
LCX: Left circumflex artery
IVUS: Intravascular ultrasound.

Acknowledgments

We thank Angela Morben, DVM, ELS, from the Edanz Group (https://en-author-services.edanzgroup.com/) for editing a draft of this manuscript.

Supplementary Materials

Supplementary 1. Video 1. Left coronary angiography (right anterior oblique caudal view) revealed a dissection at the proximal site of the LAD extending from the LMT, suggestive of type 1 spontaneous coronary artery dissection.

Supplementary 2. Video 2. The IVUS-guided rewiring technique was performed, and the third guide wire was inserted from the true lumen of the LCX to the true lumen of the LAD using a double-lumen catheter.

Supplementary 3. Video 3. The IVUS imaging after successful rewiring revealed that the third guide wire passed entirely through the true lumen from the LMT to LAD.

References

[1] S. N. Hayes, E. S. H. Kim, J. Saw et al., "Spontaneous coronary artery dissection: current state of the science: a scientific statement from the American Heart Association," *Circulation*, vol. 137, no. 19, pp. e523–e557, 2018.

[2] J. Saw, A. Starovoytov, K. Humphries et al., "Canadian spontaneous coronary artery dissection cohort study: in-hospital and 30-day outcomes," *European Heart Journal*, vol. 40, no. 15, pp. 1188–1197, 2019.

[3] J. Saw, E. Aymong, T. Sedlak et al., "Spontaneous coronary artery dissection: association with predisposing arteriopathies and precipitating stressors and cardiovascular outcomes," *Circulation Cardiovascular Interventions*, vol. 7, no. 5, pp. 645–655, 2014.

[4] M. Veerasamy, M. E. Jacoby, and R. D. Madder, "Spontaneous dissection of the left main coronary artery: case report and brief review," *Cardiovascular Revascularization Medicine*, vol. 19, no. 3, Part B, pp. 380–383, 2018.

[5] A. Main and J. Saw, "Percutaneous coronary intervention for the treatment of spontaneous coronary artery dissection,"

Interventional Cardiology Clinics, vol. 8, no. 2, pp. 199–208, 2019.

[6] R. Lee and I. Ben-Dor, "Revascularization methods in spontaneous coronary artery dissection: a focused review," *Cardiovascular Revascularization Medicine*, vol. 18, no. 7, pp. 544–548, 2017.

[7] A. S. Lobo, S. M. Cantu, S. W. Sharkey et al., "Revascularization in patients with spontaneous coronary artery dissection and ST-segment elevation myocardial infarction," *Journal of the American College of Cardiology*, vol. 74, no. 10, pp. 1290–1300, 2019.

[8] M. S. Tweet, M. F. Eleid, P. J. Best et al., "Spontaneous coronary artery dissection: revascularization versus conservative therapy," *Circulation Cardiovascular Interventions*, vol. 7, no. 6, pp. 777–786, 2014.

[9] J. Saw, "Coronary angiogram classification of spontaneous coronary artery dissection," *Catheterization and Cardiovascular Interventions*, vol. 84, no. 7, pp. 1115–1122, 2014.

[10] T. Nakashima, T. Noguchi, S. Haruta et al., "Prognostic impact of spontaneous coronary artery dissection in young female patients with acute myocardial infarction: a report from the Angina Pectoris-Myocardial Infarction Multicenter Investigators in Japan," *International Journal of Cardiology*, vol. 207, pp. 341–348, 2016.

[11] S. A. Harding, E. B. Wu, S. Lo et al., "A new algorithm for crossing chronic total occlusions from the Asia Pacific Chronic Total Occlusion Club," *JACC: Cardiovascular Interventions*, vol. 10, no. 21, pp. 2135–2143, 2017.

[12] M. M. Mahmood and D. Austin, "IVUS and OCT guided primary percutaneous coronary intervention for spontaneous coronary artery dissection with bioresorbable vascular scaffolds," *Cardiovascular Revascularization Medicine*, vol. 18, no. 1, pp. 53–57, 2017.

[13] A. Main, W. L. Lombardi, and J. Saw, "Cutting balloon angioplasty for treatment of spontaneous coronary artery dissection: case report, literature review, and recommended technical approaches," *Cardiovascular Diagnosis and Therapy*, vol. 9, no. 1, pp. 50–54, 2019.

[14] H. Sharma, V. Vetrugno, and S. Q. Khan, "Successful treatment of a spontaneous right coronary artery dissection with a 4-mm diameter cutting balloon: a case report," *European Heart Journal - Case Reports*, vol. 3, no. 4, pp. 1–6, 2019.

[15] R. Prakash, A. Starovoytov, M. Heydari, G. B. Mancini, and J. Saw, "Catheter-induced iatrogenic coronary artery dissection in patients with spontaneous coronary artery dissection," *JACC: Cardiovascular Interventions*, vol. 9, no. 17, pp. 1851–1853, 2016.

[16] J. Saw, G. B. J. Mancini, and K. H. Humphries, "Contemporary review on spontaneous coronary artery dissection," *Journal of the American College of Cardiology*, vol. 68, no. 3, pp. 297–312, 2016.

20

A Rare Complication of HVAD Outflow Thrombosis and the Importance of HVAD Waveform Analysis

John Ning and Nunzio Gaglianello

Medical College of Wisconsin, 8701 West Watertown Plank Road Milwaukee, WI 53226, USA

Correspondence should be addressed to Nunzio Gaglianello; ngaglian@mcw.edu

Academic Editor: Assad Movahed

We present a case of a 64-year-old female who was supported with an HVAD as bridge-to-transplant (BTT) who presented with a gastrointestinal (GI) bleeding and underwent esophagogastroduodenoscopy (EGD) and colonoscopy. Her waveforms changed abruptly following the procedure, and she decompensated. With various imaging modalities and hemodynamic monitoring, we felt that she had thrombus in her outflow graft, which improved following systemic heparinization. She was listed for cardiac transplantation and remained hospitalized. At the time of surgery, her outflow graft was noted to be compressed externally and pathology was consistent with platelet-fibrin thrombus deposition.

1. Introduction

In this case report, we describe a rare complication of outflow graft compression as well as our approach to analyzing HVAD waveform and use of imaging modalities that led to our differential diagnosis and management.

2. Case Presentation

64-year-old African American female with nonischemic cardiomyopathy implanted with an HVAD as a bridge to transplant, listed for cardiac transplantation as UNOS status 1B, had been doing well until the time of her hospital presentation. She was admitted to the hospital with concern for GI bleeding. Her hemoglobin was 7.9 g/dL, down from her baseline of 10.4 g/dL. Her lactate dehydrogenase (LDH) and haptoglobin were stable at presentation at 219 U/L and 64 mg/dL, respectively. The patient underwent evaluation for GI bleeding with an EGD and colonoscopy with no initial source found, so a capsule endoscopy was placed. On capsule endoscopy, the patient was found to have a jejunal bleeding. Following this, a push enteroscopy was performed with argon plasma coagulation and clipping of the arteriovenous malformation. After being transferred to the floor in a stable condition, the patient became acutely hypoxic and started having low flow alarms on her HVAD device and her waveform became less pulsatile. Her heart rate was in 120 s, mean arterial pressures were in 50 s, and she was transferred to a cardiovascular ICU for emergent intubation. She was started on a heparin drip as well as on vasopressors and inotropes for hemodynamic instability. After the transfer to the cardiovascular ICU, a bedside swan was obtained demonstrating the following hemodynamics: right atrium (RA) 13 mmHg, right ventricle 52/13 mmHg, pulmonary artery 53/28/40 mmHg, pulmonary capillary wedge pressure (PCWP) 28 mmHg, and cardiac output/cardiac index 3.0/1.6 L/min. Repeat lactate dehydrogenase and haptoglobin were 165 U/L and 48 mg/dL respectively.

3. Materials and Methods

The following are the pre-GI procedure HVAD parameters: flow 4.0 L/min, speed 2460 rpm, 2.8 watts, MAP 68 mmHg, and normal waveform pulsatility. The following are the post-GI procedure HVAD parameters: flow 2.1 L/min, speed 2400 rpm, and 2.1 watts (Figure 1). The transthoracic echocardiogram (TTE) showed a severely enlarged left ventricle with severe systolic dysfunction and severe global hypokinesis with an ejection fraction (EF) of 10-20% and moderate

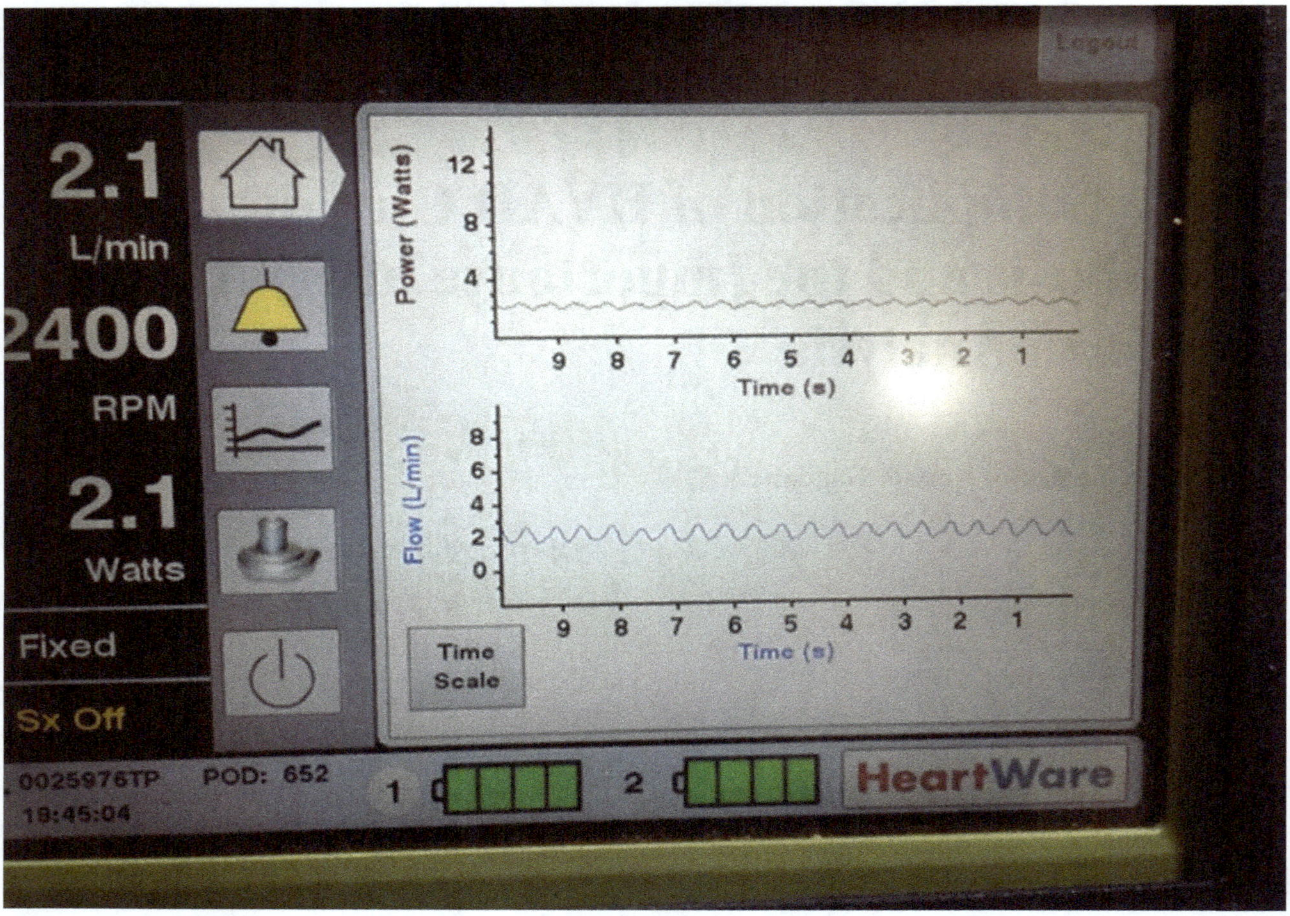

FIGURE 1: Demonstration of a low flow-low pulsatility waveform with no increase in HVAD power consumption.

right ventricular systolic dysfunction. No inflow cannula thrombus was noted. Inflow cannula velocities were normal. Outflow cannula velocities were low at <1 m/s. After the patient was stabilized, a gated computed tomography (CT) of the chest demonstrated an interval development of nearly occlusive thrombus involving the proximal half of the outflow graft with opacification of the distal half (Figure 2).

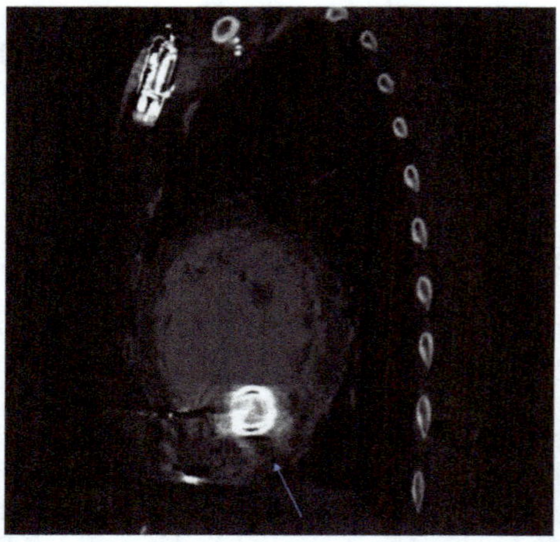

FIGURE 2: Gated CT scan of the chest with IV contrast in the sagittal plane demonstrating compression/thrombosis of the HVAD outflow graft (arrow).

4. Results

The patient's HVAD waveform improved with systemic heparinization. She was diuresed, extubated, and weaned off vasopressors and inotropes and was listed as UNOS status 1A and was successfully transplanted. At the time of transplantation and HVAD explantation, the outflow graft material was noted to be platelet-fibrin thrombus (Figures 3 and 4).

5. Discussion

Left ventricular assist devices (LVADs) serve as a bridge to transplant (BTT) and offer patients with advanced heart failure better survival and functional status and quality of life as they await heart transplantation [1]. Recently, the ENDURACE trial suggested that a small, intrapericardial, centrifugal flow LVAD was noninferior to axial flow LVAD in terms of survival free from disabling stroke or device removal for malfunction or failure [2].

A known serious complication of LVADs is the formation of thrombus within the pump impeller. Pump thrombus requiring exchange occurred at a rate of 0.04 events per patient year (EPPY) with a total suspected thrombus rate

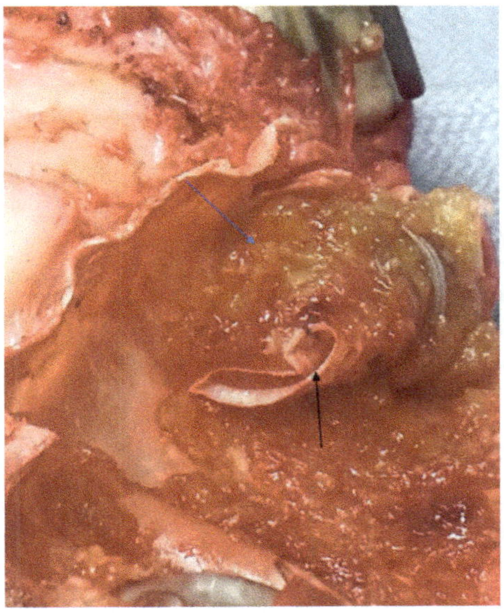

FIGURE 3: Analysis of the HVAD outflow graft at the time of cardiac transplantation demonstrating platelet-fibrin rich collection (blue arrow) causing external compression of the outflow graft (black arrow).

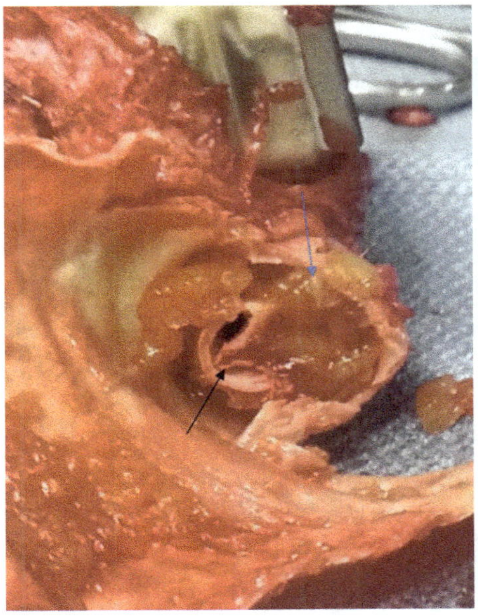

FIGURE 4: Different view of the HVAD outflow graft (black arrow) at the time of cardiac transplantation demonstrating external compression of the outflow graft by platelet-fibrin rich thrombus (blue arrow).

of 0.08 EPPY in patients implanted with an HVAD from the HeartWare BTT and CAP (Continued Access Protocol) trials [3]. This case is unique in that the thrombus formation was an external compression of fibrin-rich material that caused compression of the outflow graft. A recent study found that PTFE graft covering of the LVAD outflow graft can lead to graft occlusion and should be reconsidered a potentially harmful modification [4]. Our patient's LVAD was wrapped in polytetrafluoroethylene (PTFE) which does not breathe or leak. This leads to confinement of the outflow graft and potential external compression of the outflow graft limiting blood flow.

Interpreting the HVAD waveform and understanding changes in flows and pulsatility can help the clinician create a differential diagnosis. In this case, an abrupt change in pulsatility and flow led our group to suspect an inflow thrombus or outflow cannula thrombus/obstruction [5]. Other considerations in the setting of low flow-low pulsatility waveforms include right ventricular failure, cardiac tamponade, ventricular fibrillation, and rapid ventricular tachycardia. During the evaluation, an echocardiogram was obtained which did not demonstrate an inflow cannula thrombus or a pericardial effusion. The patient's hemodynamics from right heart catheterization were not consistent with right ventricle failure given that the RA pressure was only 13 mmHg as well as maintain a preserved PCWP:RA pressure ratio of 2:1 along with TTE findings of unchanged moderate RV systolic dysfunction.

Ultimately, a gated CT scan demonstrated compression of the outflow graft with narrowing of the outflow graft lumen. In the most common form of pump thrombosis, a clot forms on the pump rotor. This increased resistance manifests as an increase in pump power and a falsely elevated increase in pump flow. In contrast, inflow and outflow thrombosis demonstrates low pulsatility, low flow, and a drop in power as it requires less energy to maintain the set pump speed with less blood flow through the device, as demonstrated by a drop in pulsatility on the HVAD waveform and a decrease in flow.

Given the implications and severity of pump thrombosis, many clinicians have sought to find effective strategies to detect and treat pump thrombosis. Laboratory tests such as LDH and haptoglobin to detect hemolysis along with patient hemodynamics, elevated VAD power consumption, and acoustic analysis have been utilized to detect platelet thrombosis [6]. Imaging modalities such as computed tomography angiography (CTA) and intravascular ultrasound (IVUS) may also assist in the diagnosis of pump thrombosis. A recent study showed that luminal narrowing found on CTA in patients with LVAD outflow grafts was suggestive of extrinsic compression of the graft rather than intraluminal thrombus [7].

Despite advancement in the detection of pump thrombosis, there has not been a consensus on treatment modality. Treatment options such as medical therapy with thrombolytics or surgical device exchange are common; however, the variability of patient and device factors has caused the ideal treatment to be elusive. Studies suggested that the medical treatment of pump thrombosis has a low success rate and a high risk of hemorrhagic stroke and death [8]. It was found that treatment with tPA is more likely to be successful in thrombi that showed gradual development and have not reached a high percent of expected power [9]. LVAD device exchange has shown to have very low early mortality and low complication rates [10].

As the heart failure population grows and LVAD utilization increases, it is of upmost importance that HVAD waveforms are utilized and recognized by heart failure cardiologists, cardiothoracic surgeons, and intensivists to formulate a differential diagnosis to troubleshoot HVAD waveform abnormalities.

References

[1] E. A. Rose, A. C. Gelijns, A. J. Moskowitz et al., "Long-Term Use of a Left Ventricular Assist Device for End-Stage Heart Failure," *New England Journal of Medicine*, vol. 345, pp. 1435–1443, 2001.

[2] J. G. Rogers, F. D. Pagani, A. J. Tatooles et al., "Intrapericardial left ventricular assist device for advanced heart failure," *New England Journal of Medicine*, vol. 376, pp. 451–460, 2017.

[3] S. S. Najjar, M. S. Slaughter, F. D. Pagani et al., "An analysis of pump thrombus events in patients in the HeartWare ADVANCE bridge to transplant and continued access protocol trial," *The Journal of Heart and Lung Transplantation*, vol. 33, pp. 23–34, 2014.

[4] T. Alnabelsi, A. E. Shafii, J. C. Gurley, K. Dulnuan, D. D. Harris, and M. Guglin, "Left ventricular assist device outflow graft obstruction: a complication specific to polytetrafluoroethylene covering. A word of caution!," *ASAIO Journal*, vol. 65, no. 6, pp. e58–e62, 2019.

[5] J. D. Rich and D. Burkhoff, "HVAD flow waveform morphologies: theoretical foundation and implications for clinical practice," *ASAIO Journal*, vol. 63, no. 5, pp. 526–535, 2017.

[6] A. M. Scandroglio, F. Kaufmann, M. Pieri et al., "Diagnosis and treatment algorithm for blood flow obstructions in patients with left ventricular assist device," *Journal of the American College of Cardiology*, vol. 67, pp. 2758–2768, 2016.

[7] C. R. Trankle, J. D. Grizzard, K. B. Shah et al., "Left ventricular assist device outflow graft compression: incidence, clinical associations and potential etiologies," *Journal of Cardiac Failure*, vol. 25, pp. 545–552, 2019.

[8] J. M. Stulak, S. M. Dunlay, S. Sharma et al., "Treatment of device thrombus on the HeartWare HVAD: success and outcomes depend significantly on the initial treatment strategy," *Journal of Heart and Lung Transplantation*, vol. 34, pp. 1535–1541, 2015.

[9] U. P. Jorde, K. D. Aaronson, S. S. Najjar et al., "Identification and Management of Pump Thrombus in the HeartWare Left Ventricular Assist Device System: A Novel Approach Using Log File Analysis," *JACC: Heart Failure*, vol. 3, pp. 849–856, 2015.

[10] N. Moazami, C. A. Milano, R. John et al., "Pump replacement for left ventricular assist device failure can be done safely and is associated with low mortality," *The Annals of Thoracic Surgery*, vol. 95, pp. 500–505, 2013.

21

Successful Low-Dose tPA for Mechanical Mitral Valve Thrombosis in a Patient with Postinfarction Contained Left Ventricular Free Wall Rupture

James Livesay,[1] Emmanuel Isang,[1] Hassan Tahir,[1] and Raj Baljepally[1,2]

[1]Department of Medicine, University of Tennessee Graduate School of Medicine, Knoxville, TN, USA
[2]Heart Lung Vascular Institute, University of Tennessee Medical Center, Knoxville, TN, USA

Correspondence should be addressed to Raj Baljepally; rbaljepa@utmck.edu

Academic Editor: Francesco Nappi

Prosthetic valve thrombosis is a potentially life-threatening complication diagnosed by a combination of clinical features and imaging modalities, but the optimal management in high bleeding risk patients remains controversial. Current treatment options for prosthetic valve thrombosis included surgery, thrombolytic therapy, and anticoagulation. We present a very unusual case of a patient with a recent ST-elevation myocardial infarction complicated by contained left ventricle free wall rupture and mechanical mitral valve thrombosis. Deemed a high surgical risk candidate, low-dose tissue plasminogen activator was used despite significant bleeding risk from contained left ventricle free wall rupture, which resulted in resolution of the thrombus. To the best of our knowledge, this is the first report of successful thrombolytic therapy for prosthetic mechanical mitral valve thrombosis in a patient with recent postmyocardial infarction contained left ventricular free wall rupture.

1. Introduction

The most common complications after native valve replacement include prosthetic valve thrombosis (PVT), pannus formation, embolic events, bleeding, and infective endocarditis [1]. The rate of PVT is higher in patients with mechanical valves versus those with bioprosthetic valves, with an annual rate up to 5.7% in the mechanical valve group [2]. Mitral mechanical PVT is twice as common as aortic mechanical PVT, and rates of thromboembolism are higher for certain types of mechanical valves [3]. Any patient with a known mechanical valve that presents with clinical signs of valve obstruction such as a new murmur, subdued clicks, symptoms or signs of heart failure, thromboembolic events, or elevated transvalvular gradients should be evaluated for PVT. Prosthetic valve mean gradients increased by 50% from the baseline in the setting of acute presenting symptoms, and subtherapeutic anticoagulation is consistent with PVT [4]. The current management strategies for PVT include surgical intervention, thrombolytic therapy, and anticoagulation [2]. However, the best treatment option depends on many factors, including right versus left-sided valve involvement, thrombus burden, surgical risk, and patient preference.

2. Case Presentation

A 52-year-old woman with a history of chronic kidney disease status post kidney transplant, remote history of mitral valve endocarditis status post St Jude mechanical mitral valve replacement, and heart failure presented with an ST-elevation myocardial infarction. She underwent emergent left heart catheterization revealing a 100% occluded obtuse marginal branch for which percutaneous intervention with stent implantation was performed. Follow-up transthoracic echocardiogram (TTE) showed a low normal ejection fraction of 52% and normal mitral valve gradients. She was discharged home on guideline-directed medical therapy postacute myocardial infarction.

Approximately three weeks later, she presented with acute dyspnea, orthopnea, and acute hypoxic respiratory failure. Her international normalized ratio (INR) on presentation was supratherapeutic at 8.29 with a repeat the following day of 2.02. She was initially treated for a heart failure exacerbation with bilevel positive airway pressure and aggressive intravenous diuretics. A TTE was repeated given her acute clinical change, revealing a severely reduced ejection fraction of 30-35%, abnormal prosthetic mitral valve gradients, and restricted posterior valve leaflet mobility. The mitral valve max pressure gradient was 21.1 mmHg with a mean gradient across the mitral valve of 11.0 mmHg. The TTE also revealed a tricuspid regurgitation (TR) max velocity of 343.9 cm/sec, TR max PG 47.3 mmHg, RVSP 50.3 mmHg, and pressure half-time of 2.5 cm^2. PVT was diagnosed based on her acute clinical symptoms and echocardiography findings.

Incidentally, contrast TTE also revealed a posterolateral pseudoaneurysm with contrast extending into the pericardial space concerning for left ventricular free wall rupture (Figure 1). A transesophageal echocardiogram (TEE) was considered, but the patient required high levels of supplemental oxygen and therefore deemed high risk by anesthesia. Given her history of renal transplant and worsening renal function, cardiac magnetic resonance was performed instead of a CT angiogram which confirmed a contained left ventricle free wall rupture (Figure 2).

Due to mechanical mitral PVT and left ventricular pseudoaneurysm, felt to be secondary to recent myocardial infarction, cardiothoracic surgery was consulted. She was considered inoperable due to multiple factors: recent myocardial infarction on dual antiplatelet therapy, heart failure with reduced ejection fraction, acute respiratory failure, worsening renal function, prior renal transplant, and prior open-heart surgery. Management options were extremely limited, but after discussion with the patient's family, low-dose tissue plasminogen activator (tPA) was administered and infused at 25 mg over six hours. The following day, patient's dyspnea improved. She underwent a TEE showing a normally functioning mechanical mitral valve with a mean gradient across the valve of 5 mmHg. There was no evidence of thrombus and the left ventricle posterior wall pseudoaneurysm was unchanged (Figures 3 and 4).

Although her initial hospital course was complicated by renal failure requiring continuous renal replacement therapy, prolonged respiratory failure requiring high doses of supplemental oxygen, and hypotension limiting guideline-directed medical therapy, she recovered gradually with conservative management of the contained posterior wall rupture. She continued to show improvement and was discharged home following a twenty-five-day hospitalization. She was seen in the ambulatory setting two months later without complaints of dyspnea or orthopnea and an echocardiogram showing a mean mitral valve gradient of 8.9 mmHg with no pericardial effusion. Since then, she has been seen multiple times in our outpatient clinic and is doing very well.

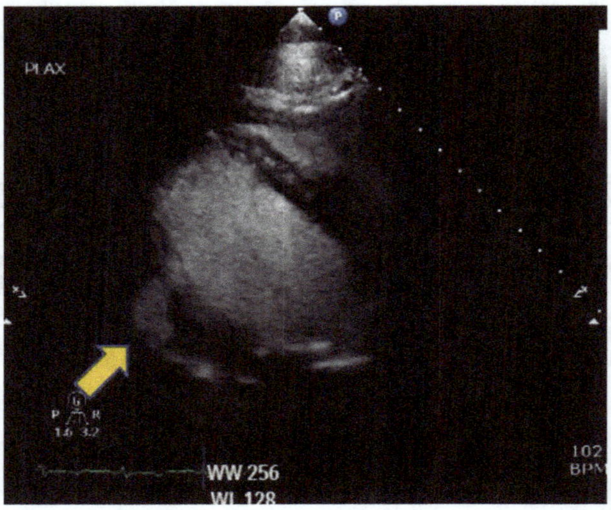

Figure 1: Parasternal long axis view of contrast leaking into the pericardial space on echocardiogram.

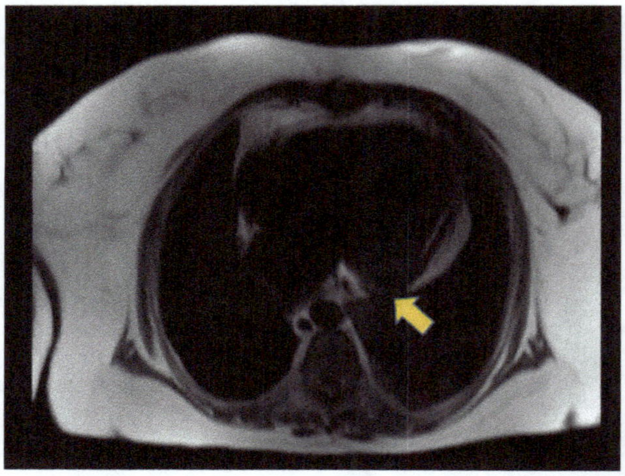

Figure 2: Cardiac magnetic resonance view of the contained left ventricle free wall rupture.

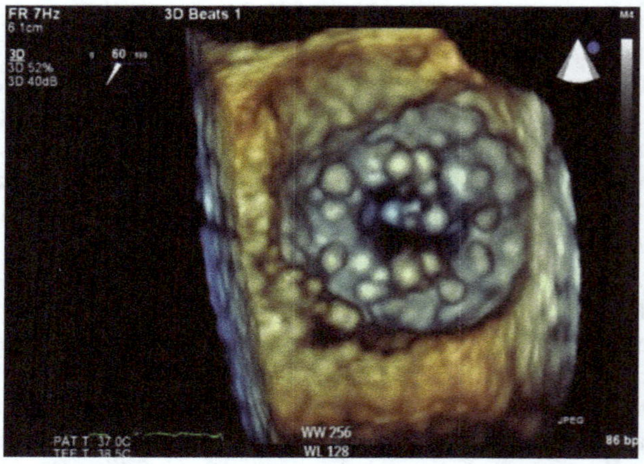

Figure 3: 3D transesophageal echocardiogram of the normally functioning mechanical mitral valve at 60 degrees following treatment with tPA.

3. Discussion

The current prevalence of mitral and aortic valve disease in the United States is approximately 2.5% in the general population and up to 10% in people 75 years or older [2]. Treatment of valvular disease includes surgical replacement such as mechanical and biological valves and, more recently,

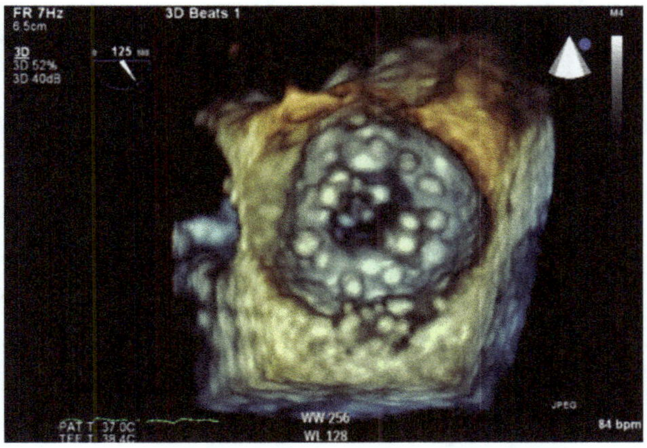

Figure 4: 3D transesophageal echocardiogram of the normally functioning mechanical mitral valve at 125 degrees following treatment with tPA.

transcatheter technology. While mechanical valves are more durable, they have a significantly elevated risk of developing thrombus with symptomatic obstructive mechanical valve thrombosis occurrence ranging from 0.3% to 1.3% per year [1]. Management of PVT remains challenging and depends on several patient factors: thrombus location, thrombus size, the patient's functional status, and surgical and bleeding risk [5].

PVT should be considered when patients present with acute symptoms, new murmur, signs of heart failure, diminished valve sounds, and thromboembolic events [1]. The exact incidence of PVT is likely underestimated as appropriate imaging is either not performed or suboptimal. TTE, TEE, fluoroscopy, and CT imaging are used to assist in diagnosing PVT [2, 4]. Thrombolytic therapy for right-sided PVT is considered if clot persists despite intravenous heparin. However, the management of left-sided PVT is more problematic. Factors that favor surgery include the availability of surgical expertise, low surgical risk, recurrent thrombus, NYHA class IV heart failure, possible pannus, and coronary artery disease requiring revascularization. While factors that favor thrombolytics include lack of available surgical expertise, high surgical risk, first-time thrombosis, NYHA class ≤ III heart failure, no coronary artery disease, and no pannus formation. [2, 4]. Other advantages of thrombolytic therapy over surgery include its ubiquitous availability and ease of use. Intravenous heparin is recommended in each case with thrombolytic therapy if valve thrombus persists [2].

Kapos and colleagues presented a case of a 52-year-old female presenting with signs of cardiac congestion. An urgent TTE revealed an elevated diastolic transmitral gradient of 21 mmHg with impaired movement of one of the disc. TEE confirmed the TTE findings, but no mass was seen. Given her symptoms and echocardiographic findings, she was diagnosed with a PVT and started on unfractionated heparin. Despite five days of therapy, the mitral stenosis remained unchanged, and she was started on low-dose-ultraslow fibrinolytic therapy [1].

Kalçik and colleagues present a case of a 57-year-old female that presented with NYHA class III dyspnea. TTE revealed an increased mean mitral transvalvular gradient of 15 mmHg with a decreased mitral valve area of 0.9 cm^2. She had no contraindications to thrombolytic therapy and was started on low-dose tPA 25 mg over the course of 25 hours (low-dose and ultraslow fibrinolytic therapy). Repeat TTE showed a decreased transvalvular gradient and relaxation in the restricted leaflet. She was discharged on oral anticoagulation and did not require surgical intervention [6].

The ultraslow PROMETEE trial evaluated the use of low-dose slow infusion of tPA (25 mg over 6 hours) in patients with mechanical PVT. Thrombolytic therapy was administered to 114 patients under TTE guidance. They found a low-dose ultraslow infusion of tPA was associated with an overall success rate of 90% and low morbidity and mortality in each NYHA class except class IV [7]. Low-dose thrombolytic therapy is a viable alternative to surgical intervention in patients with PVT but not well studied in patients at an elevated bleeding risk. Although an ultraslow tPA infusion (25 hours) is probably more appropriate in patients with higher bleeding risk, it is not an effective option in unstable patients such as ours, who require more rapid treatment. Overall, however, the benefit of thrombolytic therapy for PVT may outweigh the risk in critically ill inoperable patients, despite the elevated bleeding risk.

4. Conclusion

The optimal management option is unclear in patients presenting with both PVT and extremely high bleeding risk. Our patient is unique in that she presented with both acute respiratory failures from mechanical mitral PVT and a left ventricular free wall contained rupture after a recent ST-elevation myocardial infarction. A successful outcome in our highly unusual case illustrates that despite the extreme bleeding risk, low-dose thrombolytics are potentially lifesaving and should always be considered, especially in inoperable patients.

References

[1] I. Kapos, T. Fuchs, and F. C. Tanner, "Case report of successful low-dose, ultra-slow infusion thrombolysis of prosthetic mitral valve thrombosis in a high risk patient after redo-mitral valve replacement," *European Heart Journal-Case Reports*, vol. 4, no. 3, pp. 1–5, 2020.

[2] G. D. Dangas, J. I. Weitz, G. Giustino, R. Makkar, and R. Mehran, "Prosthetic heart valve thrombosis," *Journal of the American College of Cardiology*, vol. 68, no. 24, pp. 2670–2689, 2016.

[3] R. Roudaut, K. Serri, and S. Lafitte, "Thrombosis of prosthetic heart valves: diagnosis and therapeutic considerations," *Heart*, vol. 93, no. 1, pp. 137–142, 2007.

[4] Writing Committee Members, C. M. Otto, R. A. Nishimura et al., "2020 ACC/AHA guideline for the management of patients with valvular heart disease: executive summary: a report of the American College of Cardiology/American Heart Association Joint Committee on clinical practice guidelines,"

Journal of the American College of Cardiology, vol. 77, no. 4, pp. 450–500, 2021.

[5] M. Biteker, I. Altun, O. Basaran, V. Dogan, B. Yildirim, and G. Ergun, "Treatment of prosthetic valve thrombosis: current evidence and future directions," *Journal of clinical medicine research*, vol. 7, no. 12, pp. 932–936, 2015.

[6] M. Kalçık, M. Yesin, M. O. Gürsoy, and M. Özkan, "Obstructive prosthetic mitral valve thrombosis successfully thrombolysed with low-dose ultra-slow infusion of tissue plasminogen activator," *International Cardiovascular Forum Journal*, vol. 3, pp. 40-41, 2015.

[7] M. Özkan, S. Gündüz, O. M. Gürsoy et al., "Ultraslow thrombolytic therapy: a novel strategy in the management of PROsthetic MEchanical valve Thrombosis and the prEdictors of outcomE: the ultra-slow PROMETEE trial," *American Heart Journal*, vol. 170, no. 2, pp. 409–418.e1, 2015.

22

Isolated Native Tricuspid Valve Endocarditis in a Nonintravenous Drug User

Habtewold Shibru,[1] Ermias shenkutie Greffie,[1] Zenahbezu Abay,[1] and Oumer Abdu Muhie[2]

[1]Department of Internal Medicine, University of Gondar, Gondar, Ethiopia
[2]Department of Internal Medicine, GAMBY Teaching General Hospital, Bahir Dar, Ethiopia

Correspondence should be addressed to Oumer Abdu Muhie; umerabdu88@gmail.com

Academic Editor: Christopher S. Snyder

Infective endocarditis (IE) is a disease characterized by high morbidity and mortality. IE was first described in the mid-16th century. Right-sided infective endocarditis (RSIE) represents 5% to 10% of all IE episodes in adults. RSIE can be divided into three groups according to the underlying risk factors: intravenous drug users (IDUs), cardiac device carriers, and the "three noes" group (no left-sided IE, no IDUs, and no cardiac devices). Tricuspid valve endocarditis in nonintravenous drug users can occur in a variety of conditions including congenital heart disease, intracardiac devices, central venous catheters, and immunologically debilitated patients. Due to the rareness of isolated native nonrheumatic tricuspid valve endocarditis, here, we like to present an 18-year-old male from rural Ethiopia with the diagnosis of isolated native tricuspid valve endocarditis that was treated and cured.

1. Clinical Profile of the Patient

A previously healthy, 18-year-old male patient from Gorgora, North West Ethiopia, presented to the University of Gondar Hospital with progressive dyspnea associated with orthopnea, palpitation, bilateral leg swelling, cough productive of blood-tinged sputum, and right-sided pleuritic chest pain that lasted for a week before his visit. A week prior to the onset of the above symptoms, he had left knee joint swelling associated with high-grade fever. He noticed decreased urine amount since three days prior to admission with reddish discoloration. He had piercing injury to his right foot which formed a wound that healed by itself two months before presentation. He never had a history of intravenous drug use. He neither had a history of dental, genitourinary, or gastrointestinal procedures. He has no previous cardiac surgery.

The physical examination of this patient at presentation to the Emergency Department revealed a critically sick febrile patient in cardiopulmonary distress with low oxygen saturation. Respiratory examination showed bronchial breath sound and signs of right-side pleura effusion. Likewise, the cardiovascular examination was remarkable for raised jugular venous pulsations (JVP), displaced apical impulse, and a murmur of Tricuspid regurgitation. He also had tender hepatomegaly with a tipped spleen (3 cm below left costal margin). Musculoskeletal examination showed swollen tender right knee joint, palmar pallor, deeply dark patches on the lateral side of left foot, clubbing, and peripheral edema.

He was diagnosed with acute decompensated heart failure and severe multilobar pneumonia and was admitted to the intensive care unit and started on standard heart failure management and intravenous antibiotics. Chest radiography revealed homogenous opacity on the right hemichest. This is depicted in Figure 1. Echocardiography study showed an echogenic mobile focus attached to the anterior cusp of the tricuspid valve with moderate tricuspid regurgitation. The echocardiography result of the patient is depicted in Figure 2. Further laboratory investigations revealed leucocytosis with anemia (white cell count—32,200/μl and hemoglobin—5 gm/dl), erythrocyte sedimentation rate of 159 mm/hr, elevated blood urea nitrogen, and creatinine (190 mg/dl and 1.6 mg/dl subsequently). Urine analysis showed microscopic

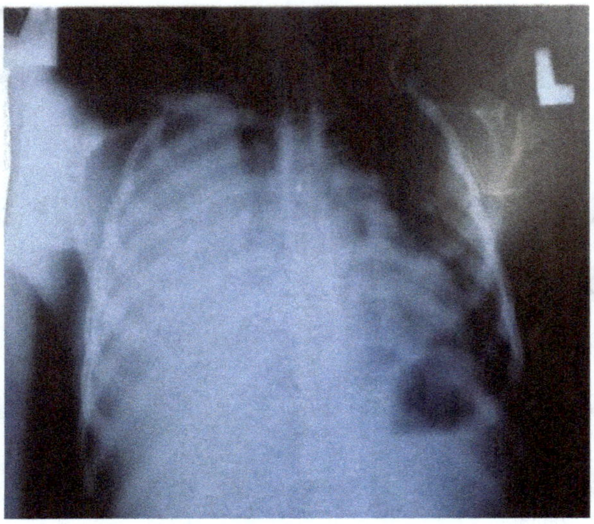

FIGURE 1: Chest roentgenography of the patient showing massive right pleural effusion.

hematuria. Rapid test for HIV infection was negative. Blood culture that was done after two doses of intravenous antibiotics showed no growth. Both pleural and joint fluid aspirate cultures showed growth of *Staphylococcus aureus* with sensitivity to several antibiotics including cloxacillin.

After the echocardiography evaluation, the patient's diagnosis was changed to tricuspid valve infective endocarditis with septic arthritis and septic pulmonary emboli. He was managed for acute heart failure and infective endocarditis with intravenous diuretics and intravenous antibiotics (ceftriaxone plus vancomycin which was later changed to cloxacillin after the antibiogram result). He also received supportive treatment with intranasal oxygen and blood transfusion. We did therapeutic pleurocentesis and arthrocentesis for him based on indications. After eight days of stay in the ICU, the patient's condition significantly improved with normalization of vital signs and improvement of cardiorespiratory status. The patient was discharged improved from the hospital in stable condition after a total of thirty days of intravenous antibiotics. The patient showed up on subsequent follow-up without any permanent cardiac sequel.

2. Discussion

Infective endocarditis (IE), first described in the mid-16th century, is a disease characterized by a high in-hospital mortality (17-30% mortality) [1–7]. IE is a microbial infection of the heart valves, intracardiac device, septal defects, mural endocardium, or rarely the subvalvular apparatus. Right-sided infective endocarditis (RSIE), IE of the tricuspid or pulmonic valve, is a rare entity accounting for 5-10% of all infective endocarditis cases. Most cases of RSIE (90%) involve the tricuspid valve [8–11]. The rarity of right-sided congenital heart diseases and rheumatic heart diseases coupled with the low pressure/low oxygen saturation on the right chambers of the heart is believed to be the reason for the lesser frequency of RSIE as compared to the left-side infective endocarditis [6, 11]. RSIE can be divided into three groups according to the underlying risk factors: intravenous drug users (IDUs), cardiac device carriers, and the "three noes" group (no left-sided IE, no IDUs, and no cardiac devices). Tricuspid valve endocarditis in nonintravenous drug users can occur in a variety of conditions including congenital heart disease, intracardiac devices, central venous catheters, and immunologically debilitated patients [5, 6, 9]. Intravenous drug use and the presence of cardiac devices (pacemakers, implantable automatic defibrillators, and central venous catheters) are the well-known risk factors for RSIE. Its occurrence in the absence of these risk factors and in otherwise normal heart is less understood. There are rare reports of RSIE following septic abortion, abscess, and septic arthritis. Globally, reports of tricuspid valve infective endocarditis (TVE) are growing because of the increasing frequency of intravenous drug use [5, 6].

Right-sided infective endocarditis usually presents with fever, persistent bacteremia, and septic emboli to the lungs. Initial presentation may comprise haemoptysis, cough, or chest pains which are related to septic emboli to the lungs. Pulmonary events occur in 80% of these cases and vary from minor atelectases to large infiltrates, pleural exudates, and cavitations. Septic shock, renal failure, and uncontrolled disseminated infection are common features of patients with RSIE without notable risk factors. Systemic emboli are rare manifestations of TVIE and, when noted, should be considered evidence of either left-sided involvement or paradoxical embolism. The peripheral stigmata of IE are not consistently present. Cardiac complications of TVE are much less common than those of left-sided endocarditis. The commonest cardiac complication of TVE is tricuspid regurgitation, the severity of which is a predictor of mortality besides vegetation size. Clinical suspicion of TVE should be raised in the presence of "tricuspid syndrome" characterized by recurrent pulmonary events, anemia, and microscopic hematuria [7, 9, 12].

Classically infective endocarditis is diagnosed using the modified Duke criteria, but the sensitivity and specificity of this criteria in right-sided endocarditis has not been studied; hence, a high index of suspicion is required for the diagnosis. A transesophageal echocardiography may be required in the detection of vegetations on the pulmonary valve and for the exclusion of left-sided valve involvement. The two most important diagnostic features of TVE are echocardiography evidence of vegetation and the presence of septic embolic phenomena. The vegetation of TVE is detected more commonly on the anterior leaflet of the valve and it is mostly large (>2 cm) due to low pressure, which enables the vegetation to grow large. Vegetation size correlates with mortality. TVE vegetations are highly mobile, which explains the higher rate of pulmonary embolic phenomenon associated with the entity [5–7, 10, 13].

Staphylococcus aureus is the commonest causative organism of isolated TVE followed by the *Candida* species, *Pseudomonas aeruginosa*, coagulase-negative *Staphylococcus*, *Corynebacterium* species, *Lactobacillus*, *Neisseria* species, and *Bacillus cereus* [9–11, 14, 15].

Medical therapy remains the mainstay of management for TVE. Intravenous antibiotics tailored to culture and

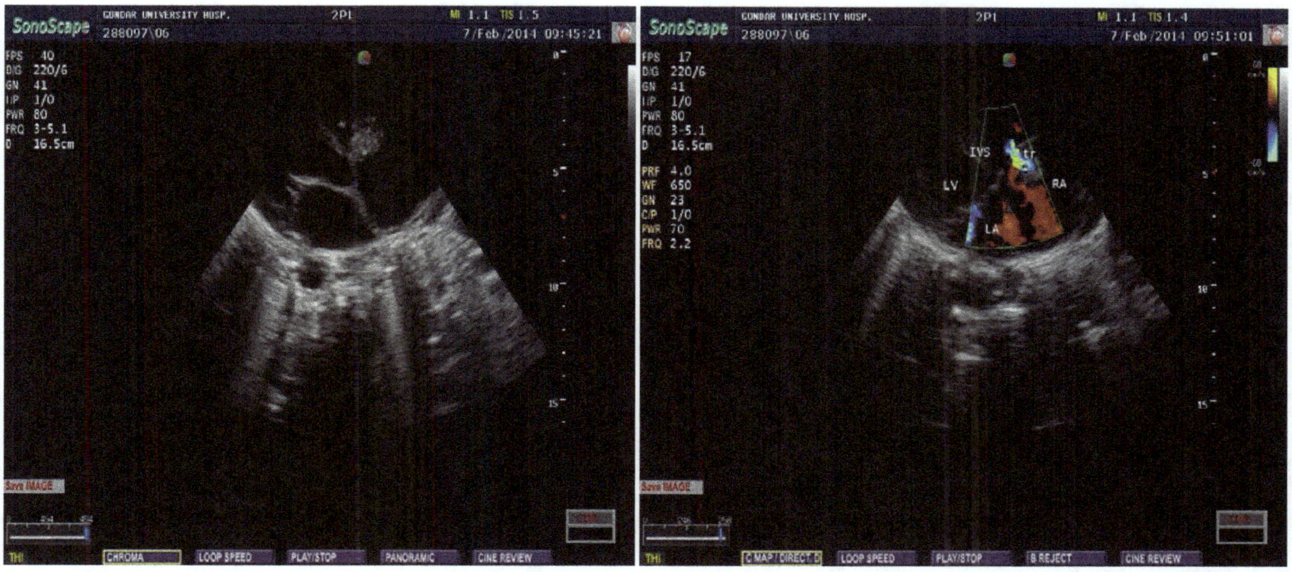

FIGURE 2: Doppler echocardiography showing an echogenic mobile focus (2.4 cm by 1.7 cm) attached to the anterior cusp of the valve (a) with moderate tricuspid regurgitation (b).

sensitivity results with initial coverage of presumed organism are the mainstay of treatment. *Staphylococcus aureus*, being the commonest cause, should always be covered with effective antibiotics. In IVDUs with underlying valve lesions and/or concomitant left-sided involvement, coverage for streptococci and enterococci should be included. The duration of antibiotics depends on the following factors: the type of organism identified, vegetation size, presence of metastatic infections, involvement of left-sided valves, involvement of prosthetic valves, and immune status of the host [7, 13].

Surgical treatment is needed in 5-16% of TVE, and it has to be considered in the following situations: (1) intractable right-sided heart failure with poor response to diuretics, (2) persistent bacteremia despite the use of appropriate antimicrobial therapy, (3) large vegetation (>20 mm) that does not diminish in size despite repeated embolism, (4) fungal endocarditis, (5) concomitant left-sided IE, and (7) prostatic valve endocarditis. Valvectomy, valve replacement, or repair are the common surgeries performed for tricuspid valve endocarditis [7, 10, 13].

As compared to left-sided endocarditis, generally, the prognosis of TVE is more favorable and many patients can be cured with medical treatment alone. Overall mortality for TVE is between 5 and 15%, but could be as high as 30% in those lacking the traditional risk factors (intravenous drug use and cardiac devices) [7, 9, 13].

3. Conclusion

The symptoms of TVE are similar to those of respiratory infection (fever, dyspnea, and pulmonary infiltration), making misdiagnosis likely. Hence, TVE should be included in the differential diagnosis of patients presenting with febrile syndrome and pulmonary manifestations even in the absence of IDUs or cardiac devices.

Consent

Informed consent was obtained from the case.

Authors' Contributions

All the authors have significant contribution to this case report.

References

[1] T. J. Cahill and B. D. Prendergast, "Infective Endocarditis," *The Lancet*, vol. 387, no. 10021, pp. 882–893, 2016.

[2] T. J. Cahill, L. M. Baddour, G. Habib et al., "Challenges in infective endocarditis," *Journal of the American College of Cardiology.*, vol. 69, no. 3, pp. 325–344, 2017.

[3] D. H. Kang, Y. J. Kim, S. H. Kim et al., "Early surgery versus conventional treatment for infective endocarditis," *New England Journal of Medicine*, vol. 366, no. 26, pp. 2466–2473, 2012.

[4] D. R. Murdoch, R. G. Corey, B. Hoen et al., "Clinical presentation, etiology, and outcome of infective endocarditis in the 21st century," *Archives of Internal Medicine*, vol. 169, no. 5, pp. 463–473, 2009.

[5] N. Raut, A. Potdar, and S. Sharma, "Tricuspid valve endocarditis in non-drug abusers: a case series from India," *Indian Heart Journal*, vol. 70, no. 4, pp. 476–481, 2018.

[6] H. Galal, O. Rifaei, M. Abdel Rahman, and H. El-Sayed, "Prevalence and characteristics of tricuspid valve endocarditis among patients presented to Ain Shams Hospital echocardiography lab; one year study," *The Egyptian Heart Journal*, vol. 70, no. 2, pp. 59–63, 2018.

[7] S. T. Hussain, J. Witten, N. K. Shrestha, E. H. Blackstone, and G. B. Pettersson, "Tricuspid valve endocarditis," *Annals of Cardiothoracic Surgery*, vol. 6, no. 3, pp. 255–261, 2017.

[8] K. Akinosoglou, E. Apostolakis, M. Marangos, and G. Pasvol, "Native valve right sided infective endocarditis," *European Journal of Internal Medicine*, vol. 24, no. 6, pp. 510–519, 2013.

[9] C. Ortiz, J. López, H. García et al., "Clinical classification and prognosis of isolated right-sided infective endocarditis," *Medicine*, vol. 93, no. 27, p. e137, 2014.

[10] R. Meel, "Right-sided infective endocarditis secondary to intravenous drug abuse," *Infective Endocarditis*, 2019.

[11] J. Swiston, S. D. Shafran, and N. Kassam, "Isolated native tricuspid valve endocarditis caused by viridans streptococcus," *Canadian Journal of Infectious Diseases*, vol. 12, no. 5, pp. 305–307, 2001.

[12] A. A. Heydari, H. Safari, and M. R. Sarvghad, "Isolated tricuspid valve endocarditis," *International Journal of Infectious Diseases*, vol. 13, no. 3, pp. e109–e111, 2009.

[13] A. Revilla, J. López, E. Villacorta et al., "Isolated right-sided valvular endocarditis in non-intravenous drug users," *Revista Española de Cardiología (English Edition)*, vol. 61, no. 12, pp. 1253–1259, 2008.

[14] S. M. Yuan, "Right-sided infective endocarditis: recent epidemiologic changes," *International Journal of Clinical and Experimental Medicine*, vol. 7, no. 1, pp. 199–218, 2014.

[15] D. P. Naidoo, "Right-sided endocarditis in the non-drug addict," *Postgraduate Medical Journal*, vol. 69, no. 814, pp. 615–620, 1993.

23

Successful Removal of a Posterior Cardiac Lipoma by Transection of the Ascending Aorta and Main Pulmonary Artery

Saeki Watanabe, Yuki Ichihara, Kozo Morita, Satoshi Saito, and Hiroshi Niinami

Tokyo Women's Medical University, Department of Cardiovascular Surgery, Kawada-cho 8-1, Shinjuku-ku, Tokyo, Japan

Correspondence should be addressed to Saeki Watanabe; s12-112ws@nms.ac.jp

Academic Editor: Takatoshi Kasai

Primary cardiac tumors are unusual, whereas lipomas are particularly rare. We successfully removed a very large posterior cardiac lipoma by transecting the ascending aorta and main pulmonary artery. Transecting both the ascending aorta and the main pulmonary artery facilitated surgical exposure and complete removal of the posterior cardiac lipoma.

1. Introduction

Primary cardiac tumors are highly unusual, and lipoma accounts for only 8.4% of these already rare tumor cases, making its occurrence extremely rare [1]. In the present case, a posterior cardiac lipoma extending into the left atrium was successfully removed by transecting the ascending aorta and main pulmonary artery, which enabled good surgical exposure and complete resection of the posterior cardiac lipoma.

2. Case Presentation

A 51-year-old woman presented with an abnormal electrocardiogram (ECG). The ECG showed abnormal Q waves. Further, transthoracic echocardiography revealed a substantial mass lesion on the posterior surface of the heart, and the patient was referred to our department for additional examinations.

She had no specific medical history, and blood tests showed no other abnormalities, including tumor-related parameters. ECG findings revealed a normal sinus rhythm with a heart rate of 69 bpm, no axis deviation, but abnormal Q waves at V1-V3. Transthoracic echocardiography showed a hyperechoic area sized 51 × 11 mm extending from the left atrium to the posterior wall of the left ventricle. Thoracoabdominal enhanced computed tomography (CT) revealed a homogeneous, large fatty mass extending from the posterior border of the main pulmonary artery to the dorsal left atrium, ascending aorta, and superior vena cava, which was penetrated by the bilateral pulmonary arteries (Figure 1). Magnetic resonance imaging (MRI) revealed that the mass showed high signal intensity on T1-weighted imaging (Figure 2), while it was suppressed on fat-suppressed imaging and showed low signal intensity. Coronary angiography revealed no significant stenosis of the coronary arteries and no obvious feeding vessels to the tumor. Since malignancy could not be completely ruled out and since the tumor was large enough to have the potential to compress the heart, we decided to resect the tumor completely.

The median sternotomy approach was used. The tumor was found to protrude into the left pericardial sac, extending from the dorsal surface of the superior vena cava, ascending aorta, and main pulmonary artery to the dorsal surface of the left atrium and left atrial appendage and was covered with a capsule. Total resection of the tumor by dissection of the ascending aorta and main pulmonary artery under cardiac arrest was decided. Cardiopulmonary bypass from the right femoral artery with removal from the bilateral vena cava was initiated. After the ascending aorta was cross-clamped, the ascending aorta was transected to remove the tumor from the posterior surface of the heart, and the portion on the back of the ascending aorta was dissected. Subse-

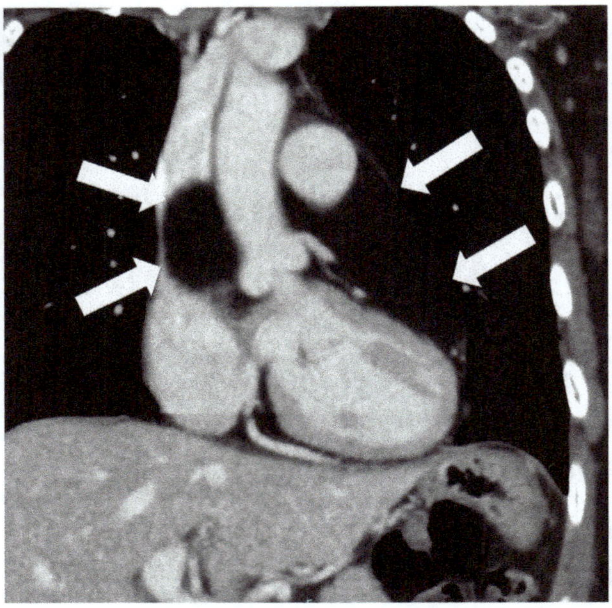

FIGURE 1: Preoperative enhanced computed tomography image. A mass on the posterior surface of the ascending aorta and main pulmonary artery is shown.

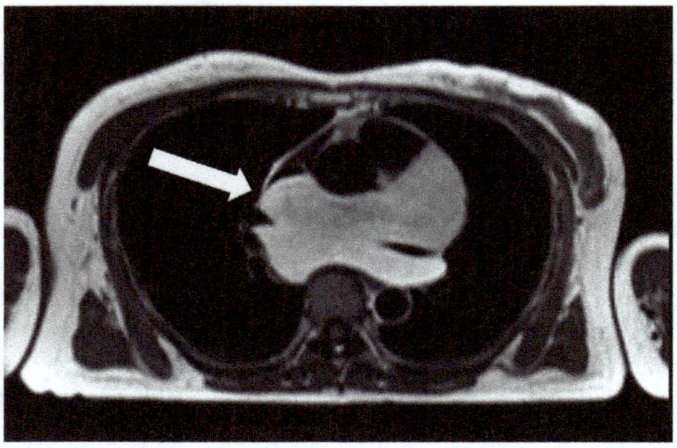

FIGURE 2: Preoperative magnetic resonance imaging findings. Arrows indicate mass.

quently, when the main pulmonary artery was transected and the heart was removed, good exposure was obtained, and the tumor was found to be widespread on the posterior surface of the heart (Figure 3). Dissection was performed from the left atrial ceiling to the transverse pericardial sinus, and the tumor was removed as a single mass. The size was 12.5 × 7 × 4 cm (Figure 4), and an intraoperative rapid diagnosis showed no malignant component. The operation time was 294 min, with an extracorporeal circulation time of 126 min and an aortic cross-clamp time of 59 min.

Pathological findings included hyperplasia of mature adipocytes, with no hyperplasia of lipoblasts showing atypia, thus indicating a lipoma (Figure 5).

The patient was extubated on the same day as the surgery, the postoperative course was uneventful, and she was discharged from the hospital on day 12. The postoperative pathological diagnosis was lipoma.

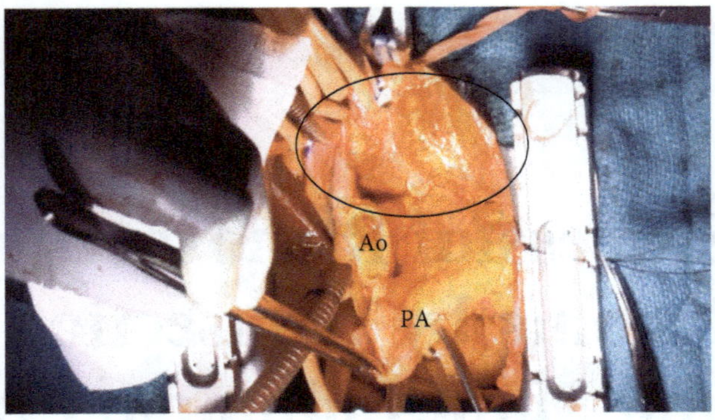

FIGURE 3: Operative image. The ascending aorta and main pulmonary artery were transected, and a mass was found on the posterior surface of the heart.

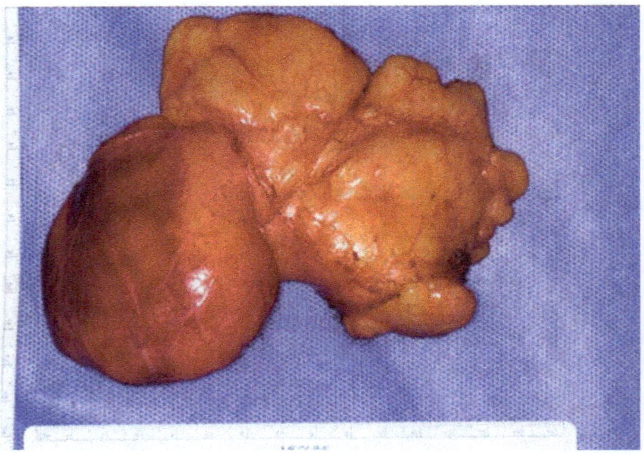

FIGURE 4: Image of the extracted mass.

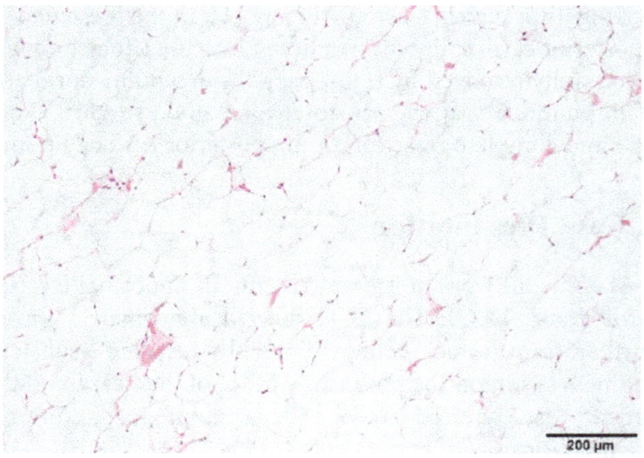

FIGURE 5: Pathological findings. The tumor was formed by hyperplasia of mature adipocytes.

3. Discussion

Primary cardiac tumors are rare, with an overall prevalence of 0.17% to 0.19% [2]. Approximately 75% of these tumors are benign, while lipoma accounts for approximately 8.4% of the cases [1]. Most lipomas are asymptomatic and often found incidentally, although depending on the site of origin, they may be symptomatic [3].

Although there were no clinical symptoms in the present case, it was decided to intervene surgically because of ECG abnormalities, a possibility of future arrhythmia, a high possibility of clinical symptoms due to its extensive presence on the posterior surface of the heart, previous reports of sudden death due to a lipoma [4], an inability to obtain a biopsy specimen from the tumor on the posterior surface of the heart, and the possibility of liposarcoma that could not be completely ruled out. Since lipomas are benign and the risk of recurrence is reported to be low [3], partial resection may be chosen if the risk of complications from tumor resection outweighs the risk of recurrence [5]. However, there are also reports of residual symptoms due to a remaining tumor and recurrence of a liposarcoma following partial resection [6], thus making complete resection desirable.

In the present case, a widespread tumor had developed on the posterior surface of the heart, and there was a concern that it might compress the organ and cause heart failure symptoms in the future. MRI findings with high signal intensity on T1- and T2-weighted images and low signal intensity on fat-suppressed images suggested the diagnosis of benign lipoma [7], while the possibility of liposarcoma could not be completely ruled out. In addition, considering that the patient was 51 years old and in an otherwise good condition, complete resection was the goal.

As mentioned earlier, the tumor was extensively widespread and was considered difficult to remove with complete resection using minimally invasive surgery. Li and Gao reported 60 (26.3%) robot-assisted tumor resections and 12 (5.3%) small right anterior lateral thoracotomy resections of primary cardiac tumors [8]; however, the minimally invasive approach was not suitable for this case because of tumor size and morphological extension. The tumor extended from the posterior margin of the superior vena cava, ascending aorta, and main pulmonary artery to the dorsal side of the left atrium, and a good surgical exposure was obtained only by transecting the ascending aorta and main pulmonary artery, thus making it possible to perform a complete resection. The ascending aorta and the main pulmonary arteries were reconstructed without any complications.

The methods used for resection in the present case are rarely employed. No residual tumor was found after the operation, and two years later, there was no recurrence.

In conclusion, complete resection of a widespread lipoma on the posterior surface of the heart was successfully performed by transecting the ascending aorta and main pulmonary artery, followed by tumor removal.

Consent

The patient has provided permission to publish the case details, and their identity has been protected.

References

[1] N. Ozaki, N. Mukohara, M. Yoshida, and T. Shida, "Cardiac lipoma in the interventricular septum–a case report," *The Thoracic and Cardiovascular Surgeon*, vol. 54, no. 5, pp. 356-357, 2006.

[2] W. Shengjun, P. Teng, Y. Zhou, and Y. Ni, "A rare case report of giant epicardial lipoma compressing the right atrium with septal enhancement," *Journal of Cardiothoracic Surgery*, vol. 10, no. 1, pp. 1–3, 2015.

[3] C. M. Steger, "Intrapericardial giant lipoma displacing the heart," *International Scholarly Research Notices*, vol. 2011, Article ID 243637, 4 pages, 2011.

[4] K. Ashar and K. H. van Hoeven, "Fatal lipoma of the heart," *The American Journal of Cardiovascular Pathology*, vol. 4, no. 1, pp. 85–90, 1992.

[5] J. D'Souza, R. Shah, A. Abbass, J. R. Burt, A. Goud, and C. Dahagam, "Invasive cardiac lipoma: a case report and review of literature," *BMC Cardiovascular Disorders*, vol. 17, no. 1, pp. 1–4, 2017.

[6] K. Shibata, Y. Koga, T. Onitsuka et al., "Primary liposarcoma of the mediastinum–a case report and review of the literature," *The Japanese Journal of Surgery*, vol. 16, no. 4, pp. 277–283, 1986.

[7] S. Domoto, K. Nakano, K. Kodera et al., "Cardiac lipoma originating from the left ventricular apex diagnosed using the magnetic resonance imaging fat suppression technique: report of a case," *Surgery Today*, vol. 40, no. 9, pp. 871–873, 2010.

[8] S. Li and C. Gao, "Surgical experience of primary cardiac tumor: single-institution 23-year report," *Medical Science Monitor*, vol. 23, pp. 2111–2117, 2017.

24

ST-Elevation Myocardial Infarction (STEMI) in a Patient with Moyamoya Disease

James Livesay and Jeffrey Johnson

Department of Medicine, University of Tennessee Graduate School of Medicine, Knoxville, TN, USA

Correspondence should be addressed to Jeffrey Johnson; jhjohnso@utmck.edu

Academic Editor: Man-Hong Jim

Moyamoya disease is a rare condition that is primarily reported in Asian populations, characterized by stenoocclusive intracranial angiopathy with small, fragile, and multiple collateral vessel formation. Extracranial complications, mainly abnormalities within the renal vasculature, have been described; however, there are very few case reports of cardiovascular complications in patients with Moyamoya disease. We report a 26-year-old Caucasian female with known Moyamoya disease who presented with both typical and atypical chest pain, mimicking symptoms of a previous non-ST-elevation myocardial infarction. Approximately six months prior to the current hospital admission, she underwent coronary angiography requiring percutaneous coronary intervention (PCI) with two drug-eluting stents to the right coronary artery (RCA) for a critical stenosis. Despite medical management, our patient developed inferior lead ST-elevations leading to a repeat left heart catheterization which showed clinically significant stenosis of the first obtuse marginal branch. Development of significant coronary artery stenosis in a short period of time demonstrates the clinical significance of minimal atherosclerosis in the setting of underlying fibrocellular thickening as seen in patients with Moyamoya disease. Clinicians need to be aware of the possibility of coronary involvement in addition to intracranial vascular complications in patients with Moyamoya disease and take appropriate measures to prevent or delay the development of atherosclerosis in these arteries.

1. Introduction

Moyamoya disease is a rare condition, primarily reported in Japanese and other Asian populations, best described by stenoocclusive changes in the internal carotid arteries and developed collateral vasculature [1]. These patients typically present at a young age with intracranial features such as ischemic or hemorrhagic strokes, and the occurrence of extracranial vascular dysfunction is exceptionally rare [2]. Reports of extracranial dysfunction in a patient with Moyamoya disease have mostly involved the renal vasculature leading to chronic kidney disease, while coronary artery involvement is extremely uncommon. The pathology of Moyamoya disease involves fibrocellular thickening of the vessel wall, and in this patient population, even minimal atherosclerosis can rapidly lead to significant stenosis of the coronary arteries [2]. Our patient, with known Moyamoya disease, presented with recurrent chest pain and stenosis in several coronary arteries that was successfully treated with multiple drug-eluting stents.

2. Case Presentation

A 26-year-old Caucasian female with known Moyamoya disease presented with a chief complaint of right-sided chest pain and numbness radiating to her right arm mimicking symptoms of a previous non-ST-elevation myocardial infarction.

Six months prior, the patient underwent coronary angiography remarkable for a critical lesion of the right distal coronary artery (Figure 1). At that time, she underwent successful percutaneous intervention with two drug-eluting stents to the distal right coronary artery (Figure 2). She had multiple other comorbidities including coronary artery disease, restrictive cardiomyopathy, hyperlipidemia, chronic kidney disease stage IV, anemia of chronic disease, recurrent pneumonia, immunoglobulin deficiency, osteoporosis, and

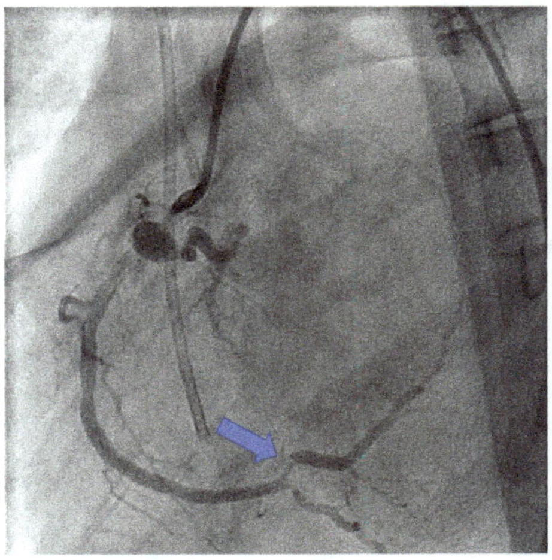

FIGURE 1: Previous critical RCA stenosis before stent placement.

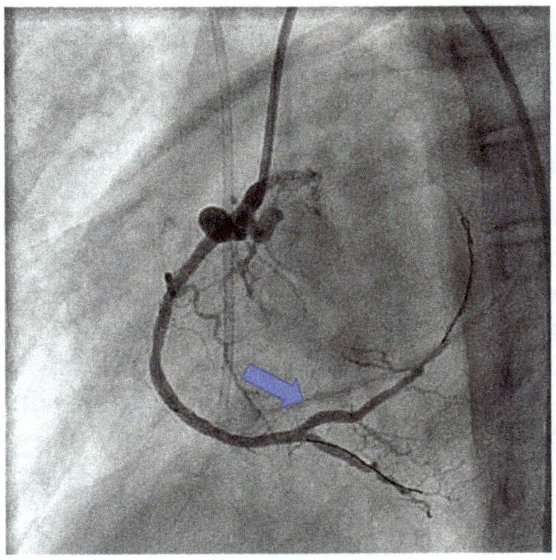

FIGURE 2: Previous critical RCA stenosis after stent placement.

history of cerebral vascular disease. In the months leading up to this admission, she suffered multiple noncardiac complications including symptomatic anemia, pneumonia with hemoptysis, and lower extremity ulcerations. She closely followed with hematology requiring Procrit for hemoglobin levels less than 7.0 g/dL with notable improvement in fatigue and weakness. She was also referred to dermatology for suspicious lower extremity lesions that were biopsied and felt to be autoimmune with intentions on starting IVIG.

Upon this admission, her initial troponin was 0.12 ng/mL which continued to rise to a maximum of 0.79 ng/mL over the first 24 hours; however, no specific EKG changes were noted. Given her rising troponin, presenting symptoms, and recently diagnosed coronary artery disease, she was started on guideline-directed medical therapy for acute coronary syndrome including heparin and beta blockade with as needed nitroglycerin, which provided significant improvement in symptoms. Due to the initial resolution of symptoms with medical management and associated high-morbidity conditions, we deferred left heart catheterization. Other

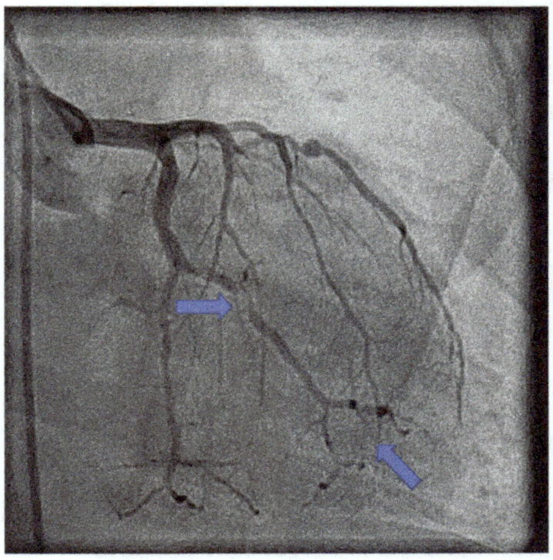

FIGURE 3: Stenosis of the obtuse marginal branch before stent placement. Distal obtuse marginal shows a string of bead appearance.

significant initial labs included a 62 mg/dL BUN, 4.52 mg/dL creatinine, 23.0 mEq/L anion gap, 9.4 g/dL hemoglobin, 29.6% hematocrit, 18.2 white blood cell count, and 394 platelet count. A bedside echocardiogram was preformed revealing a normal left ventricular size with moderately reduced function with an LVEF of 40-45% along with mild global hypokinesis.

Over the subsequent 72 hours, she continued to have intermittent angina and her cardiac biomarkers began to climb, but serial EKGs did not display any signs of ST-segment changes. During this time, we obtained daily complete blood cell counts revealing a declining hemoglobin, and over time, a fall in her blood pressure was noted. Ultimately, we made a diagnosis of a type II non-ST-elevation myocardial infarction, believed to be secondary to demand ischemia. Therefore, we began blood transfusions to maintain a hemoglobin greater than 8.0 g/dL providing a resolution of anginal type symptoms.

Despite continued medical management and improvement in her hemoglobin level, our patient again developed persistent recurrent angina. On hospital day nine, she developed angina not relieved by nitroglycerin, and a repeat EKG revealed inferior lead ST-elevations consistent with acute ST-elevation myocardial infarction. She underwent left heart catheterization remarkable for 90% stenosis of the first obtuse marginal branch (Figure 3), which was revascularized with a third drug-eluting stent (Figure 4). Diagnostic catheterization also revealed new 40-50% restenosis of her previous distal RCA stent (Figure 5) and noncritical stenosis of the first diagonal branch (Figure 6).

During this prolonged hospitalization, our patient suffered further complications including superficial femoral artery ischemia requiring intervention, acute on chronic renal failure, and sepsis secondary to pneumonia. Due to her worsening overall condition and multiple comorbidities, our patient elected to go home with hospice and ultimately passed away.

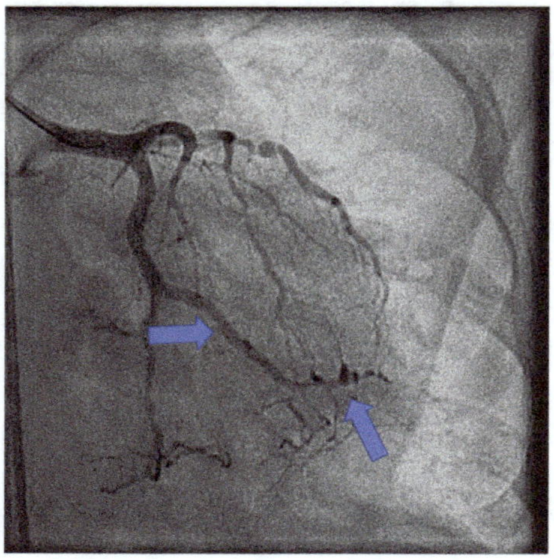

FIGURE 4: Stenosis of the obtuse marginal branch after stent placement. Distal obtuse marginal shows a string of bead appearance.

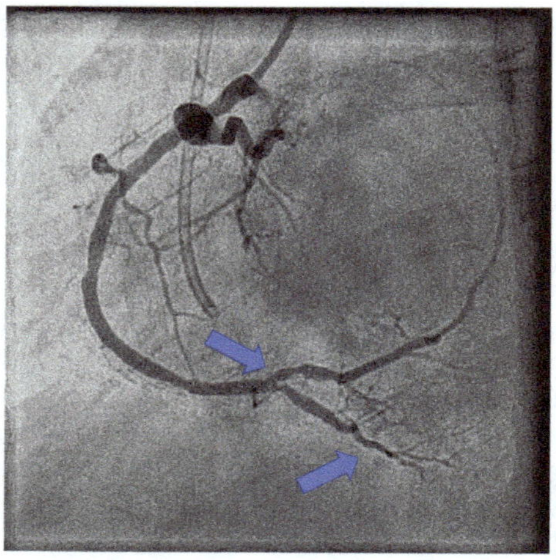

FIGURE 5: Restenosis of a previously placed RCA stent. Distal RCA shows a string of bead appearance.

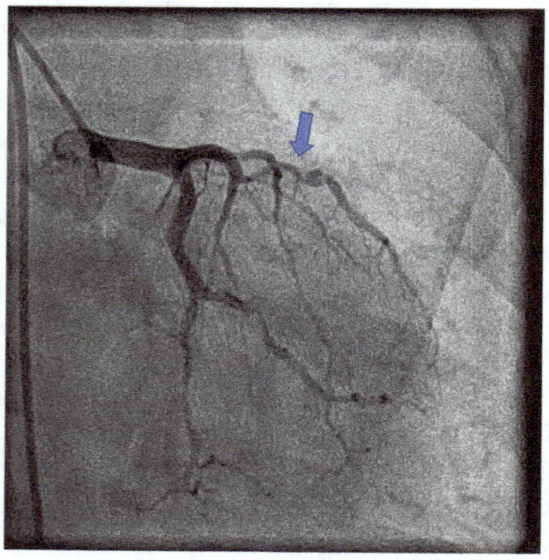

FIGURE 6: Stenosis of the first diagonal branch demonstrating multivessel involvement.

3. Discussion

Moyamoya disease is a rare disease that occurs in the Asian population, most often clinically manifested as an ischemic or hemorrhagic stroke at a young age. Cases of coronary artery disease secondary to Moyamoya disease are exceedingly rare with one article noting only 12 documented cases [3].

Choi and colleagues describe a patient with known Moyamoya disease that presented with recurrent chest pain aggravated by stress and relieved by nitroglycerin. This patient was diagnosed with variant angina after receiving two doses of ergonovine revealing 95% stenosis of the proximal LAD along with fibrous plaque occupying 33% of the coronary lumen [2]. A case reported by Komiyama and colleagues demonstrates a 56-year-old female that presented with angina with secondary to clinically significant LAD disease treated initially with balloon angioplasty followed by CABG several months later for restenosis [4].

Fibrocellular thickening of the intima and proliferative smooth muscle cell growth are the primary causes of arterial occlusion in Moyamoya disease. Nam and colleagues performed a retrospective study and postulated that symptomatic coronary heart disease is most likely the result of small atherosclerosis due to underlying endothelial proliferation [1]. Another study used intravascular ultrasound (IVUS) and virtual histology (VH) to evaluate a critical proximal LAD lesion in a 20-year-old Korean male with known Moyamoya disease. IVUS and VH revealed a homogenous, eccentric, echogenic intimal thickening composed of fibrous tissue with no mid or distal intimal thickening. Stenotic lesions seen in individuals with Moyamoya disease are distinctly different when compared to lesions seen in patients with CAD from atherosclerosis as there is minimal lipid pooling and no calcium deposition [5].

Our patient's coronary angiography showed several areas where the vessel resembles a string of beads, which is best seen in the distal OM branch and distal RCA (Figures 3, 4, and 5). The string of bead appearance has been previously described in other vessels such as the peripheral pulmonary, renal, and carotid arteries as a direct result of intimal thickening [6]. This distinct pattern helps clinicians distinguish CAD in Moyamoya disease from CAD in the setting of atherosclerosis using coronary angiography.

A recent study, using genetic analysis, found an association with homozygosity for *RNF213* p.Arg4810Lys and multiple extracranial vasculopathies. The p.Arg4810Lys variant, commonly found in the Eastern Asian population, is thought to cause the classic intracranial vasculopathy when in the heterozygous state. However, individuals that possess the homozygous variant seem to develop systemic vasculopathy and more severe symptoms [6]. The link between the RNF variant, p.Arg4810Lys, and Moyamoya disease has potential to be a screening tool for the risk of systemic disease and disease severity.

To the best of our knowledge, there are no other documented cases of coronary artery disease in a Caucasian female with Moyamoya disease. In this case, we were able to carefully track our patient's CAD progression from the time of her original NSTEMI, secondary to a critical RCA lesion, to her STEMI only six months later. Repeat coronary angiography revealed an unexpected critical lesion in a completely different vessel, the first distal obtuse marginal artery, along with mild RCA restenosis.

Regarding our patient's disease progression, she was originally diagnosed with Moyamoya disease at a young age after a typical presentation of a cerebral vascular accident requiring coiling by interventional radiology. Her disease continued to advance to include chronic renal failure, peripheral vascular disease, and finally coronary artery disease. As demonstrated from previous studies, even minimal atherosclerosis can lead to critical vascular lesions in a Moyamoya patient [1]. Therefore, we believe patients with the diagnosis of Moyamoya disease, especially with any extracranial features, should be counseled on their risk of heart disease. Clinicians following patients with Moyamoya disease should consider aggressive medical management to prevent plaque progression as minimal atherosclerosis can drastically increase this patient population's morbidity and mortality.

4. Conclusion

Extracranial vascular complications in patients with Moyamoya disease are rare but can have a significant impact on a patient's overall morbidity and mortality. Our patient was initially diagnosed with Moyamoya disease after presenting with cerebral vasculature complications and went on to develop multiple extracranial complications ultimately leading to death. Clinicians should be aware of the cardiovascular complications seen in Moyamoya patients and assess for the potential benefit of aggressive medical management in preventing coronary plaque progression. It is crucial that these patients are counseled on their risk of ischemic heart disease and informed about the optimal timing for cardiovascular medical evaluation.

References

[1] T. M. Nam, K. I. Jo, J. Y. Yeon, S. C. Hong, and J. S. Kim, "Coronary heart disease in Moyamoya disease: are they concomitant or coincidence?," *Journal of Korean Medical Science*, vol. 30, no. 4, pp. 470–474, 2015.

[2] W. Choi, Y. N. Kim, and K. H. Kim, "Variant angina in Moyamoya disease–a correlative etiology and different presentation: a case report," *Journal of Medical Case Reports*, vol. 9, no. 1, p. 86, 2015.

[3] M. Komiyama, M. Nishikawa, T. Yasui, M. Otsuka, and K. Haze, "Moyamoya disease and coronary artery disease -case report," *Neurologia Medico-Chirurgica*, vol. 41, no. 1, pp. 37–41, 2001.

[4] M. Komiyama, T. Ishikawa, S. Takanashi, and Y. Shimizu, "Minimal invasive direct coronary artery bypass in Moyamoya disease," *Interactive Cardiovascular and Thoracic Surgery*, vol. 2, no. 1, pp. 65 67, 2003.

[5] J. H. Lee, T. J. Youn, Y. E. Yoon et al., "Coronary artery stenosis in Moyamoya disease: tissue characterization by 256-slice multi-detector CT and virtual histology," *Circulation*, vol. 127, no. 20, pp. 2063–2065, 2013.

[6] S. A. Chang, J. S. Song, T. K. Park et al., "Nonsyndromic peripheral pulmonary artery stenosis is associated with homozygosity of RNF213 p.Arg4810Lys regardless of co-occurrence of Moyamoya Disease," *Chest*, vol. 153, no. 2, pp. 404–413, 2018.

Chest Pain in a Psychiatric Patient Due to Clozapine-Induced Myopericarditis

James L. Laws,[1] Esther Kim,[2] Rebecca Hung,[2] JoAnn Lindenfeld,[2] and Richa Gupta[3]

[1]*Department of Internal Medicine, Vanderbilt University Medical Center, Nashville, Tennessee, USA*
[2]*Department of Cardiovascular Medicine, Vanderbilt University Medical Center, Nashville, Tennessee, USA*
[3]*Department of Cardiovascular Medicine, MedStar Washington Hospital Center, Washington, DC, USA*

Correspondence should be addressed to Richa Gupta; richa.gupta@medstar.net

Academic Editor: Assad Movahed

Drug-induced myocarditis is a rare, but underrecognized complication of clozapine therapy for schizophrenia. We present a case of clozapine-induced myocarditis with recovery of cardiac function after drug cessation and summarize the literature to highlight the variable presentation of this condition.

1. Case Presentation

A 29-year-old man presented from a psychiatric hospital with 2 days of sudden onset, progressive chest pain, and troponin elevation after recently initiating clozapine therapy.

The patient had a history of alcohol abuse and treatment-resistant schizoaffective disorder with multiple suicide attempts. After intentional ingestion of acetaminophen and lithium, he was involuntarily hospitalized for intensive treatment, including initiation of clozapine therapy.

The differential diagnosis included acute coronary syndrome, myopericarditis from viral or drug-induced etiology, pulmonary embolism, and pneumonia. The patient first noted substernal chest pain worse with deep inspiration 8 days after clozapine initiation. Symptoms worsened over the following two days. Electrocardiogram (EKG) demonstrated ST elevations most prominent in V2-V3 (Figure 1). Serum labs were notable for leukocytosis and elevated troponin, brain natriuretic peptide, and inflammatory markers (Table 1).

Chest pain persisted, and he was transferred to the cardiology service. Cardiovascular exam was notable for tachycardia without murmurs or rubs. He had no peripheral edema or elevated jugular venous pressure. Lungs were clear. Cardiac magnetic resonance (CMR) imaging showed global hypokinesis with a left ventricular (LV) ejection fraction (EF) of 45% (Figure S1) and subtle late gadolinium enhancement of the epicardial lateral wall and lateral pericardium with abnormal parametric mapping (Figure 2) consistent with myopericarditis. Respiratory viral panel was negative. Clozapine was discontinued. Metoprolol was initiated for impaired LV function with colchicine and ibuprofen for pericarditis with prompt symptomatic relief. Repeat EKG showed resolution of ST-elevation and no arrhythmic events on telemetry. He was discharged back to the psychiatric hospital with planned cardiology follow-up for echocardiogram and repeat laboratory testing.

2. Discussion

Myocarditis was suspected based on a clinical syndrome of chest pain and elevated troponin in the setting of a known causative medication and low pretest probability for coronary artery disease. CMR confirmed the diagnosis by the updated Lake Louise Criteria [1]. This case meets the ESC definition of myocarditis, as a clinical syndrome supported by laboratory and imaging findings [2]. Endomyocardial biopsy (EMB), long considered the gold standard for diagnosis, is not indicated unless histology would alter treatment as with certain fulminant subtypes like giant cell myocarditis.

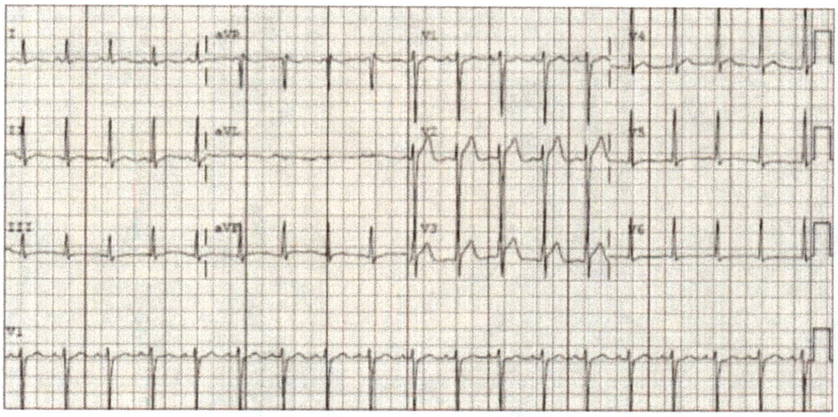

(a)

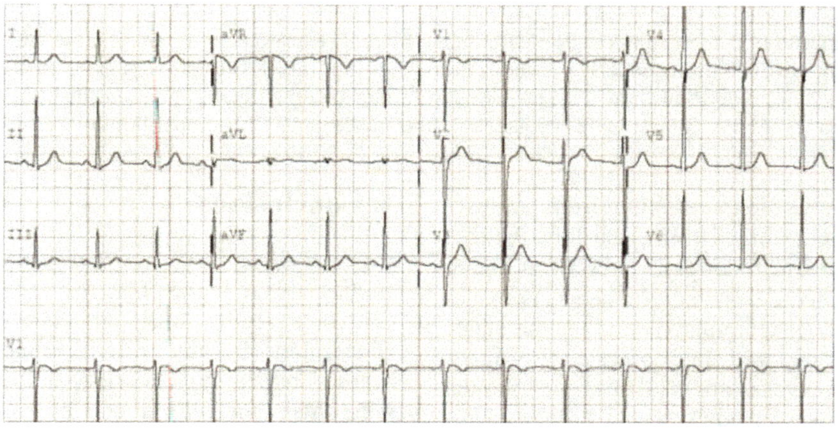

(b)

Figure 1: Electrocardiogram on presentation (a) showed sinus tachycardia (heart rate 111 beats per minute), ST elevations most prominent in leads V2-V3 with inferolateral T wave flattening. Baseline EKG (b) showing less prominent ST elevations in V2-V3 consistent with early repolarization without inferolateral T wave flattening.

Table 1: Lab values at presentation to emergency department and at 7-day follow-up appointment.

(a)

Lab	At presentation	7 d follow-up
White blood cell count (cells/μL)	14.9	—
Absolute eosinophils (cells/μL)	0.06	—
C-reactive protein (μg/mL)	173.0	5.1
Erythrocyte sedimentation rate (mm/hr)	64	5
Brain natriuretic peptide (pg/mL)	311	33

(b)

	Presentation	4 h	Discharge (2 d)
Troponin-I (ng/mL, normal<0.03)	0.49	0.37	0.05

Clozapine-induced myocarditis (CIM) is a drug-related myocarditis with variable presentation ranging from mild symptoms to fulminant myocarditis. The mechanism of toxicity to cardiomyocytes is unclear. In animal models, clozapine induces serum catecholamine excess that causes cardiac inflammation and myocyte apoptosis through tumor necrosis factor-alpha-mediated pathways [3]. At autopsy, histologic specimens from CIM patients have shown either lymphocytic infiltrate resulting from cytotoxic-mediated inflammation or eosinophilic infiltrate consistent with a hypersensitivity myocarditis, suggesting multiple mechanisms of injury [4].

The true incidence of CIM is difficult to ascertain due to underdiagnosis of subclinical or mild presentations and may be underrecognized; thus, a high index of suspicion is required [5]. Shortness of breath and tachycardia (67% and 58%, respectively) are the most common symptoms, though nonspecific [6]. In one cohort, 13% of patients ultimately diagnosed with CIM had normal cardiac biomarkers. Ronaldson and colleagues proposed a monitoring program based on review of suspected cases using serial troponin and C-reactive protein measurements over a 4-week initiation period [7]. No prospectively validated algorithms exist, however, and monitoring practices vary by institution. While some patients may present with a classic syndrome of myocarditis prompting additional evaluation, sudden cardiac death may be the initial presentation, highlighting the importance of monitoring [8].

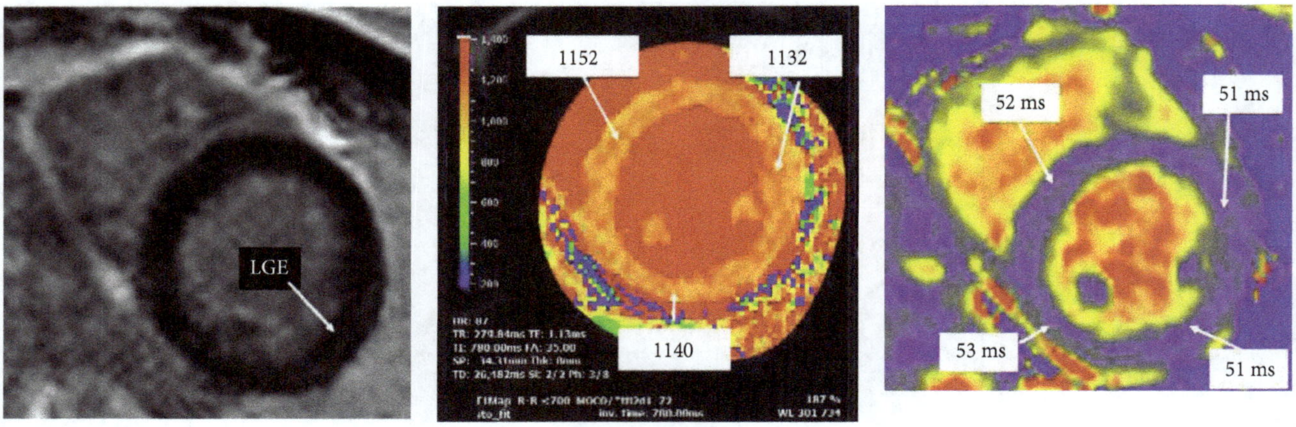

(a) (b) (c)

FIGURE 2: Tissue characterization on presenting cardiac MRI. Subtle stripe of epicardial LGE noted in the lateral wall (a). The native T1 relaxation time is diffusely elevated throughout the myocardium (ULN for this 1.5 Tesla magnet is 1010 ms), suggestive of diffuse inflammation (b). The native T2 relaxation time is mildly elevated throughout the myocardium and highest in the inferior wall (ULN: 50 ms), suggestive of edema (c). Abbreviations: LGE: late gadolinium enhancement; ULN: upper limit of normal.

Cardiovascular complications resulting from antipsychotic medications are not limited to myocarditis. Patients with schizophrenia treated with antipsychotics are at higher risk of sudden unexplained death than the general population [8]. Cardiovascular, pulmonary, and hematologic causes have been implicated with high prevalence of myocardial infarction (53%), myocarditis (6%), and a substantial proportion remaining unexplained (12%) [9]. Early recognition of angina and myocardial injury should prompt further evaluation and intervention crucial to preventing sudden cardiac death.

When CIM is suspected, cardiology consultation should be obtained with inpatient monitoring for arrhythmia and heart failure. Aside from drug withdrawal, no specific treatment for CIM has been identified. Patients with LV systolic dysfunction warrant guideline-directed medical therapy (GDMT) in the absence of contraindications. Close cardiology follow-up and repeat echocardiography after clozapine cessation and initiation of GDMT should be individualized.

Intriguingly, published literature reports cases of clozapine reinitiation in patients with severe schizophrenia refractory to alternate antipsychotics despite prior drug withdrawal due to CIM. Rechallenge with clozapine can be successfully achieved with intensive monitoring with swift discontinuation of the drug for any sign of myocardial injury [10]. In one case, serial CMR was used to monitor for disease recurrence and allowed the patient to safely remain on clozapine therapy [11]. Thus, individualized shared decision-making between patient, cardiology, and psychiatry is the key to optimize both cardiac and psychiatric outcome for these patients.

3. Follow-Up

The patient was not reinitiated on clozapine and instead was treated with lithium and electroconvulsive therapy. Repeat echocardiography 2 weeks later demonstrated recovery of LV function (Figure S2).

4. Conclusions

Patients with schizoaffective disorders treated with antipsychotics are at higher risk for sudden unexplained death. CIM is a rare but likely an underrecognized complication of clozapine therapy and a mechanism of sudden cardiac death. Treating psychiatrists and consulting cardiologists must maintain high index of suspicion for CIM with withdrawal of clozapine in the acute setting to reduce poor outcomes. In the long term, care must be patient-centered with consideration of underlying psychiatric and cardiovascular disease severity.

5. Learning Objectives

(i) To recognize the clinical presentation of drug-induced myocarditis, associated with the use of clozapine

(ii) To illustrate the role of noninvasive testing in diagnosis of clozapine-induced myocarditis

(iii) To understand the importance of a multidisciplinary approach involving both psychiatry and cardiology specialists in managing clozapine-induced myocarditis

References

[1] V. M. Ferreira, J. Schulz-Menger, G. Holmvang et al., "Cardiovascular magnetic resonance in nonischemic myocardial inflammation: expert recommendations," *Journal of the American College of Cardiology*, vol. 72, no. 24, pp. 3158–3176, 2018.

[2] A. L. P. Caforio, S. Pankuweit, E. Arbustini et al., "Current state of knowledge on aetiology, diagnosis, management, and therapy of myocarditis: a position statement of the European Society of Cardiology Working Group on Myocardial and

Pericardial Diseases," *European Heart Journal*, vol. 34, no. 33, pp. 2636–2648, 2013.

[3] J.-F. Wang, J.-Y. Min, T. G. Hampton et al., "Clozapine-induced myocarditis: role of catecholamines in a murine model," *European Journal of Pharmacology*, vol. 592, no. 1–3, pp. 123–127, 2008.

[4] J. G. Kilian, K. Kerr, C. Lawrence, and D. S. Celermajer, "Myocarditis and cardiomyopathy associated with clozapine," *The Lancet*, vol. 354, no. 9193, pp. 1841–1845, 1999.

[5] K. J. Ronaldson, P. B. Fitzgerald, and J. J. McNeil, "Clozapine-induced myocarditis, a widely overlooked adverse reaction," *Acta Psychiatrica Scandinavica*, vol. 132, no. 4, pp. 231–240, 2015.

[6] B. L. Bellissima, M. D. Tingle, A. Cicović, M. Alawami, and C. Kenedi, "A systematic review of clozapine-induced myocarditis," *International Journal of Cardiology*, vol. 259, pp. 122–129, 2018.

[7] K. J. Ronaldson, P. B. Fitzgerald, A. J. Taylor, D. J. Topliss, and J. J. McNeil, "A new monitoring protocol for clozapine-induced myocarditis based on an analysis of 75 cases and 94 controls," *The Australian and New Zealand Journal of Psychiatry*, vol. 45, no. 6, pp. 458–465, 2011.

[8] K. J. Li, A. P. Greenstein, and L. E. Delisi, "Sudden death in schizophrenia," *Current Opinion in Psychiatry*, vol. 31, no. 3, pp. 169–175, 2018.

[9] P. Ifteni, C. U. Correll, V. Burtea, J. M. Kane, and P. Manu, "Sudden unexpected death in schizophrenia: autopsy findings in psychiatric inpatients," *Schizophrenia Research*, vol. 155, no. 1–3, pp. 72–76, 2014.

[10] K. N. Knoph, R. J. Morgan 3rd., B. A. Palmer et al., "Clozapine-induced cardiomyopathy and myocarditis monitoring: a systematic review," *Schizophrenia Research*, vol. 199, pp. 17–30, 2018.

[11] V. Chow, I. Feijo, J. Trieu, J. Starling, and L. Kritharides, "Successful rechallenge of clozapine therapy following previous clozapine-induced myocarditis confirmed on cardiac MRI," *Journal of Child and Adolescent Psychopharmacology*, vol. 24, no. 2, pp. 99–101, 2014.

Radiation-Induced Left Main Coronary Artery Stenosis in a Patient with Atretic Internal Mammary Arteries

Siddhant Dogra, Asha M. Mahajan, Albert Jung, Michael Attubato, Muhamed Saric, and Alan Shah

Leon H. Charney Division of Cardiology, Department of Medicine, New York University School of Medicine, 530 First Avenue, Skirball 9U, New York, NY10016, USA

Correspondence should be addressed to Alan Shah; alan.shah@nyulangone.org

Academic Editor: Assad Movahed

Coronary artery disease (CAD) is a known potential complication of thoracic radiation treatment that typically affects the proximal segments of the coronary arteries, requiring coronary artery bypass grafting (CABG). We present a case of acute coronary syndrome occurring in a 57-year-old man with prior thoracic radiation therapy following resection of a chest wall chondrosarcoma. Coronary angiogram demonstrated significant areas of stenosis in the left main coronary artery (LMCA) and ostial left anterior descending (LAD) coronary artery. The patient was also found to have atretic bilateral internal mammary arteries as a consequence of his radiation therapy, rendering them unsuitable as grafts. Percutaneous coronary intervention (PCI) was thus performed with a successful outcome. To our knowledge, this is the first case of radiation-induced CAD of the LMCA with atretic internal mammary arteries treated successfully with PCI.

1. Introduction

Radiation therapy can play a critical role in treatment of cancers involving the chest such as breast cancer, lung cancer, lymphoma, and other thoracic-related cancers. However, radiation therapy does pose a risk of damaging pulmonary and cardiovascular tissues. Radiation-induced cardiovascular disease can manifest as acute or constrictive pericarditis, aortic disease, valvular disease, heart failure, arrhythmias, and vasculopathy involving both microvascular and macrovascular structures, including coronary artery disease (CAD). The injury can either be acute or develop years after treatment [1]. Studies in patients receiving radiation therapy suggest a dose-response relationship between radiation exposure and incidence of cardiovascular complications [2]. Radiation-induced CAD tends to affect the left main coronary artery (LMCA) or proximal left anterior descending (LAD) artery, making a patient more favorable for coronary artery bypass grafting (CABG) [3]. However, radiation may also damage the internal mammary arteries. In this report, we describe to our knowledge the first case of a patient with radiation-induced LMCA disease with atretic left and right internal mammary arteries treated successfully with percutaneous coronary intervention (PCI).

2. History of Presentation and Medical History

A 57-year-old man presented to his outpatient cardiologist with two weeks of exertional left-sided chest pain and decrease in exercise tolerance from a baseline of 20 blocks to 1 block. The pain was described as pressure in a band-like region across his chest, brought on by exertion and relieved after 5-10 minutes of rest. His history was significant for high-grade dedifferentiated chest wall chondrosarcoma involving the left ribs that was resected three years earlier (Figures 1(a) and 1(b)). The internal mammary arteries were isolated and protected perioperatively. The patient subsequently received one cycle of adjuvant high-dose ifosfamide with mesna complicated by worsening renal function. This was followed by thoracic radiation treatment of 60 Gray total delivered in 30 fractions. He then was started on pazopanib daily complicated by hypertension and hypothyroidism.

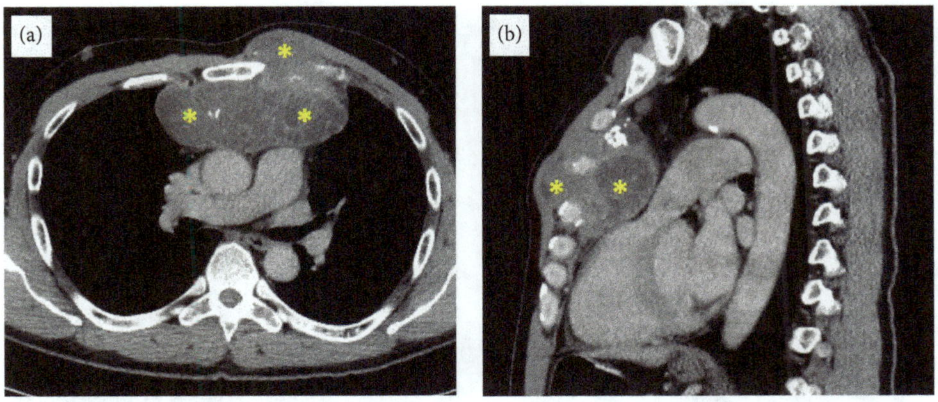

(a) (b)

Figure 1: Chest wall chondrosarcoma on prior CT scan. CT scan of chest wall chondrosarcoma in (a) transverse and (b) sagittal planes marked by asterisks.

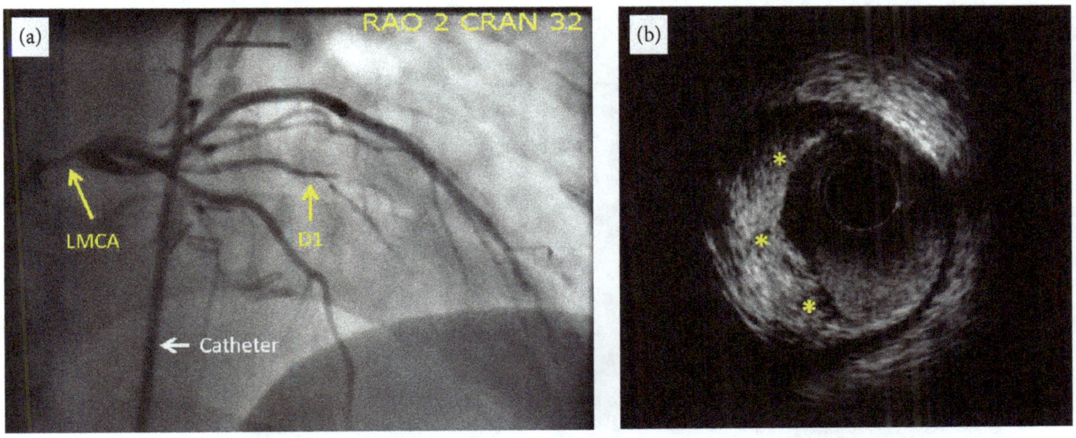

(a) (b)

Figure 2: Initial coronary angiogram of left coronary system. Coronary angiogram showing the stenotic lesion in the (a) left internal mammary artery (LMCA) and first diagonal branch (D1) and (b) IVUS of LMCA lesion showing significant plaque (noted by yellow asterisks).

3. Investigation

The patient experienced chest pain walking to the exam room and was sent to the emergency department for further evaluation. His electrocardiogram showed normal sinus rhythm with new T-wave inversions in the anterior and lateral leads as well as poor R wave progression. Two successive troponins were elevated at 0.13 and 0.11 ng/mL. A transthoracic echocardiogram showed severe hypokinesis in the LAD distribution with a new mildly reduced ejection fraction of 40%.

Coronary angiogram showed significant LMCA stenosis extending into the ostial segment of the LAD artery with 90% stenosis, which was further evaluated by intravascular ultrasound (IVUS) noting significant plaque (Figures 2(a) and 2(b)). There were also stenotic lesions in the first diagonal branch. The right coronary artery, left circumflex artery, and ramus intermedius artery displayed minimal luminal abnormalities. Given the patient's history of chest radiation therapy, angiography of the internal mammary arteries was performed and demonstrated diminutive, possibly occluded vessels (Figures 3(a) and 3(b)).

4. Management

PCI was performed on the mid-LMCA to ostial LAD lesion. After prestent dilatation, a 3.5 × 20 mm Promus ELITE drug-eluting stent was successfully delivered (Figures 4(a) and 4(b)). Poststent balloon dilatation was performed, and IVUS confirmed good stent apposition and expansion. The decision was made to medically manage the first diagonal branch disease. The patient was discharged on aspirin 81 mg daily, ticagrelor 90 mg twice daily, and atorvastatin 80 mg daily in addition to continuing his home medications.

5. Follow-Up

Three months postdischarge, the patient was doing well, asymptomatic, and back to his baseline exercise tolerance.

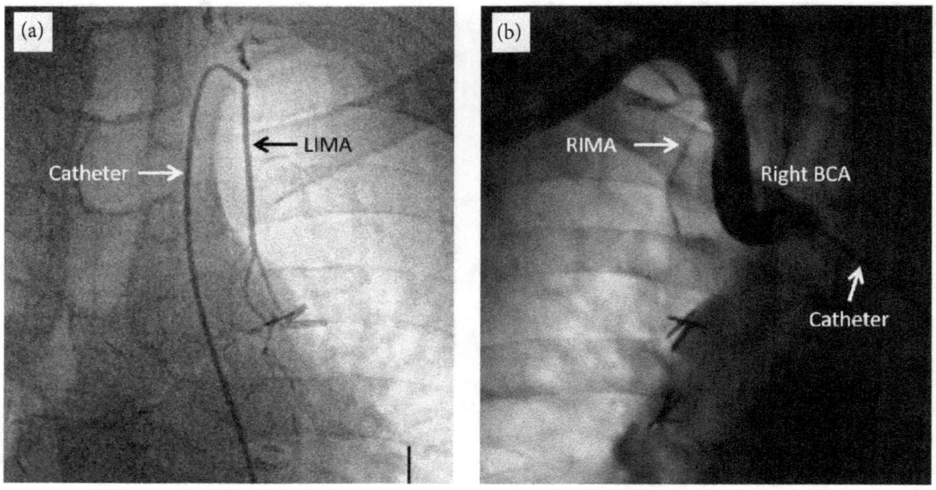

(a) (b)

Figure 3: Coronary angiogram of internal mammary arteries. Coronary angiogram of the (a) left internal mammary artery (LIMA) and the (b) right internal mammary artery (RIMA) coming just off of the right brachiocephalic artery (BCA).

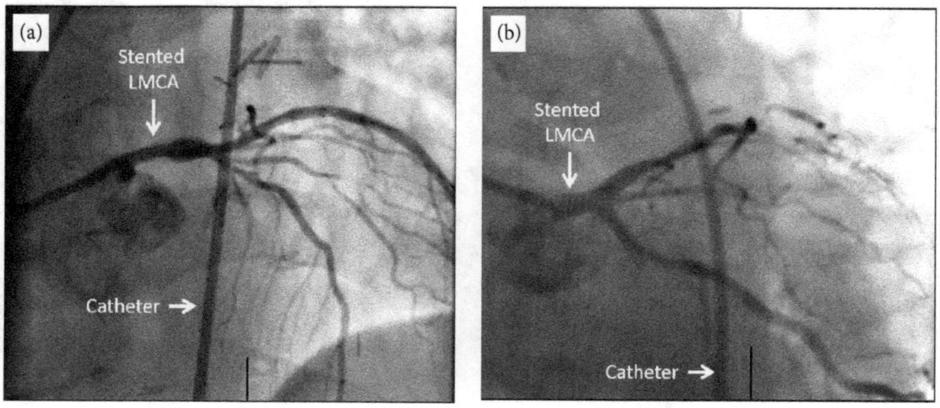

(a) (b)

Figure 4: Coronary angiogram of LMCA lesion after PCI. (a, b) Coronary angiogram of LMCA lesion after stent placement.

6. Discussion

Cardiovascular disease and cancer together are the top two leading causes of mortality worldwide and share significant common characteristics including overlap in risk factors as well as pathophysiologic components ranging from genetic to inflammatory. Moreover, numerous cancer treatments have been demonstrated to be cardiotoxic, including chemotherapeutic agents such as doxorubicin and newer targeted immunotherapies. Combination with radiation can increase the risk of cardiac toxicities. As cancer therapies have improved, cancer survival rates have significantly increased. As the number of cancer survivors grows, practitioners must be aware of the links between cancer treatment and development of future cardiac complications [4].

Radiation therapy can affect both pulmonary and cardiovascular structures and function. Patients can develop pulmonary toxicities such as radiation-induced fibrosis or pleural effusions, which can be both acute and chronic. Pulmonary hypertension can develop as a consequence of this injury. They can develop vasculopathy which can involve both macrovascular and microvascular structures. There is a risk of developing aortic calcification which can complicate surgical options. CAD and microvascular disease can lead to both angina and ischemic cardiomyopathy. Patients can develop both acute and chronic pericarditis, pericardial effusions, and constrictive pericarditis. Valvular heart disease usually presents as progressive thickening and calcification which can affect the valvular structure, the subvalvular apparatus, and the aortomitral curtain. The aortic and mitral valves are more commonly affected, and symptomatic disease can develop 10 to 20 years later [5]. Conduction defects including atrial fibrillation, atrioventricular block, and ventricular arrhythmias can also occur. Finally, radiation can cause myocardial dysfunction due to diffuse fibrosis and can lead to heart failure [6, 7].

Thoracic radiation treatment can lead to accelerated CAD, even in patients without typical risk factors. Patients with radiation-induced CAD tend to present at a younger age than the general population. They commonly have LMCA and/or proximal LAD lesions since these structures are more anterior and central and thus likely exposed to more radiation than distal vessel segments [1, 3]. Radiation-induced CAD is thought to be driven by increased inflammatory cytokine production and inflammatory cell recruitment leading to accelerated intimal plaque formation. Furthermore, radiation induces fibrosis of the media and adventitia in the vessel wall. Inflammatory marker concentration and risk of vessel injury increase proportionally to cumulative radiation dose [1].

Radiation-induced CAD management in terms of medical therapy and revascularization remains the same as that of atherosclerotic CAD. However, revascularization decisions can become challenging as radiation can damage the internal mammary arteries that are more favorable to use especially for left main and LAD disease [1, 8]. Some concern exists about whether the internal mammary arteries should be used as grafts even if they appear undamaged due to potential radiation-induced atherosclerosis. It has been reported that the use of healthy internal mammary arteries is not associated with early graft failure up to one year [9]. However, there was a reported case of a patient with radiation-induced CAD who underwent CABG using the internal mammary arteries and decompensated immediately postoperatively. Emergent angiography showed suboccluded arterial grafts, which were explanted and replaced by saphenous vein grafts. Pathological analysis of the arterial grafts showed significant atherosclerotic plaque and fibrosis [10]. In addition, among patients with radiation-induced CAD who undergo surgery, there is higher risk of postoperative complications such as poor wound healing and higher mortality up to 10 years compared to CABG patients with no history of radiation therapy [11]. PCI is an appealing alternative as it has been shown to be noninferior to CABG for LMCA disease among patients with low-intermediate SYNTAX scores [12]. However, mortality is reportedly higher in patients who undergo PCI for radiation-induced CAD compared to those without radiation exposure at up to 12 years, and there is debate about whether restenosis rates may be higher [13].

Given our patient's significant LMCA stenosis with bifurcation involvement to the LAD and low disease burden in other vessels, it would be most appropriate to pursue CABG based on the 2017 ACC/AHA Appropriate Use Criteria [14]. However, our patient had atretic left and right internal mammary arteries due to radiation, making them unfavorable grafts. In addition, he would have had increased risk of sternal wound infection given this would have been his second sternotomy in the setting of prior radiation therapy. Ultimately, our patient underwent PCI to the lesion with an excellent angiographic result.

7. Conclusion

CAD is one possible consequence of thoracic radiation treatment. The cardiovascular team should evaluate both pulmonary and cardiovascular complications of radiation in order to determine the best revascularization strategy that will lead to a good long-term patency as well as reduce comorbidities of the revascularization procedure. While CABG is commonly used, patients may have radiation damage to the internal mammary arteries. PCI is an available option in the treatment of these patients.

Abbreviations

CAD: Coronary artery disease
CABG: Coronary artery bypass grafting
LMCA: Left main coronary artery
PCI: Percutaneous coronary intervention
LAD: Left anterior descending
IVUS: Intravascular ultrasound
D1: First diagonal branch
LIMA: Left internal mammary artery
RIMA: Right internal mammary artery
BCA: Brachiocephalic artery

References

[1] S. W. Yusuf, S. Sami, and I. N. Daher, "Radiation-induced heart disease: a clinical update," *Cardiology Research and Practice*, vol. 2011, Article ID 317659, 9 pages, 2011.

[2] K. M. Menezes, H. Wang, M. Hada, and P. B. Saganti, "Radiation matters of the heart: a mini review," *Frontiers in Cardiovascular Medicine*, vol. 5, article 83, 2018.

[3] N. Borges and S. R. Kapadia, *Radiation-induced CAD: incidence, diagnosis, and management outcomes*May 2018, https://www.acc.org/latest-in-cardiology/articles/2018/05/24/01/44/radiation-induced-cad.

[4] T. M. Okwuosa, S. Anzevino, and R. Rao, "Cardiovascular disease in cancer survivors," *Postgraduate Medical Journal*, vol. 93, no. 1096, pp. 82–90, 2017.

[5] E. J. Flores-Umanzor, M. Hernández-Enríquez, G. Caldentey, R. San Antonio, and C. Paré, "Radiation-induced cardiac valve disease," *American Journal of Medicine*, vol. 130, no. 3, pp. e99–e100, 2017.

[6] M. Y. Desai, S. Windecker, P. Lancellotti et al., "Prevention, diagnosis, and management of radiation-associated cardiac disease: JACC scientific expert panel," *Journal of the American College of Cardiology*, vol. 74, no. 7, pp. 905–927, 2019.

[7] H. M. Chang, T. M. Okwuosa, T. Scarabelli, R. Moudgil, and E. T. H. Yeh, "Cardiovascular complications of cancer therapy: best practices in diagnosis, prevention, and management: part 2," *Journal of the American College of Cardiology*, vol. 70, no. 20, pp. 2552–2565, 2017.

[8] F. Otsuka, K. Yahagi, K. Sakakura, and R. Virmani, "Why is the mammary artery so special and what protects it from atherosclerosis?," *Annals of Cardiothoracic Surgery*, vol. 2, no. 4, pp. 519–526, 2013.

[9] G. Nasso, C. Canosa, C. M. de Filippo et al., "Thoracic radiation therapy and suitability of internal thoracic arteries for myocardial revascularization," *Chest*, vol. 128, no. 3, pp. 1587–1592, 2005.

[10] N. Amabile, A. Veugeois, K. Zannis, and C. Caussin, "Radiotherapy-induced vascular damage in mammary arterial graft: correlations between optical coherence tomography and pathology," *European Heart Journal*, vol. 37, no. 6, p. 567, 2016.

[11] W. Wu, A. Masri, Z. B. Popovic et al., "Long-term survival of patients with radiation heart disease undergoing cardiac sur-

gery: a cohort study," *Circulation*, vol. 127, no. 14, pp. 1476–1485, 2013.

[12] G. W. Stone, J. F. Sabik, P. W. Serruys et al., "Everolimus-eluting stents or bypass surgery for left main coronary artery disease," *The New England Journal of Medicine*, vol. 375, no. 23, pp. 2223–2235, 2016.

[13] G. W. Reed, A. Masri, B. P. Griffin, S. R. Kapadia, S. G. Ellis, and M. Y. Desai, "Long-term mortality in patients with radiation-associated coronary artery disease treated with percutaneous coronary intervention," *Circulation Cardiovascular Interventions*, vol. 9, no. 6, 2016.

[14] M. R. Patel, J. H. Calhoon, G. J. Dehmer et al., "ACC/AATS/AHA/ASE/ASNC/SCAI/SCCT/STS 2017 appropriate use criteria for coronary revascularization in patients with stable ischemic heart disease: a report of the American College of Cardiology Appropriate Use Criteria Task Force, American Association for Thoracic Surgery, American Heart Association, American Society of Echocardiography, American Society of Nuclear Cardiology, Society for Cardiovascular Angiography and Interventions, Society of Cardiovascular Computed Tomography, and Society of Thoracic Surgeons," *Journal of the American College of Cardiology*, vol. 69, no. 17, pp. 2212–2241, 2017.

Recurrent Acute Coronary Syndromes in a Patient with Idiopathic Thrombocytopenic Purpura

Nikolaos Iakovis, Andrew Xanthopoulos, Aikaterini Chamaidi, Michail Papamichalis, Apostolos Dimos, Filippos Triposkiadis, and John Skoularigis

Department of Cardiology, University General Hospital of Larissa, Larissa, Greece

Correspondence should be addressed to Andrew Xanthopoulos; andrewvxanth@gmail.com

Academic Editor: Hajime Kataoka

A 53-year-old man was admitted to a peripheral hospital with the diagnosis of acute myocardial infarction without ST elevation. Due to the concomitant presence of first-diagnosed thrombocytopenia (platelet count 50.000/μL), it was decided to be treated conservatively with clopidogrel. Five days later, he developed an acute myocardial infarction with ST elevation (STEMI) and was transferred to our department for primary percutaneous coronary intervention (PCI). Coronary angiography revealed three-vessel disease. The left anterior descending lesion was considered culprit, and PCI was successfully performed using a drug-eluting balloon. This approach was considered safer due to the risk of intolerance of prolonged dual antiplatelet therapy in case of stent implantation. Indeed, four days later, aspirin was discontinued, and the patient remained only on clopidogrel due to a platelet fall. Meanwhile, idiopathic thrombocytopenic purpura (ITP) was diagnosed by hematology consultation, and specific ITP treatment was initiated. Seven days following the procedure, the patient was transferred to the Hematology clinic, where a continuous rise of platelet count up to 115.000/μL while on clopidogrel was observed, and he was discharged from the hospital asymptomatic. Unfortunately, twenty days later, the patient died of a lung infection. In ITP patients with STEMI, primary PCI with drug-eluting balloon angioplasty may be a reasonable approach.

1. Introduction

Idiopathic thrombocytopenic purpura (ITP) is an autoimmune disorder characterized by a low platelet count predisposing to bleeding but paradoxically associated with increased risk of acute coronary syndromes (ACS) [1–3]. Herein, we report the case of a 53-year-old man with first-diagnosed ITP and recurrent ACS, treated with stentless primary percutaneous coronary intervention and antiplatelet drug administration.

2. Case Presentation

A 53-year-old man was admitted to a peripheral hospital with the diagnosis of acute myocardial infarction without ST elevation (NSTEMI) [4]. Due to the concomitant presence of first-diagnosed thrombocytopenia (platelet count (PLT) 50.000/μL, visual estimate), it was decided to be treated conservatively with single antiplatelet therapy (clopidogrel 75 mg). Five days later, he developed an acute anterolateral myocardial infarction with ST elevation (STEMI) and was transferred to our department for primary percutaneous coronary intervention (PCI) (time from STEMI diagnosis to wire crossing ≈105 min). The patient had a history of untreated hyperlipidemia and unrecognized diabetes mellitus (HbA1c = 11, 4%). On admission, his blood pressure was 100/75 mmHg and heart rate 100 beats per minute. On auscultation, first and second heart sounds were normal, and a third heart sound was audible. The lung examination was unremarkable. The 12-lead electrocardiogram revealed ST segment elevation in anterolateral and precordial leads. The peripheral blood smear revealed PLT of 55.000/μL (visual estimate). A transthoracic echocardiogram demonstrated anteroapical and lateral wall hypokinesis and severely reduced systolic function (ejection fraction ≈ 35%). The patient was immediately transferred to the catheterization

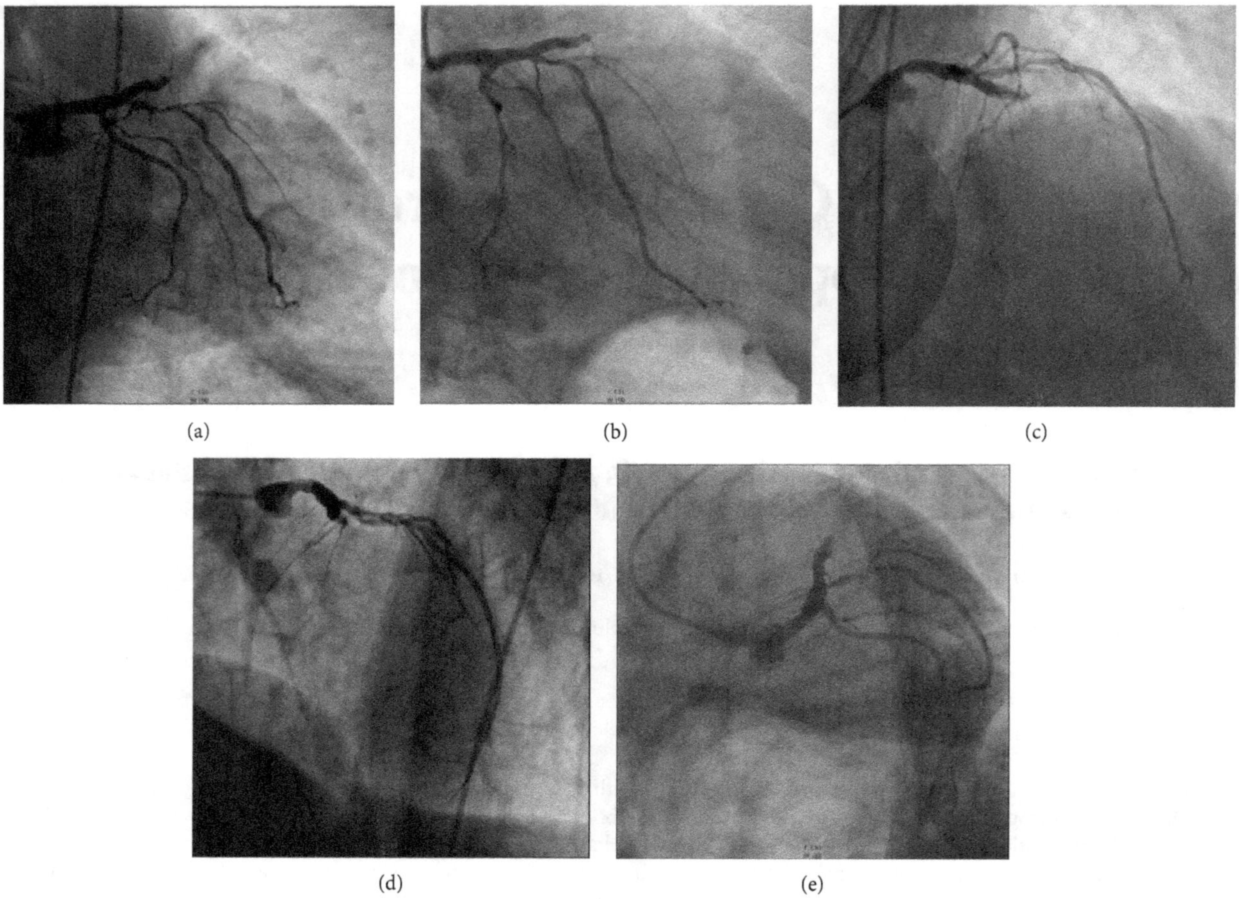

FIGURE 1: A total occlusion of the left anterior descending coronary artery (LAD), high-grade proximal stenosis in the first diagonal branch (90%), and a diffuse atherosclerotic left circumflex coronary artery (LCx) are depicted in RAO caudal (a, b), RAO cranial (c), LAO cranial (d), and LAO caudal (e) projections. RAO = right anterior oblique; LAO = left anterior oblique.

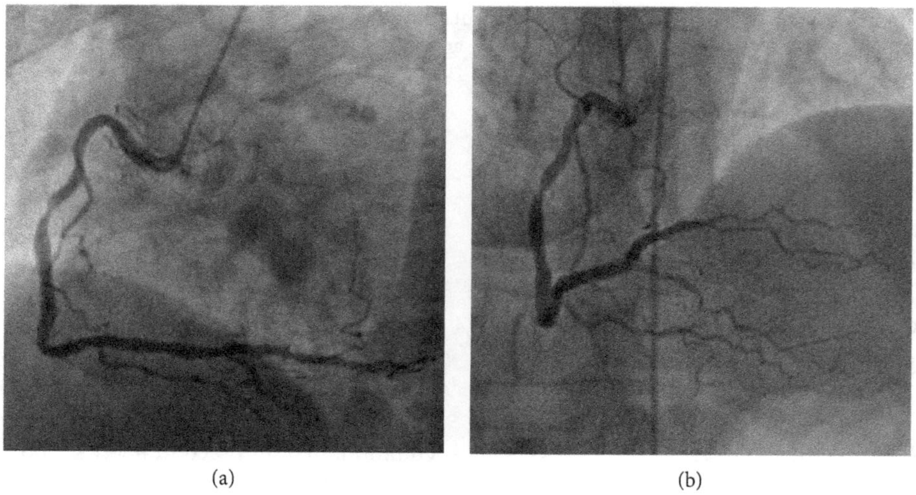

FIGURE 2: A moderate-severe stenosis (70%) in the middle dominant right coronary artery (RCA) is shown in LAO caudal (a) and RAO cranial (b) projections. RAO = right anterior oblique; LAO = left anterior oblique.

laboratory, where aspirin 80 mg and clopidogrel 300 mg were administered orally prior to coronary angiography. The right femoral artery was accessed with a 6 French sheath. Coronary angiography revealed a total occlusion of the left anterior descending artery (LAD), high-grade proximal stenosis in the first diagonal branch (90%), diffuse atherosclerosis of the left circumflex coronary artery (LCx), and moderate-severe stenosis (70%) in the middle of a dominant right coronary artery (RCA) (Figures 1 and 2). The LAD lesion was considered culprit, and PCI was performed. During the

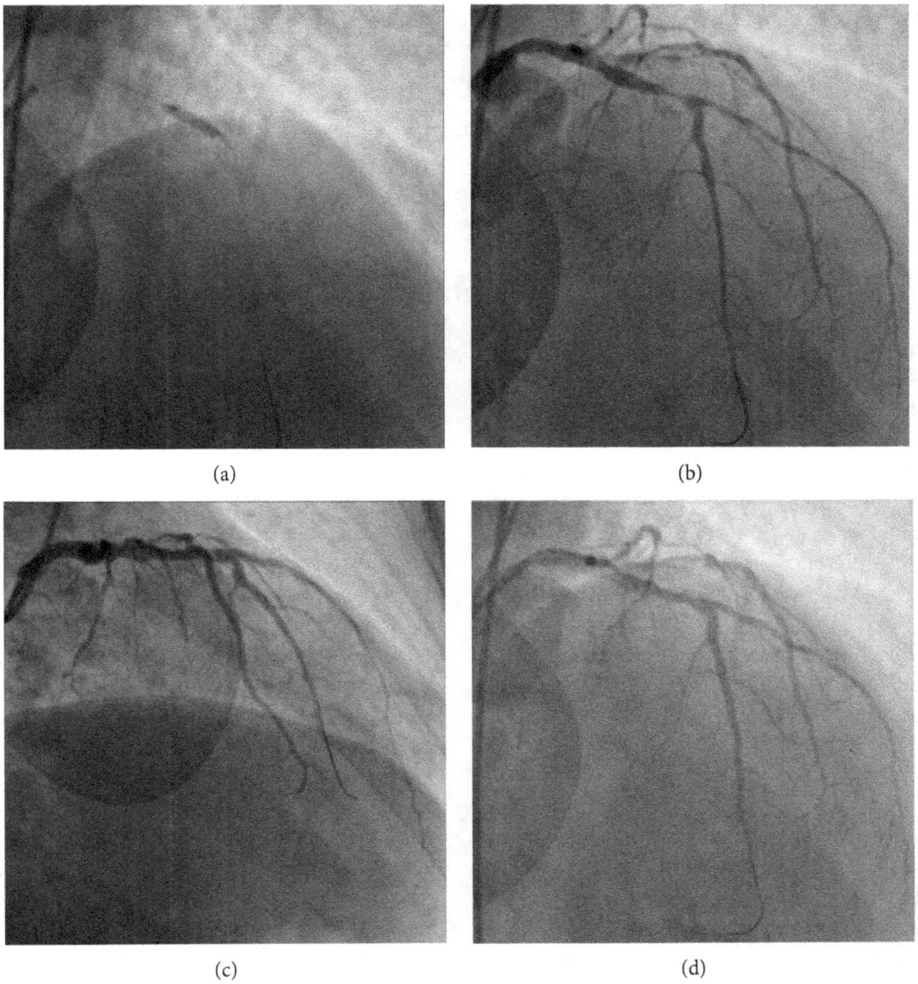

FIGURE 3: Left coronary angiogram in a RAO cranial projection showing (a) dilatation of the LAD culprit lesion with drug-eluting balloon, (b) post predilatation of the lesion using a SC Artimes balloon, and (c, d) successful drug-eluting balloon angioplasty with a TIMI grade II flow. TIMI = thrombolysis in myocardial infarction study group; RAO = right anterior oblique.

procedure, bivalirudin was administered intravenously. An ADROIT® Guiding Catheter XB 3.5 6F (Cordis Corporation, USA) and a BMW guide wire (Abbott Laboratories, USA) were used, and successful crossing of the total LAD occlusion was achieved. Subsequently, predilatation of the lesion using a balloon SC Artimes 1.5 × 12 mm at 16 Atm was done, resulting in a TIMI grade II flow. Subsequently, multiple dilatations of the LAD lesion with a drug-eluting balloon 3.5 × 15mm (Blue Medical Paclitaxel-Eluting Balloon at 6 Atm) were performed (Figure 3). Additionally, due to the presence of thrombotic material and no-reflow phenomenon, eptifibatide (a glycoprotein IIb/IIIa inhibitor) and adenosine were administered intracoronary. Following the procedure, the patient was treated with dual antiplatelet therapy (DAPT), aspirin (100 mg/day), and clopidogrel (75 mg/day), but four days later, aspirin was discontinued due to a platelet fall (from 52.000/μL to 16.000/μL). No minor or major bleeding was detected. Meanwhile, by requested hematology consultation and through examination of peripheral blood smear, exclusion of alternative disorders and bone marrow findings, the diagnosis of ITP was made (Table 1) [5–7]. Recommended ITP treatment included the intravenous infusion of γ-globulin (IG) for three days and the administration of steroids (methylprednisolone, initially 60 mg/day and subsequently 40 mg/day) as well as romiplostim (500 mcg sc weekly), to increase platelet count (Table 2).

TABLE 1: Differential diagnosis of idiopathic thrombocytopenic purpura.

Differential diagnosis
Idiopathic (unknown etiology)
Pseudothrombocytopenia
Renal or liver disease
Myelodysplastic syndrome, acute leukemia
Aplastic anemia
Genetic diseases that cause thrombocytopenia
Thrombotic thrombocytopenic purpura
Heparin-induced thrombocytopenia
Infection (i.e., HIV, HCV, and Helicobacter pylori)

HIV: human immunodeficiency virus; HCV: hepatitis C virus.

Seven days following the procedure, the patient was transferred to the Hematology clinic, where a continuous

TABLE 2: Platelet count and idiopathic thrombocytopenic purpura treatment during hospitalization.

	1st day post PCI	2nd day post PCI	3rd day post PCI	4th day post PCI	5th day post PCI	6th day post PCI	16th day post PCI*
PLT	52.000	32.000	47.000	56.000	16.000	22.000	115.000
Antiplatelet therapy	Aspirin Clopidogrel	Aspirin Clopidogrel	Aspirin Clopidogrel	Aspirin Clopidogrel	Clopidogrel	Clopidogrel	Clopidogrel
ITP treatment	IVIG	IVIG	IVIG			Steroids Romiplostim	Steroids

*Hospital discharge. PCI: percutaneous coronary intervention; PLT: platelets; ITP: idiopathic thrombocytopenic purpura; IVIG: intravenous immunoglobulin.

rise of platelet count until the sixteenth day at the level of 115.000/μL was observed, and the patient was discharged from the hospital stable and asymptomatic. The follow-up visit for the cardiac reevaluation of the patient was scheduled 30 days postdischarge. Treatment at discharge included methylprednisolone (40 mg/day), clopidogrel (75 mg/day), bisoprolol (5 mg/day), atorvastatin (40 mg/day), ramipril (2.5 mg/day), eplerenone (50 mg/day), furosemide (40 mg/day), ivabradine (5 mg/day), metformin (850 mg/day), and insulin glargine (40 U/day).

20 days after his discharge, the patient was readmitted to the Hematology clinic due to lung infection. During his hospitalization, he became septic and died a few days later.

3. Discussion

ITP is an autoimmune disorder, most commonly seen in females. It is characterized by a low platelet count due to autoantibody-mediated platelet destruction and suppression of platelet production that predispose to bleeding. Given the critical role of platelets in atherothrombosis, the prevalence of coronary artery disease in ITP seems to be low. However, ITP may be associated with increased risk of thrombotic events, including acute coronary syndromes (ACS) that may be related to endothelial damage caused by antigenic mimicry between larger and more adhesive platelets and endothelial cells. In addition, it can be related to ITP treatment with steroids that induce metabolic changes and an hypercoagulable state, or intravenous immunoglobulin that may result in expansion of plasma volume and increase in blood viscosity [8].

In general, the optimal management of STEMI includes timely revascularization of the culprit lesion with PCI and stent (s) implantation, followed by DAPT (i.e., acetylsalicylic acid and a thienopyridine derivative). However, antiplatelet therapy is not recommended, and avoidance of PCI is advised when the platelet count is below 50.000/μL, due to high bleeding risk [1].

So far, no recommendations exist regarding the selection and duration of antiplatelet therapy and whether or not to implant a stent in the culprit vessel, as relatively few cases of PCI have been reported in ACS patients and concomitant ITP [3]. In ACS patients with thrombocytopenia undergoing PCI, second-generation drug-eluting stents are preferable to bare-metal stents, and radial approach is generally preferred to femoral, due to evidence of a lower risk of bleeding, as well as easy hemostatic compression [1, 9]. Due to limited data, in stented patients with ACS who have a platelet count of ≤100.000/μL but ≥50.000/μL, DAPT with aspirin and clopidogrel is recommended for short time—1 month—followed by a single antiplatelet agent, with clopidogrel being the treatment of choice [10]. Less is known regarding stentless PCI, although a strategy of single antiplatelet treatment has been proposed [2].

Furthermore, periprocedural supportive treatment to increase platelet counts, platelet transfusion, intravenous IG, and steroids has been used to reduce bleeding complications [8].

In our case, we decided to proceed with primary PCI using a drug-eluting balloon, as we could not predict the patient's tolerance and response to prolonged DAPT required following stent implantation, given that the patient was recently diagnosed with thrombocytopenia. The stentless approach is also supported by the recent REVascularization with paclitaxEL-coated balloon Angioplasty versus drug-eluting stenting in acute myocardial infarcTION (REVELATION) trial which demonstrated that in the setting of STEMI, the drug-coated balloon strategy was noninferior to drug-eluting stent in terms of fractional flow reserve assessed at 9 months and seemed to be safe and feasible [11]. Regarding the access site of the procedure, despite the theoretical advantages of the radial, excellent results have also been reported with the transfemoral approach [3]. Notably, in patients undergoing primary PCI without cardiogenic shock who are treated with bivalirudin (as in our case), the differences in mortality or bleeding rates related to the access site are negligible [12]. Bivalirubin, a direct thrombin inhibitor, was used as an alternative to heparin since it is the only agent proved to be safe in cases with thrombocytopenia [13].

The no-reflow phenomenon that the patient suffered is a devastating complication, and the results of several pharmacological therapies are generally unsatisfactory. In our case, adenosine and the glycoprotein IIb/IIIa inhibitor eptifibatide were administered, as the intracoronary use of the latter appears to be safe [14, 15].

In ITP patients with STEMI, primary PCI with drug-eluting balloon angioplasty is a reasonable approach that can be safely and successfully applied, if platelet count and bleeding risk are carefully monitored.

Abbreviations

ITP: Idiopathic thrombocytopenic purpura
ACS: Acute coronary syndromes
STEMI: ST elevation myocardial infarction
NSTEMI: Non-ST elevation myocardial infarction
PCI: Percutaneous coronary intervention

LAD: Left anterior descending artery
LCx: Left circumflex artery
RCA: Right coronary artery
DAPT: Dual antiplatelet therapy
IVIG: Intravenous immunoglobulin.

References

[1] C. P. McCarthy, G. Steg, and D. L. Bhatt, "The management of antiplatelet therapy in acute coronary syndrome patients with thrombocytopenia: a clinical conundrum," *European Heart Journal*, vol. 38, no. 47, pp. 3488–3492, 2017.

[2] S. Fujino, S. Niwa, K. Fujioka et al., "Primary percutaneous coronary intervention by a stentless technique for acute myocardial infarction with idiopathic thrombocytopenic purpura: a case report and review of the literature," *Internal Medicine*, vol. 55, no. 2, pp. 147–152, 2016.

[3] C. H. Lee and U. Kim, "Revascularization for patients with idiopathic thrombocytopenic purpura and coronary artery disease," *Korean Circulation Journal*, vol. 44, no. 4, pp. 264–267, 2014.

[4] M. Roffi, C. Patrono, J. P. Collet et al., "2015 ESC guidelines for the management of acute coronary syndromes in patients presenting without persistent ST-segment elevation: task force for the management of acute coronary syndromes in patients presenting without persistent ST-segment elevation of the European Society of Cardiology (ESC)," *European Heart Journal*, vol. 37, no. 3, pp. 267–315, 2016.

[5] F. Rodeghiero, R. Stasi, T. Gernsheimer et al., "Standardization of terminology, definitions and outcome criteria in immune thrombocytopenic purpura of adults and children: report from an international working group," *Blood*, vol. 113, no. 11, pp. 2386–2393, 2009.

[6] N. Cooper and W. Ghanima, "Immune thrombocytopenia," *The New England Journal of Medicine*, vol. 381, no. 10, pp. 945–955, 2019.

[7] A. Matzdorff and B. Wörmann, "Diagnostik und Therapie der Immunthrombozytopenie," *DMW - Deutsche Medizinische Wochenschrift*, vol. 143, no. 15, pp. 1076–1081, 2018.

[8] M. P. Lambert and T. B. Gernsheimer, "Clinical updates in adult immune thrombocytopenia," *Blood*, vol. 129, no. 21, pp. 2829–2835, 2017.

[9] M. Valgimigli, A. Patialiakas, A. Thury et al., "Zotarolimus-eluting versus bare-metal stents in uncertain drug-eluting stent candidates," *Journal of the American College of Cardiology*, vol. 65, no. 8, pp. 805–815, 2015.

[10] D. L. Bhatt, A. T. Hirsch, P. A. Ringleb, W. Hacke, and E. J. Topol, "Reduction in the need for hospitalization for recurrent ischemic events and bleeding with clopidogrel instead of aspirin," *American Heart Journal*, vol. 140, no. 1, pp. 67–73, 2000.

[11] N. S. Vos, N. D. Fagel, G. Amoroso et al., "Paclitaxel-coated balloon angioplasty versus drug-eluting stent in acute myocardial infarction: the REVELATION randomized trial," *JACC: Cardiovascular Interventions*, vol. 12, no. 17, pp. 1691–1699, 2019.

[12] J. Mallidi, J. Ulahannan, V. K. Chaubey et al., "Comparison of clinical outcomes: bivalirudin with transfemoral access versus heparin with transradial access in patients with ST segment elevation myocardial infarction," *Critical Pathways in Cardiology*, vol. 18, no. 3, pp. 130–134, 2019.

[13] A. Cuker, G. M. Arepally, B. H. Chong et al., "American Society of Hematology 2018 guidelines for management of venous thromboembolism: heparin-induced thrombocytopenia," *Blood Advances*, vol. 2, no. 22, pp. 3360–3392, 2018.

[14] X. Zhou, X. Wu, H. Sun, and J. Li, "Efficacy and safety of eptifibatide versus tirofiban in acute coronary syndrome patients: a systematic review and meta-analysis," *Journal of Evidence-Based Medicine*, vol. 10, no. 2, pp. 136–144, 2017.

[15] A. J. Deibele, L. K. Jennings, J. E. Tcheng, C. Neva, A. D. Earhart, and C. M. Gibson, "Intracoronary eptifibatide bolus administration during percutaneous coronary revascularization for acute coronary syndromes with evaluation of platelet glycoprotein IIb/IIIa receptor occupancy and platelet function: the intracoronary eptifibatide (ICE) trial," *Circulation*, vol. 121, no. 6, pp. 784–791, 2010.

28

Brugada Syndrome Caused by Autonomic Dysfunction in Multiple Sclerosis

Michel Ibrahim,[1] **Garly Saint-Croix**,[1] **and Rosario Colombo**[2]

[1]*Department of Internal Medicine, Jackson Memorial Hospital/University of Miami Hospital, Miami, FL, USA*
[2]*Department of Cardiovascular Medicine, Jackson Memorial Hospital, Miami, FL, USA*

Correspondence should be addressed to Michel Ibrahim; ibrahimichel@gmail.com

Academic Editor: Domingo A. Pascual-Figal

Only one case report has previously described a patient with multiple sclerosis and a type 1 Brugada pattern on the electrocardiogram. Patients with multiple sclerosis have several neurological deficits including sensory symptoms, acute or subacute motor weakness, gait disturbance, and balance problems that may lead to an increased risk of falls. Concurrent autonomic dysfunction and neurologic consequences of multiple sclerosis may precipitate both mechanical falls and falls with loss of consciousness. While mechanistically different, the type 1 Brugada pattern presents similarly with syncope due to an insufficient cardiac output during dysrhythmia. In such patients, intracardiac defibrillators have shown to prevent sudden cardiac death in patients with the Brugada syndrome. In light of these similarly presenting but unique clinical entities, MS patients who develop a syncopal event in the setting of a spontaneous type I Brugada pattern pose a diagnostic and therapeutic dilemma. This case illustrates an approach to the risks and benefits of an ICD placement in an MS patient with the type 1 Brugada pattern.

1. Introduction

The Brugada syndrome (BruS) is an autosomal dominant genetic disorder with variable expression characterized by typical electrocardiogram (ECG) findings with an increased risk of ventricular arrhythmias and sudden cardiac death [1]. It is essential to distinguish BruS and Brugada sign (BrS) which are two terms distinguishable by the presence or absence of symptoms. Patients with BrS are asymptomatic and have no other clinical criteria. This distinction aids in decision-making for appropriate management.

Multiple sclerosis (MS) is a chronic disease that leads to the diffuse destruction of the nervous tissue [2]. Its associations with cardiac complications have been extensively described [3]: these lesions may ultimately affect regulation of the cardiac autonomic nervous system (ANS), thus causing orthostatic signs and symptoms. MS can also present with gait instability, neuropathic pain, ataxia, and weakness, which all may increase the risk for falls.

We describe a case of a patient with multiple sclerosis presenting to the hospital after experiencing an episode of questionable syncope and ST segment elevation on the ECG that was found to have BrS.

2. Brugada Syndrome Diagnosis Criteria

BruS is diagnosed in symptomatic patients with a pseudo right bundle branch block and ST segment abnormality characteristic of type 1 morphology with a 2 mm or more elevation in the leads V1 and V2 on the ECG (Figure 1). This may occur either spontaneously or in patients with type 2 or 3 patterns during a provocative drug test with intravenous administration of class I antiarrhythmic drugs. Documented ventricular fibrillation or polymorphic VT, syncope of a probable arrhythmic cause, or a family history of sudden cardiac death [4, 5] together with a spontaneous or induced type I Brugada pattern make the diagnosis of BruS.

3. Autonomic Dysfunction in Multiple Sclerosis

Dysfunction of the autonomic nervous system can cause lightheadedness, dizziness, orthostatic intolerance, tachycardia or

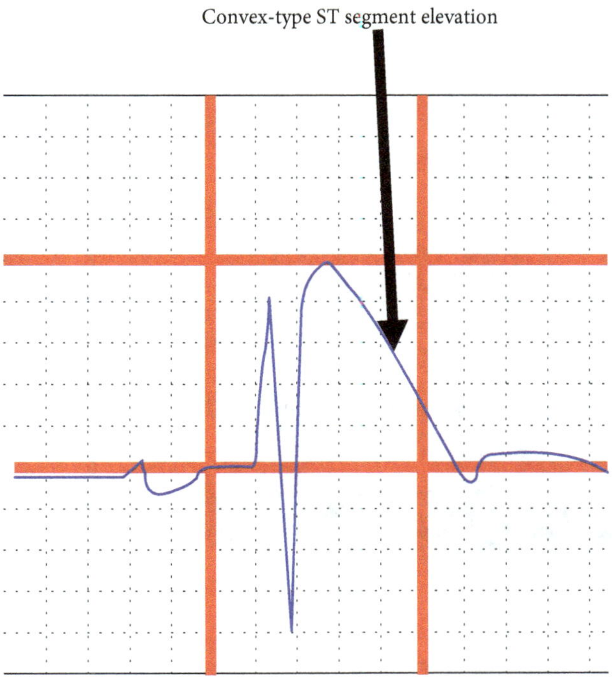

FIGURE 1: Type 1 Brugada pattern on the ECG.

bradycardia, blood pressure fluctuations, and bowel or bladder dysfunction. In MS, cardiovascular dysfunction is mainly due to ANS dysfunction from overall demyelinating plaque burden in the medulla disrupting reflex pathways from higher cortical centers. Alternatively, there may be interference as the descending autonomic pathways course through the brainstem and spinal cord [6]. ANS dysfunction explains the orthostatic symptoms including syncope, near syncope, and orthostatic hypotension that have previously been reported in MS patients [7, 8]. Cardiovascular abnormalities may be clinical or subclinical and can also lead to sudden death in some cases [7].

4. Brugada Pattern and Multiple Sclerosis

In our literature search, there has been only one previously reported case of the type 1 Brugada pattern on the ECG in an asymptomatic patient with multiple sclerosis [9]. The authors stipulated that the only abnormality that could be linked to such an ECG finding is the dysfunction of the autonomic nervous system (ANS), due to lesions in the brain and spine. There is evidence that an imbalance between the sympathetic and parasympathetic nervous systems contributes significantly to the pathophysiology of the Brugada syndrome [10].

5. Case Presentation

This is a 60-year-old right-handed man with past medical history of relapsing-remitting multiple sclerosis diagnosed 20 years ago with prior beta interferon treatment for 8 years and with chronic left residual hemiparesis who presented to the emergency room after experiencing generalized weakness followed by a fall to the ground with apparent loss of consciousness. While the patient reported no loss of consciousness, he did not have memory of the events surrounding the fall. EMS was called and patient was airlifted to the nearest percutaneous intervention-capable center after the ECG showed a ST segment elevation in the leads V1 to V3, so the ST segment elevation myocardial infarction (STEMI) alert was activated. In the emergency department, the patient was without chest pain. Upon further questioning, he denied any family history of heart disease including no cardiomyopathy, heart failure, arrhythmias, or premature or sudden cardiac death. Vitals demonstrated mild tachycardia to 105 beats per minute and a temperature of 38 degrees Celsius, and labs revealed a negative troponin level. Ultimately, the ST segment elevation myocardial infarction (STEMI) alert was cancelled due to the high clinical suspicion of the type 1 Brugada pattern in a syncopal patient with anteroseptal ST elevations without chest pain. Workup for the febrile episode revealed positive serology for influenza B. Oseltamivir was started and the patient completed 5 days of treatment. The patient was no longer febrile and his tachycardia had resolved, but he continued to show a persistent type 1 Brugada pattern on the ECG during the entire hospitalization course as seen below (Figure 2). The patient subsequently went for a transthoracic echocardiogram which demonstrated a normal left and right ventricular function and no structural abnormalities. He also underwent coronary angiography, which revealed nonobstructive coronary artery disease.

Ultimately, the primary concern was to elucidate, whether the patient's initial clinical presentation represented an episode of arrhythmogenic syncope induced by the underlying Brugada syndrome, as this would lead to a recommendation for implantation of a cardiac defibrillator. Electrophysiology service was consulted and felt that the mechanism of his fall was mechanical and not related to a true syncopal event. They recommended an outpatient follow-up for consideration of an event monitor or loop recorder.

6. Discussion

The differential diagnosis for BrS includes several conditions that can lead to Brugada-like ECG abnormalities including acute myocardial ischemia or infarction, various central and autonomic nervous system abnormalities, and viral and febrile states among others [3, 11]. Defective myocardial sodium channels reduce sodium inflow currents, thereby reducing the duration of normal action potentials [12]. Febrile states have been reported to unmask a Brugada-like ST segment elevation secondary to reduced sodium influx at a high temperature [13]. Acute myocardial infarction or ischemia in the right ventricular outflow tract produces a ST segment elevation mimicking the Brugada syndrome probably due to the depression of $I_{Ca\text{-}L}$ and the activation of I_KATP during ischemia [14]. Also, a sympathetic and parasympathetic tone imbalance may unmask the Brugada pattern on the ECG [15, 16] which may support our theory that autonomic nervous dysfunction is a possible culprit.

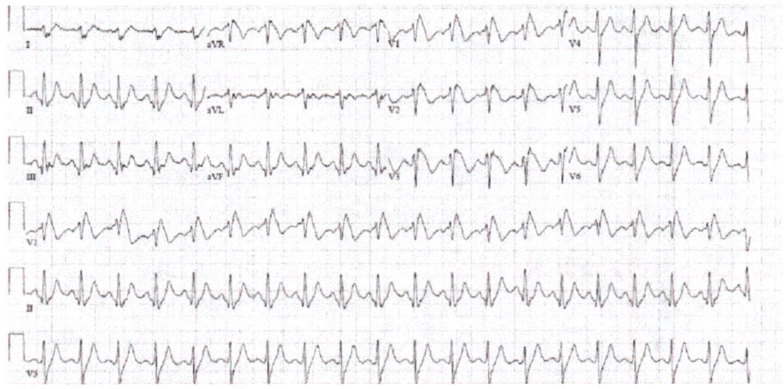

FIGURE 2: ECG: Brugada pattern. Right bundle branch block and ST segment elevation in V1 and V2.

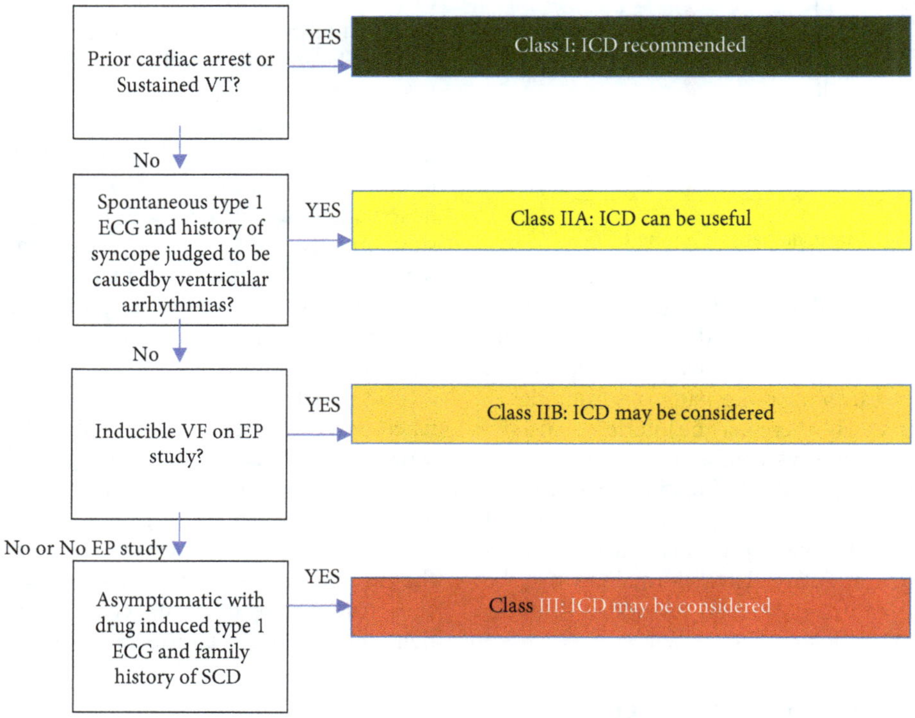

FIGURE 3: ICD in the Brugada syndrome algorithm. Consensus recommendations for ICDs in patients diagnosed with the Brugada syndrome [8].

Our patient has several different conditions that could cause him to have a ST segment elevation in V1 to V3. One of the first important ones is an acute coronary syndrome which was ruled out initially with negative serial troponin levels and definitively with a normal coronary angiogram. The patient was febrile, but he continued to have evidence of the type 1 Brugada pattern on the ECG despite improvement in his temperature and treatment for influenza. Patient's history was somewhat unclear due to loss of consciousness from arrhythmogenic syncope. Consideration can be made for an electrophysiology study; if an arrhythmia was induced, ICD implantation would be a class IIB recommendation [2]. Had the patient consciousness been secondary to an arrhythmia in the setting of the Brugada pattern on the ECG, ICD would be a class IIA recommendation [2] (Figure 3. ICD in the Brugada syndrome algorithm). Thus, it is important to be able to distinguish arrhythmogenic causes of syncope from other causes, particularly in the setting of multiple sclerosis as management and prognosis of such a patient will highly depend on this determination.

Although this patient's fever and influenza had been resolved, the classic Brugada pattern on the ECG has not been resolved. In our review, the abnormality that could be linked to the stated ECG finding is the dysfunction of the autonomic nervous system related to multiple sclerosis. Our patient did not yet have genetic testing for BruS and had no family history of sudden cardiac death. Additionally, our patient did not receive drugs with sodium channel blocking effects. In the setting of the asymptomatic Brugada syndrome, no ICD placement is recommended [17]. It is important to note that an AICD placement does not come free of risks and the patient was spared an unnecessary procedure.

Further investigation is needed in cases where the diagnostic criteria of BruS fall short, especially in patients with a typical type 1 BrS but the mechanism of syncope is in question. In our case, the patient was advised to follow closely with the electrophysiology service. But there are other modalities who have shown to be useful in such cases. In one study, the intracardiac loop recorder has shown to contribute to the exclusion of ventricular arrhythmia as a mechanism of atypical syncope in patients with electrocardiographic evidence of the type 1 Brugada pattern [18]. Continuous cardiac monitoring assists in risk stratification in patients with suspected BruS and may help to inform the possible decision for ICD implantation.

7. Conclusion

In summary, there is evidence that anatomical and/or functional abnormalities of the ANS can provoke ECG changes like BruS; however, the clinical significance for these patients needs further clarification. Due to the significant autonomic dysfunction that accompanies patients with multiple sclerosis, the formal diagnosis of the Brugada syndrome may prove more difficult. The prognostic significance of isolated BruS in multiple sclerosis patients remains a matter of considerable debate. In a patient like ours where the etiology of syncope is an unclear manifestation of BrS type 1, the ECG must be carefully investigated with a close follow-up, and more recently developed modalities of arrhythmia detection such as implantable loop recorders may prove to be useful towards confirming a diagnosis of the Brugada syndrome.

Disclosure

The authors have confirmed that this article is unique and not under consideration or published in any other publications.

Authors' Contributions

MI and RC conceived and designed the experiments. MI and GS analyzed the data. MI wrote the first draft of the manuscript. MI, RC, and GS contributed to the writing of the manuscript. MI and RC agree with the manuscript results and conclusions. MI, GS, and RC jointly developed the structure and arguments for the paper. RC made critical revisions and approved the final version. All authors reviewed and approved the final manuscript.

Acknowledgments

We would like to acknowledge Garly Saint-Croix, MD, for his contributions in editing this manuscript.

References

[1] A. Sarkozy, A. Sorgente, T. Boussy et al., "The value of a family history of sudden death in patients with diagnostic type I Brugada ECG pattern," *European Heart Journal*, vol. 32, no. 17, pp. 2153–2160, 2011.

[2] B. Hemmer, M. Kerschensteiner, and T. Korn, "Role of the innate and adaptive immune responses in the course of multiple sclerosis," *Lancet Neurology*, vol. 14, no. 4, pp. 406–419, 2015.

[3] W. Shimizu, "Acquired forms of the Brugada syndrome," *Journal of Electrocardiology*, vol. 38, no. 4, pp. 22–25, 2005.

[4] S. G. Priori, A. A. Wilde, M. Horie et al., "HRS/EHRA/APHRS expert consensus statement on the diagnosis and management of patients with inherited primary arrhythmia syndromes: document endorsed by HRS, EHRA, and APHRS in May 2013 and by ACCF, AHA, PACES, and AEPC in June 2013," *Heart Rhythm*, vol. 10, no. 12, pp. 1932–1963, 2013.

[5] S. G. Priori, C. Blomstrom-Lundqvist, A. Mazzanti et al., "2015 ESC Guidelines for the management of patients with ventricular arrhythmias and the prevention of sudden cardiac death: the Task Force for the management of patients with ventricular arrhythmias and the prevention of sudden cardiac death of the European Society of Cardiology (ESC) endorsed by: Association for European Paediatric and Congenital Cardiology (AEPC).," *European Heart Journal*, vol. 36, no. 41, pp. 2793–2867, 2015.

[6] J. Seze, T. Stojkovic, J. Y. Gauvrit et al., "Cardiac repolarization abnormalities in multiple sclerosis: spinal cord mri correlates," *Muscle & Nerve*, vol. 23, no. 8, pp. 1284–1286, 2000.

[7] K. Kanjwal, B. Karabin, Y. Kanjwal, and B. P. Grubb, "Autonomic dysfunction presenting as postural orthostatic tachycardia syndrome in patients with multiple sclerosis," *International Journal of Medical Sciences*, vol. 7, pp. 62–67, 2010.

[8] R. A. Marrie, N. Reider, J. Cohen et al., "A systematic review of the incidence and prevalence of cardiac, cerebrovascular, and peripheral vascular disease in multiple sclerosis," *Multiple Sclerosis*, vol. 21, no. 3, pp. 318–331, 2015.

[9] M. A. Babaee Bigi, A. Aslani, and A. Aslani, "Significance of cardiac autonomic neuropathy in risk stratification of Brugada syndrome," *Europace*, vol. 10, no. 7, pp. 821–824, 2008.

[10] E. Gialafos, E. Andreadou, P. Kokotis et al., "Brugada sign in a multiple sclerosis patient: relation to autonomic nervous system dysfunction and therapeutic dilemmas," *International Journal of Cardiology*, vol. 202, pp. 652-653, 2016.

[11] C. Antzelevitch, P. Brugada, M. Borggrefe et al., "Brugada syndrome: report of the second consensus conference," *Heart Rhythm*, vol. 2, no. 4, pp. 429–440, 2005.

[12] G. X. Yan and C. Antzelevitch, "Cellular basis for the Brugada syndrome and other mechanisms of arrhythmogenesis associated with ST-segment elevation," *Circulation*, vol. 100, no. 15, pp. 1660–1666, 1999.

[13] C. Antzelevitch and R. Brugada, "Fever and Brugada syndrome," *Pacing and Clinical Electrophysiology*, vol. 25, no. 11, pp. 1537–1539, 2002.

[14] H. Kataoka, "Electrocardiographic patterns of the Brugada syndrome in right ventricular infarction/ischemia," *The American Journal of Cardiology*, vol. 86, no. 9, article 1056, 2000.

[15] K. Mizumaki, A. Fujiki, T. Tsuneda et al., "Vagal activity modulates spontaneous augmentation of ST elevation in the daily life of patients with Brugada syndrome," *Journal of Cardiovascular Electrophysiology*, vol. 15, no. 6, pp. 667–673, 2004.

[16] K. Matsuo, T. Kurita, M. Inagaki et al., "The circadian pattern of the development of ventricular fibrillation in patients with Brugada syndrome," *European Heart Journal*, vol. 20, no. 6, pp. 465–470, 1999.

[17] S. G. Priori, A. A. Wilde, M. Horie et al., "Executive summary: HRS/EHRA/APHRS expert consensus statement on the diagnosis and management of patients with inherited primary arrhythmia syndromes," *EP Europace*, vol. 15, no. 10, pp. 1389–1406, 2013.

Peripherally Embolizing Aortic Thrombus: The Work-Up, Management, and Outcome of Primary Aortic Thrombus

Ramy Mando,[1] Robert Gemayel,[2] Ashish Chaddha,[3] Julian J. Barbat,[3] and Elvis Cami[3]

[1]*Department of Internal Medicine, Beaumont Health System, Royal Oak, MI, USA*
[2]*Michigan State University College of Osteopathic Medicine, Lansing, MI, USA*
[3]*Department of Cardiovascular Medicine, Beaumont Health System, Royal Oak, MI, USA*

Correspondence should be addressed to Ramy Mando; ramy.mando@beaumont.org

Academic Editor: Ming-Ren Chen

Background. Primary aortic thrombus is an uncommon entity and not frequently reported in the literature. Herein, we discuss the presentation and management of a patient with a primary thoracic mural thrombus. *Case Summary.* A 46-year-old female with past medical history of tobacco dependence presented for low-grade fever and sudden onset, severe right upper quadrant abdominal pain with associated nausea and vomiting. Computed tomography (CT) revealed an intraluminal polypoid filling defect arising from the isthmus of the aorta projecting into the proximal descending aorta and findings consistent with infarction of the spleen and right kidney. Infectious, autoimmune, hematologic, and oncologic work-up were all unyielding. The patient was started on heparin and later transitioned to apixaban 5 mg twice a day and 81 mg of aspirin daily. She was also counseled regarding smoking cessation. Two months follow-up CT revealed resolution of the thrombus. Patient had no further thromboembolic complications. *Discussion.* We present a unique case of primary aortic thrombus. To our knowledge, this is the first reported case managed successfully with a NOAC. This diagnosis is one of exclusion and through work-up should be completed. Our aim is to raise awareness of this condition and successful management with apixaban in low-risk patients.

1. Background

Aortic mural thrombi are uncommon and typically associated with severe atherosclerosis or the presence of an aneurysm. Even more uncommon is the formation of a primary aortic thrombus with no infectious, neoplastic, traumatic, autoimmune, or hypercoagulable triggers responsible for thrombus formation. To date, there is no consensus on the management of this condition; however, options include anticoagulation, thrombolytics, aortic surgery, and thromboaspiration. Herein, we describe a rare case of primary aortic thrombus presenting with systemic embolization to the lower extremities, kidney, and spleen. This is one of the first cases in the literature describing effective management of this condition with a direct oral anticoagulant.

2. Introduction

Thrombi in the thoracic aorta are most commonly associated with severe atherosclerosis or aortic aneurysm [1, 2]. Primary thrombus of the aorta in the absence of aneurysm, moderate-to-severe atherosclerosis, hypercoagulability, malignancy, infections, or autoimmune conditions is exceedingly rare [2–4]. Management of primary aortic thrombus is not well defined at this time [5, 6]. Herein, we describe the rare case of a thoracic aortic thrombus with peripheral embolization presenting as abdominal pain and lower extremity pain. This is one of the first cases in the literature describing the use of direct oral anticoagulants in the management of primary aortic thrombi. We aim to raise awareness of this condition and summarize pathophysiology as well as current treatment options available to us.

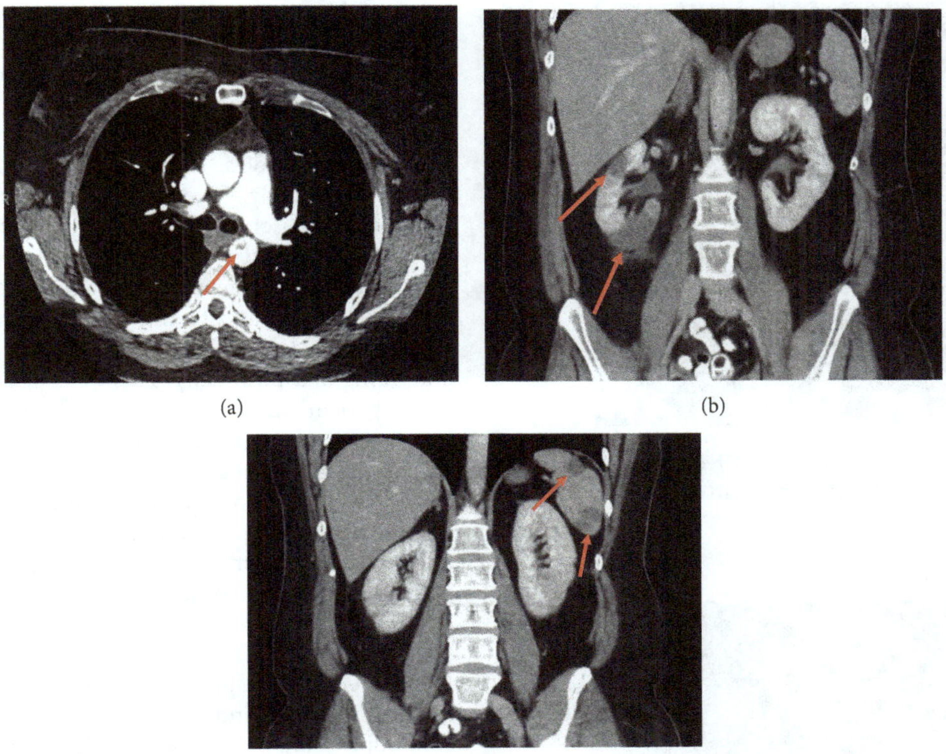

Figure 1: CT of the abdomen and pelvis revealing a mass in the descending thoracic aortia (a) with wedge-shaped infarctions in the right kidney (b) and spleen (c) consistent with an embolic phenomona.

3. Case Description

3.1. Presentation and Initial Evaluation. A 46-year-old female with past medical history of tobacco dependence presented for low-grade fever and sudden onset of severe right upper quadrant abdominal pain with associated nausea and vomiting. Computed tomography (CT) completed in the emergency department revealed an intraluminal polypoid filling defect arising from the isthmus of the aorta projecting into the proximal descending aorta and findings consistent with infarctions of the spleen and right kidney (Figures 1(a)–1(c)). Given the fever, there was a concern for sepsis so she was started on broad-spectrum antibiotics. Heparin has also initiated cardioembolic phenomena of unclear etiology; however, it was later discontinued to prevent hemorrhagic transformation of the existing infarcts. The patient was admitted for further evaluation.

3.2. Inpatient Evaluation. A transthoracic echocardiogram showed no findings to suggest valvular or cardiac source of embolus (Figure 2). An agitated saline bubble contrast study was performed with no evidence of intracardiac shunting (Figure 3). A transesophageal echocardiogram was then completed and revealed a large echogenic mobile mass attached to the wall of the descending thoracic aorta (Figures 4(a) and 4(b)). Bilateral lower extremity arterial Dopplers were obtained and revealed severe popliteal-tibial arterial disease in the left lower extremity (Figure 5).

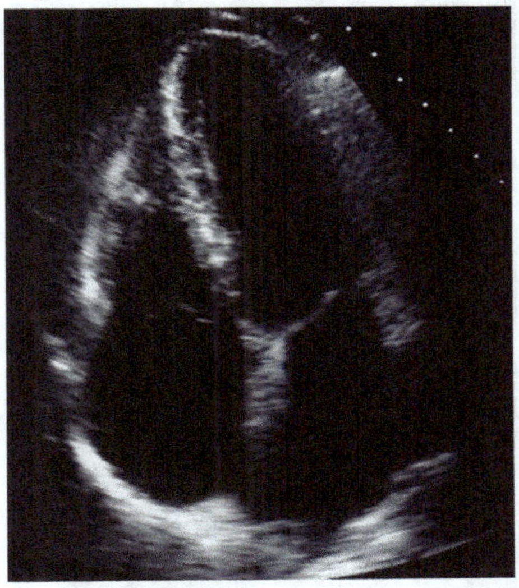

Figure 2: Apical four-chamber view of the heart with no evidence of a source of thrombosis.

Work-up for other organic causes was extensive. Infectious work-up was negative and included testing for bacterial infection, fungal infection, HIV, Bartonella henselae antibody, Coxiella burnetii antibodies, Leptospira antibodies, syphilis, aspergillus galactomannan antigen, and histoplasma antigen. Hypercoagulability work-up was also unremarkable and included DRVVT screening for lupus anticoagulant,

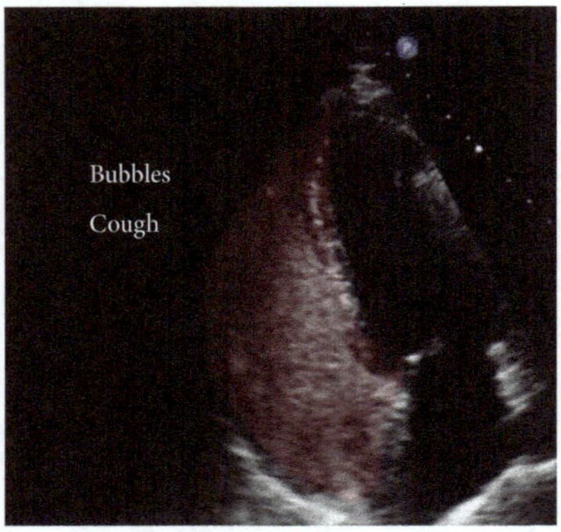

FIGURE 3: Agitated saline (highlighted in red) in the right heart revealing no crossover into the left heart consistent with no intracardiac shunts.

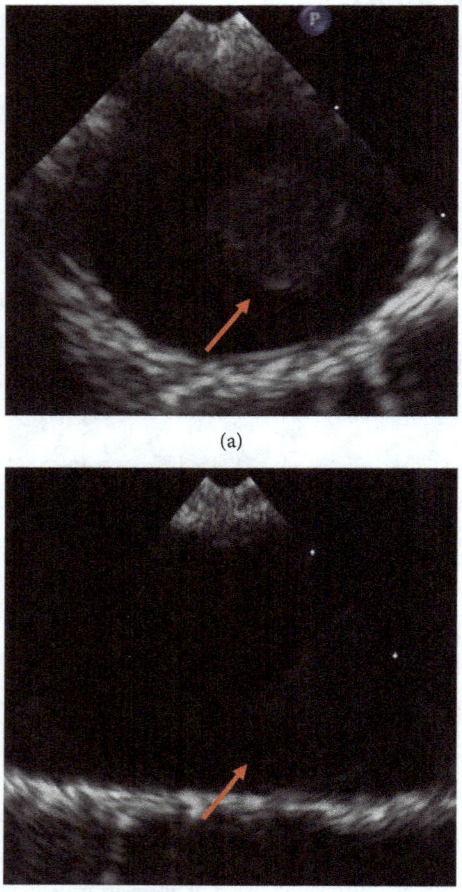

(a)

(b)

FIGURE 4: (a) Transesophageal echocardiogram (transverse view) of a large mass attached to the wall of the descending thoracic aorta. (b) Transesophageal echocardiogram (longitudinal view) of the large mobile mass attached to the aortic wall.

anticardiolipin antibodies (×2), homocysteine levels, paroxysmal nocturnal hemoglobinuria screening, Protein C and S activity, antithrombin mutations, and factor V Leiden and prothrombin genotyping. Autoimmune work-up was also unyielding and included testing for antinuclear antibody, antineutrophil cytoplasmic antibody, antidouble-stranded DNA antibody, rheumatoid factor, cyclic citrullinated peptide, Sjogren antibody, myeloperoxidase antibodies, proteinase 3 autoantibodies, complement levels, Smith antibody, and RNP antibody. Given that there are no acute threat to limb or organ ischemia, the largely negative work-up, and no straight-forward mechanism to remove the aortic thrombus, we decided to manage the patient medically with close outpatient follow-up. She was started on heparin while inpatient which was transitioned to apixaban 5 mg twice a day and 81 mg of aspirin daily. This was done primarily because of the patient's preference to avoid frequent INR checks. A board-certified hematologist agreed with the use of apixaban with monthly outpatient follow-up to ensure patient compliance and clinical improvement. Patient was also counseled regarding smoking cessation. Catheter-based or surgical thromboembolectomy would have been considered if the patient would have developed acute limb ischemia or threatened organ.

3.3. One-Month Follow-Up. At one month, the patient was seen in the clinic and denied symptoms of chest, back, or abdominal pain. She denied significant pain at rest or with exertion and did not exhibit any nonhealing wounds in either of her lower extremities. She noted being able to walk roughly one-quarter of a mile without symptoms prior to resting. She reported adherence with her daily aspirin and twice-daily Eliquis. At this time, arterial computed tomography of the abdomen and pelvis was repeated which revealed complete resolution of the filling defect involving the aortic isthmus and proximal descending aorta. There was no CT evidence to suggest vacuities. The spleen exhibited a lobulated superior margin with volume loss and the right kidney demonstrated a lobulated appearance of the right lower pole compatible with scarring from the previous infarct (Figure 6). The patient was instructed to continue with her antithrombotic regimen and follow-up in one month.

3.4. Two-Month Follow-Up. At this time, the patient no longer expressed having any symptoms of LE pain, swelling, or claudication. She reported being able to resume her daily activities with no limitations. Findings of the CTA were discussed with the patient at her two-month follow-up, and she was encouraged to continue with activity as tolerated. At this time, given the resolution of the mass after anticoagulation, it was felt that it was most likely an aortic thrombus. With regards the duration of therapy, we felt that this was likely unprovoked, and given it was arterial, we decided to continue anticoagulation for at least 12 more months pending further hematologic evaluation.

4. Discussion

Arterial thrombus is a rare clinical entity, particularly in the absence of aneurysm or severe atherosclerosis. The incidence of embolic events is higher in mobile pedunculated thrombi when compared to those that are layered and

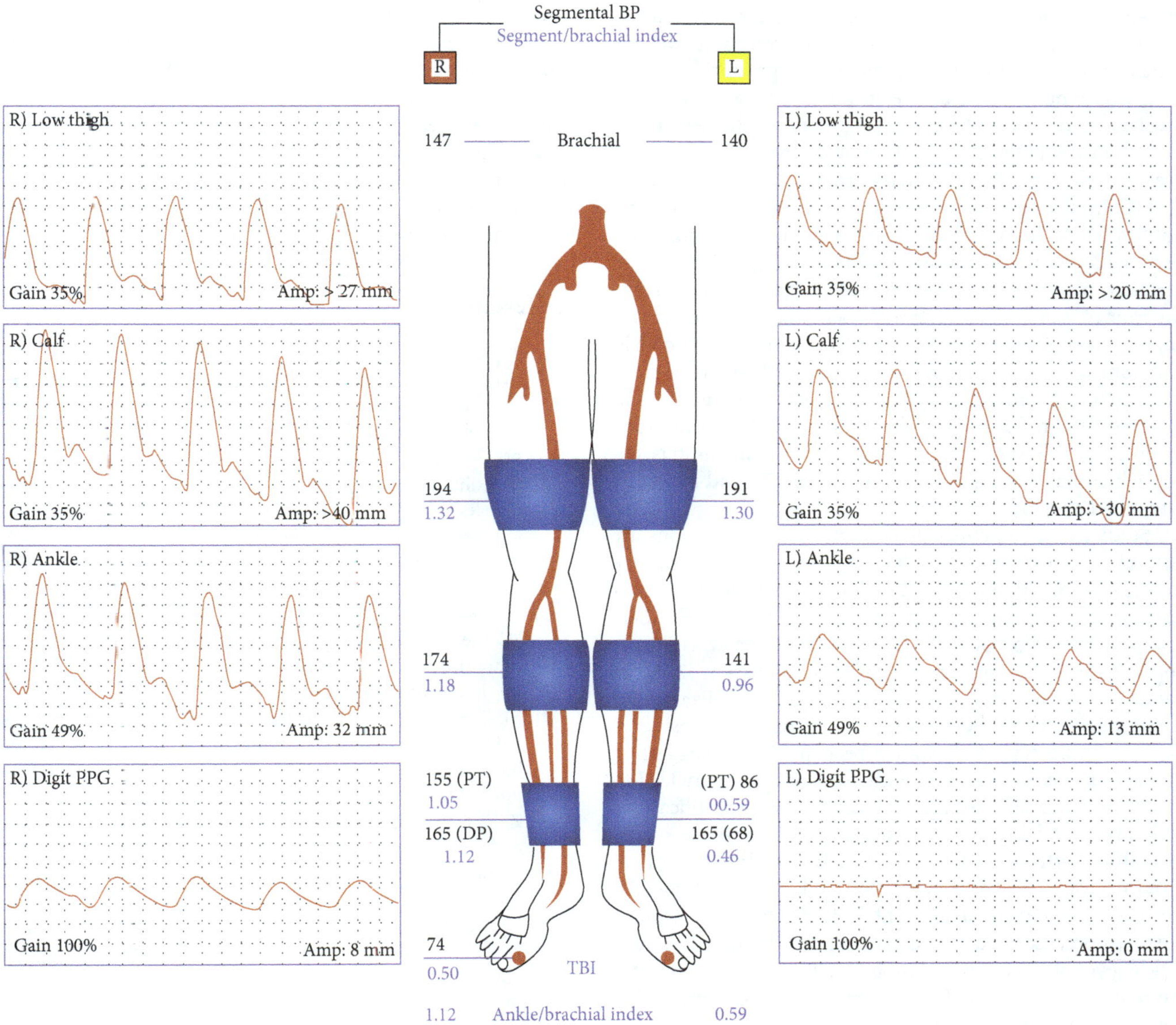

FIGURE 5: Lower extremity arterial Doppler with significant flow limitations in the left lower extremity consistent with diffuse obstructive atherosclerotic obstructive disease in the left posterior tibial artery, peroneal artery, and anterior tibial artery. The waveforms of the right lower extremity are normal multiphasic Doppler waveforms. In the left extremity, we see dampened monophasic Doppler flow signals in the area of the left posterior tibial artery and dorsalis pedis artery. Diminished pulse volume recordings were seen in the left ankle. Flat line, nonpulsatile flow signals were seen in the digits of the left foot.

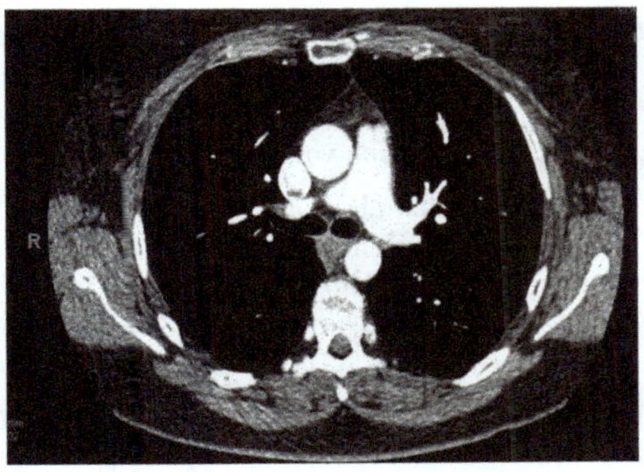

FIGURE 6: CT obtained for follow-up which reveals resolution of previously noted thrombus of the thoracic aorta.

immobile (73% versus 12% risk of embolization, respectively) [7]. The most common manifestation includes consequences related to thromboembolic phenomena, as seen in our patient [2]. These complications are serious; therefore, early detection and management of their causes are imperative to patient care.

Aortic thrombi are typically secondary to aneurysmal disease, dissection, or severe atherosclerosis [5]. Alternative pathologies which may predispose one to being at risk for arterial thrombosis should always be investigated in efforts of preventing future thrombi and their sequela. Potential causes include trauma, malignancy, hypercoagulable states (factor V Leiden mutation, polycythemia, antithrombin III deficiency, protein C and/or S deficiency, etc.) and autoimmune disorders [2, 8–10]. Other risk factors including the presence of microscopic atherosclerotic disease (difficult to exclude clinically), smoking, and oral contraceptive use should also be addressed in patients as appropriate.

Distal embolization of the thrombus causes symptoms specific to the affected organ. Thromboembolic seeding to the renal vasculature can lead to acute kidney injury and failure depending on the renal mass distal to the blocked artery [11]. Complications of seeding to the spleen include, but are not limited to, left upper quadrant pain, anemia, leukocytosis, splenic pseudocyst, abscess, or hemorrhage [12]. Any of the four major types of acute mesenteric ischemic (acute superior mesenteric artery thromboembolic occlusion, mesenteric arterial thrombosis, mesenteric venous thrombosis, and nonocclusive mesenteric ischemia) are all potential complications of thrombus seeding to the colonic vasculature and can lead to significant morbidity and mortality [13]. Emboli seeding to the lower extremities can lead to acute limb ischemia which has an amputation rate of 13-15% and mortality rate of 9-12% [14].

Studies and guideline-directed management options are currently limited, and there have not been any prospective trials addressing therapeutic strategies. Options for treatment include anticoagulation, aortic surgery, thrombolytic therapy, and thromboaspiration [1, 15, 16]. The most common approach to initial management is anticoagulation [2, 5]. In patients with recurrence of distal arterial embolization or persistence of thrombus, aortic surgery may be considered [5, 17, 18]. Several studies have been published suggesting that aggressive management with aortic surgery may lead to less recurrence of distal embolization and complications including distal limb amputation particularly those in the ascending aorta or aortic arch [1, 2, 5, 19]. In our patient, given her vastly negative evaluation and lack of risk factors, we choose to purse management with apixaban and aspirin. Furthermore, there was significant concern for distal embolization given its location and mobility. To our knowledge, we are reporting one of the first case treated successfully with a non-vitamin K–dependent oral anticoagulant.

Our patient is unique in that a very extensive evaluation was unsuccessful in identifying the etiology of arterial thrombus formation. Our working diagnoses were broad throughout the case and included endocarditis, paradoxical embolism, cardiac neoplasm, and all potential causes of aortitis. After excluding infectious sources through an extensive evaluation and autoimmune conditions which may have led to aortitis, we decided to treat the patient empirically with apixaban and low-dose aspirin. Fortunately, our patient's thrombus resolved, and she experienced no residual symptoms at two months follow-up.

5. Conclusion

Primary aortic thrombus is a rare entity which has been previously described in the literature. It is a diagnosis of exclusion, and infectious, malignant, hypercoagulable, and autoimmune causes must be excluded. With regards to treatment, some studies recommend aggressive management to prevent risk of thrombus recurrence and arterial embolization while others recommend more conservative, less invasive medical management; however, there is no expert consensus or guidelines to direct therapy or its duration at this time. Given the lack of standardized guidelines at this time, we recommend a patient-specific approach which considers anticipated adherence to medications and follow-up, risk factors, results of laboratory work-up, and risk of further embolization. In low-risk patients, we propose that the use of a direct factor Xa inhibitors for oral anticoagulation may be an acceptable alternative to coumadin.

References

[1] T. Laperche, C. Laurian, R. Roudaut, and P. G. Steg, "Mobile thromboses of the aortic arch without aortic debris. A transesophageal echocardiographic finding associated with unexplained arterial embolism," *Circulation*, vol. 96, no. 1, pp. 288–294, 1997.

[2] N. Tsilimparis, U. Hanack, G. Pisimisis, S. Yousefi, C. Wintzer, and R. I. Ruckert, "Thrombus in the non-aneurysmal, non-atherosclerotic descending thoracic aorta—an unusual source of arterial embolism," *European Journal of Vascular and Endovascular Surgery*, vol. 41, no. 4, pp. 450–457, 2011.

[3] H. Verma, N. Meda, S. Vora, R. K. George, and R. K. Tripathi, "Contemporary management of symptomatic primary aortic mural thrombus," *Journal of Vascular Surgery*, vol. 60, no. 6, pp. 1524–1534, 2014.

[4] M. E. Morris, E. L. Galinanes, W. K. Nichols, C. B. Ross, and J. Chauvupun, "Thoracic mural thrombi: a case series and literature review," *Annals of Vascular Surgery*, vol. 25, no. 8, pp. 1140.e17–1140.e21, 2011.

[5] Z. Y. Fayad, E. Semaan, B. Fahoum, M. Briggs, A. Tortolani, and M. D'Ayala, "Aortic mural thrombus in the normal or minimally atherosclerotic aorta," *Annals of Vascular Surgery*, vol. 27, no. 3, pp. 282–290, 2013.

[6] A. Maloberti, F. Oliva, B. De Chiara, and C. Giannattasio, "Asymptomatic aortic mural thrombus in a minimally atherosclerotic vessel," *Interactive Cardiovascular and Thoracic Surgery*, vol. 22, no. 3, pp. 371–373, 2016.

[7] D. G. Karalis, K. Chandrasekaran, M. F. Victor, J. J. Ross Jr., and G. S. Mintz, "Recognition and embolic potential of intraaortic atherosclerotic debris," *Journal of the American College of Cardiology*, vol. 17, no. 1, pp. 73–78, 1991.

[8] M. S. Chimenti, E. Ballanti, P. Triggianese, and R. Perricone, "Vasculitides and the complement system: a comprehensive review," *Clinical Reviews in Allergy & Immunology*, vol. 49, no. 3, pp. 333–346, 2015.

[9] E. Reinhold-Keller, K. Herlyn, R. Wagner-Bastmeyer, and W. L. Gross, "Stable incidence of primary systemic vasculitides over five years: results from the German vasculitis register," *Arthritis and Rheumatism*, vol. 53, no. 1, pp. 93–99, 2005.

[10] S. F. Agolini, K. T. Shah, J. J. Goodreau, T. M. McLoughlin Jr., and M. C. Sinclair, "Splenic infarction caused by a large thoracic aortic thrombus," *Journal of Vascular Surgery*, vol. 26, no. 6, pp. 1069–1072, 1997.

[11] N. Koivuviita, R. Tertti, M. Heiro, I. Manner, and K. Metsarinne, "Thromboembolism as a cause of renal artery occlusion and acute kidney injury: the recovery of kidney function after two weeks," *Case Reports in Nephrology and Dialysis*, vol. 4, no. 1, pp. 82–87, 2014.

[12] M. T. Jaroch, T. A. Broughan, and R. E. Hermann, "The natural history of splenic infarction," *Surgery*, vol. 100, pp. 743–750, 1986.

[13] M. J. Sise, "Acute mesenteric ischemia," *The Surgical Clinics of North America*, vol. 94, no. 1, pp. 165–181, 2014.

[14] J. L. Eliason, R. M. Wainess, M. C. Proctor et al., "A national and single institutional experience in the contemporary treatment of acute lower extremity ischemia," *Annals of surgery*, vol. 121, pp. 76–84, 2003.

[15] P. Lozano, F. T. Gomez, J. Julia, E. M-Rimbau, and F. Garcia, "Recurrent embolism caused by floating thrombus in the thoracic aorta," *Annals of Vascular Surgery*, vol. 12, no. 6, pp. 609–611, 1998.

[16] D. Hausmann, D. Gulba, K. Bargheer, J. Niedermeyer, K. A. Comess, and W. G. Daniel, "Successful thrombolysis of an aortic-arch thrombus in a patient after mesenteric embolism," *The New England Journal of Medicine*, vol. 327, no. 7, pp. 500-501, 1992.

[17] C. M. Larsen and S. L. Mulvagh, "Cardio-oncology: what you need to know now for clinical practice and echocardiography," *Echo Research and Practice*, vol. 4, no. 1, pp. R33–R41, 2017.

[18] T. L. Hahn, M. C. Dalsing, A. P. Sawchuk, D. F. Cikrit, and S. G. Lalka, "Primary aortic mural thrombus: presentation and treatment," *Annals of Vascular Surgery*, vol. 13, no. 1, pp. 52–59, 1999.

[19] E. M. Choukroun, L. M. Labrousse, F. P. Madonna, and C. Deville, "Mobile thrombus of the thoracic aorta: diagnosis and treatment in 9 cases," *Annals of Vascular Surgery*, vol. 16, no. 6, pp. 714–722, 2002.

30

A Case of Spontaneous Coronary Artery Dissection in a Patient with Severe Anorexia Nervosa

Jessica O'Neil,[1] **Soumyaa Mazumder**,[2] **Danita Yoerger Sanborn**,[1,3] **and Samantha Wu**[1,4]

[1]*Department of Medicine, Massachusetts General Hospital, Massachusetts, USA*
[2]*Harvard Medical School, Massachusetts, USA*
[3]*Department of Cardiology, Massachusetts General Hospital, Massachusetts, USA*
[4]*Hospital Medicine Unit Massachusetts General Hospital, Massachusetts, USA*

Correspondence should be addressed to Jessica O'Neil; joneil@mgh.harvard.edu

Academic Editor: Tong Liu

There are a variety of cardiac complications of anorexia nervosa including arrythmias, valvopathies, and myopathies. Spontaneous coronary artery dissection (SCAD) has not been widely reported among this patient population. This case report describes a middle-aged female with severe anorexia nervosa, who presented after being found unconscious, and was later diagnosed with SCAD. A literature review revealed one previous case of SCAD in a patient with anorexia nervosa and prompted a discussion of a series of possible predisposing factors for SCAD in this patient population. Patients with anorexia nervosa may be at increased risk for SCAD due to their complex nutritional and endocrine imbalances. This case highlights a possible underdiagnosed cardiac complication of anorexia nervosa.

1. Introduction

SCAD is a significant cause of acute coronary syndrome (ACS) in young and middle-aged women, accounting for nearly a quarter of ACS in women under the age of 50 [1]. Although advances in intracoronary imaging have helped increase the recognition of SCAD, it continues to be underdiagnosed [2]. SCAD has primarily been associated with predisposing arteriopathies (e.g., fibromuscular dysplasia and connective tissue disorders), high-stress conditions (e.g., intense exercise and significant emotional stress), and hormonal triggers (e.g., pregnancy). There has been little reported about the connection between SCAD and AN. AN is an illness marked by several nutritional and endocrine imbalances. It is associated with a number of cardiovascular complications including arrhythmias, heart failure, valvular disease, and sudden cardiac death [3]. This case raises the question of whether SCAD is an underappreciated diagnosis amongst patients with AN and may contribute to the high rate of cardiac morbidities in this population.

2. Case Presentation

A 55-year-old woman with a severe anorexia nervosa (AN) was found unresponsive for an unknown period of time with hypoglycemia (POCT glucose 14 mg/dL) and hypothermia (90.2°F). Her mentation and temperature normalized with intravenous dextrose and rewarming. She did not recall the events leading up to her presentation. She denied suicidal ideation or intentional ingestion. She reported previous mild dyspnea on exertion but denied chest pain. A few weeks prior to her presentation her father passed away leading to significant emotional stress. She was diagnosed with AN at age 18 which was primarily restrictive subtype; however, she did report prior episodes of purging. Her medical history also included hypothyroidism, for which she was on 125 mcg levothyroxine daily, hyponatremia, and iron deficiency anemia. On examination, she weighed 35 kg with a body mass index (BMI) of 12. Cardiac exam revealed regular rate and rhythm, normal S1 and S2, no murmurs, and no jugular venous distension. There was pitting edema to her ankles

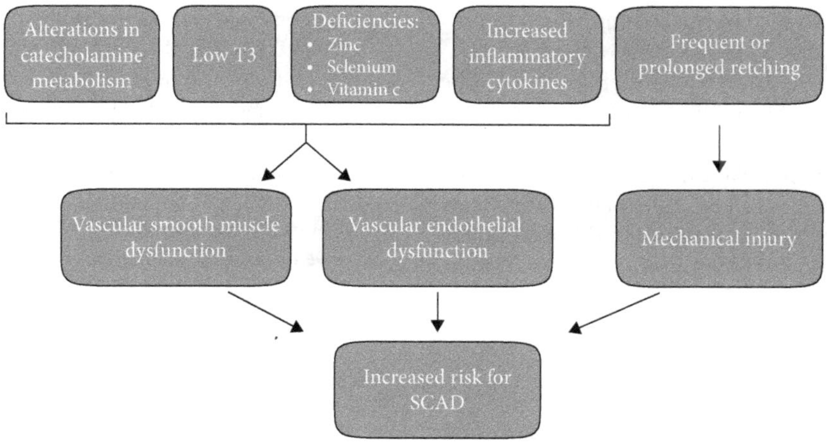

FIGURE 1: Hypothesized stressors predisposing to SCAD in patients with severe anorexia nervosa.

bilaterally. She was also noted to have gingival swelling and a petechial rash over her lower extremities, raising clinical concern for scurvy.

Laboratory values revealed hypomagnesemia (1.5 mmol/L), hypocalcemia (6.5 mgl/dL), and hypoalbuminemia (2.7 g/dL). Serum creatinine was 0.84 mg/dL. Thyroid-stimulating hormone (TSH) was within normal limits (1.27 uIU/mL) and triiodothyronine (T3) was at the lower bound of the normal range (76 ng/dL) though free thyroxine (FT4) was elevated to 3.3 ng/dL. This was attributed to a supratherapeutic dose of levothyroxine. Vitamin C (0.3 mg/dL) and 25-OH vitamin D (21.9 ng/mL) levels were low. Investigation also demonstrated an elevation in high sensitivity troponin elevated to 129 ng/L peaking to 364 ng/dL. ECG revealed Q-waves and ST elevation in leads V1-V3 c/w a septal infarct, new compared to an ECG from 4 months prior. Transthoracic echocardiogram (TTE) revealed an ejection fraction of 52% with akinesis of the septum at the midventricular level and hypokinesis of the apical septum. There was moderate mitral regurgitation. These abnormalities were new compared to a TTE from 2 years prior. A computed tomography coronary angiogram showed no atherosclerosis but demonstrated a linear hypodensity within the proximal segment of the first septal perforator artery and abrupt tapering of the vessel 5 mm from the origin consistent with SCAD. Cardiology was consulted and recommended conservative therapy with initiation of aspirin, metoprolol, and cardiac rehabilitation.

3. Discussion

SCAD is caused by the formation of an intramural hematoma (IMH) within the coronary artery wall that compresses the true lumen leading to ischemia. There are two leading theories describing of how the IMH arises: (1) it develops from damage to the vascular endothelium (possibly from an intimal tear), allowing blood to pool in a false lumen, or (2) the IMH forms following a spontaneous rupture of the vasa vasorum within the arterial wall [4]. There has been one previously reported case of SCAD in a patient with AN [5]. Sedham et al. postulated that hormonal imbalances in anorexia may contribute to poor smooth muscle development, leading to increased risk for arterial dissection. Vascular endothelial dysfunction is hypothesized to play a role in SCAD. A number of endocrine functions frequently altered in severe anorexia, support vascular endothelial health. Derangements in the hypothalamic-pituitary-thyroid axis often manifest in severe anorexia nervosa with low triiodothyronine (T3). T3 enhances endothelial and smooth muscle function and low T3 levels have a demonstrated association with cardiovascular disease [6]. However, thyroid function tests in this patient were confounded by a supratherapeutic levothyroxine dose. Significant changes in catecholamine metabolism have been observed in patients with AN when weight is 20% below ideal body weight [7]. Catecholamine surges have been previously implicated in the pathophysiology of SCAD. In fact, Chow et al. proposed that surges in catecholamines lead to vascular myointimal dysplasia and this may underlie the association observed between emotional stress and SCAD [8]. Additionally, estradiol levels are also often blunted in AN, and estradiol is protective of the vascular endothelium in several animal models [9].

A number of micronutrients often deficient in AN are important for vascular endothelial health. Zinc and selenium deficiencies are common in patients with severe anorexia [10] and have both been implicated as a mediator of inflammation in endothelial function [6, 11]. Vitamin C also has a well-established role in the development and maintenance of endothelial cells and the vascular basement membrane [12]. Recent studies have shown that patients with AN generally have increased inflammatory cytokines [13, 14]. This state of increased inflammation could lead to endothelial dysfunction, weakening the vascular intimal layer and predisposing to the development of SCAD. Finally, patients with AN may be at risk to mechanical injury to the vasculature. Prolonged retching, a behavior observed in patients with purging subtypes of eating disorders, has been identified as a precipitating factor in SCAD cases [15].

Figure 1 summarizes the proposed endocrine, nutritional, and physical stressors present in patients with severe anorexia that may predispose this population to SCAD. Considering our patient, it is possible that her preceding emotional and physical stress triggered her development of SCAD though she may have been predisposed to this injury due to her state of chronic severe malnutrition, endocrine dysregulation, and history of purging leading to a compromised vascular endothelium. This case adds to the one previously reported case of SCAD in AN. Further studies will be needed to understand whether patients with AN may be at increased risk for SCAD and may contribute to the high cardiac comorbidities in this population. Better understanding the relationship between AN and SCAD could inform treatment strategies aimed at the prevention of this potentially life-threatening cardiovascular complication.

References

[1] J. Saw, E. Aymong, G. B. Mancini, T. Sedlak, A. Starovoytov, and D. Ricci, "Nonatherosclerotic coronary artery disease in young women," *The Canadian Journal of Cardiology*, vol. 30, no. 7, pp. 814–819, 2014.

[2] A. Yip and J. Saw, "Spontaneous coronary artery dissection-a review," *Cardiovascular Diagnosis and Therapy*, vol. 5, no. 1, pp. 37–48, 2015.

[3] B. Jáuregui-Garrido and I. Jáuregui-Lobera, "Sudden death in eating disorders," *Vascular Health and Risk Management*, vol. 8, pp. 91–98, 2012.

[4] S. N. Hayes, E. S. H. Kim, J. Saw et al., "Spontaneous coronary artery dissection: current state of the science: a scientific statement from the American Heart Association," *Circulation*, vol. 137, no. 19, pp. e523–e557, 2018.

[5] D. Sedhom, E. Hiltner, C. Patel, and J. Prister, "Spontaneous coronary artery dissection in an anorexic patient: a rare and challenging case," *American Journal of Respiratory and Critical Care Medicine*, vol. 197, p. A3449, 2018.

[6] R. Napoli, V. Guardasole, V. Angelini et al., "Acute effects of triiodothyronine on endothelial function in human subjects," *The Journal of Clinical Endocrinology and Metabolism*, vol. 92, no. 1, pp. 250–254, 2007.

[7] H. A. Gross, C. R. Lake, M. H. Ebert, M. G. Ziegler, and I. J. Kopin, "Catecholamine metabolism in primary anorexia nervosa," *The Journal of Clinical Endocrinology and Metabolism*, vol. 49, no. 6, pp. 805–809, 1979.

[8] L. T. C. Chow and M. B. C. Y. Chow, "Coronary artery myointimal dysplasia in patients with pheochromocytoma—possible causal relationship: pathophysiology and clinical implication with reference to Takotsubo cardiomyopathy and spontaneous coronary dissection," *Cardiovascular Pathology*, vol. 37, pp. 45–53, 2018.

[9] T. Tolbert and S. Oparil, "Cardiovascular effects of estrogen," *American Journal of Hypertension*, vol. 14, no. 11, pp. S186–S193, 2001.

[10] M. Hanachi, M. Dicembre, C. Rives-Lange et al., "Micronutrients deficiencies in 374 severely malnourished anorexia nervosa inpatients," *Nutrients*, vol. 11, no. 4, p. 792, 2019.

[11] P. J. Little, R. Bhattacharya, A. E. Moreyra, and I. L. Korichneva, "Zinc and cardiovascular disease," *Nutrition*, vol. 26, no. 11-12, pp. 1050–1057, 2010.

[12] A. W. Ashor, M. Siervo, J. Lara, C. Oggioni, S. Afshar, and J. C. Mathers, "Effect of vitamin C and vitamin E supplementation on endothelial function: a systematic review and meta-analysis of randomised controlled trials," *The British Journal of Nutrition*, vol. 113, no. 8, pp. 1182–1194, 2015.

[13] M. Solmi, N. Veronese, A. Favaro et al., "Inflammatory cytokines and anorexia nervosa: a meta-analysis of cross-sectional and longitudinal studies," *Psychoneuroendocrinology*, vol. 51, pp. 237–252, 2015.

[14] B. Dalton, I. C. Campbell, R. Chung, G. Breen, U. Schmidt, and H. Himmerich, "Inflammatory markers in anorexia nervosa: an exploratory study," *Nutrients*, vol. 10, no. 11, p. 1573, 2018.

[15] M. Velusamy, M. Fisherkeller, M. E. Keenan, F. J. Kiernan, and D. B. Fram, "Spontaneous coronary artery dissection in a young woman precipitated by retching," *The Journal of Invasive Cardiology*, vol. 14, no. 4, pp. 198–201, 2002.

31

An Unusual Case of Ventricular Tachycardia in a Young Patient Associated with Cannabis Use

Parth J. Sampat,[1] Sana Riaz,[1] Maneesh Bisen,[1] and Robert Carhart[2]

[1]*Department of Medicine, SUNY Upstate Medical University, Syracuse, NY, USA*
[2]*Department of Cardiology, SUNY Upstate Medical University, Syracuse, NY, USA*

Correspondence should be addressed to Parth J. Sampat; sampatp@upstate.edu

Academic Editor: Christopher S. Snyder

Marijuana has become the most widely used illicit drug in the United States. Approximately 43.5 million Americans aged 12 or above have reported the use of marijuana in the last year. The use of cannabinoids and its relationship with cardiac effects are not well known. Many types of arrhythmias have been noted with the use of cannabis products with atrial fibrillation being the most common arrhythmia associated with the use of cannabis. We present a case of a 36-year-old male who presented with pounding chest pain, dyspnea, and diaphoresis following marijuana use. He was found to be in ventricular tachycardia which responded to amiodarone. Workup done was negative for any structural disease, and cardiac catheterization was negative for coronary artery disease. He was ultimately discharged on metoprolol. In this report, we focus on how marijuana can be associated with many arrhythmias including ventricular tachycardia with focus on mechanisms by which it can occur. We believe a detailed social history with screening for cannabis use can identify more cases of arrhythmias that can be potentially associated with marijuana use.

1. Introduction

Marijuana has become the most used illicit substance in the United States [1]. Approximately 43.5 million Americans aged 12 or above have reported the use of marijuana in the last year [1]. Cannabinoids have various cardiovascular effects and involve the autonomic function in central and peripheral nervous systems and its direct effect on the myocardium [2]. There have been reports of multiple types of arrhythmias with the use of marijuana [3]. In one study, the prevalence of any type of arrhythmia with the use of marijuana has been found to be 4.66%, with atrial fibrillation having highest prevalence with the use of marijuana and ventricular tachycardia being associated 0.69% of the times [4]. In another paper, it was found that 2.7 percent of marijuana users developed arrhythmia [5]. There have also been reported cases of Brugada pattern on EKG with marijuana use [6–9]. A few cases of ventricular tachycardia and cardiac arrest have also been associated with marijuana use [10–14]. We present a case of a patient who presented with ventricular tachycardia in the setting of marijuana use and found to have no other cause of ventricular tachycardia.

2. Case Presentation

A 36-year-old male with past medical history most significant for morbid obesity, obstructive sleep apnea, and marijuana use disorder presented to the hospital with complaints of pounding chest pain and shortness of breath. He was sitting on his couch and smoking marijuana, after which he developed a pounding sensation in his chest, dyspnea, and diaphoresis that lasted approximately 30 seconds after which emergency medical service was called. His symptoms had resolved by the time he reached the hospital. After reaching the emergency room, his symptoms returned, and he was found to be in a monomorphic wide-complex tachycardia at a ventricular rate of 240 beats per minute (Figure 1) and was saturating at 89% at room air. His blood pressure was 133/84 mmHg and had

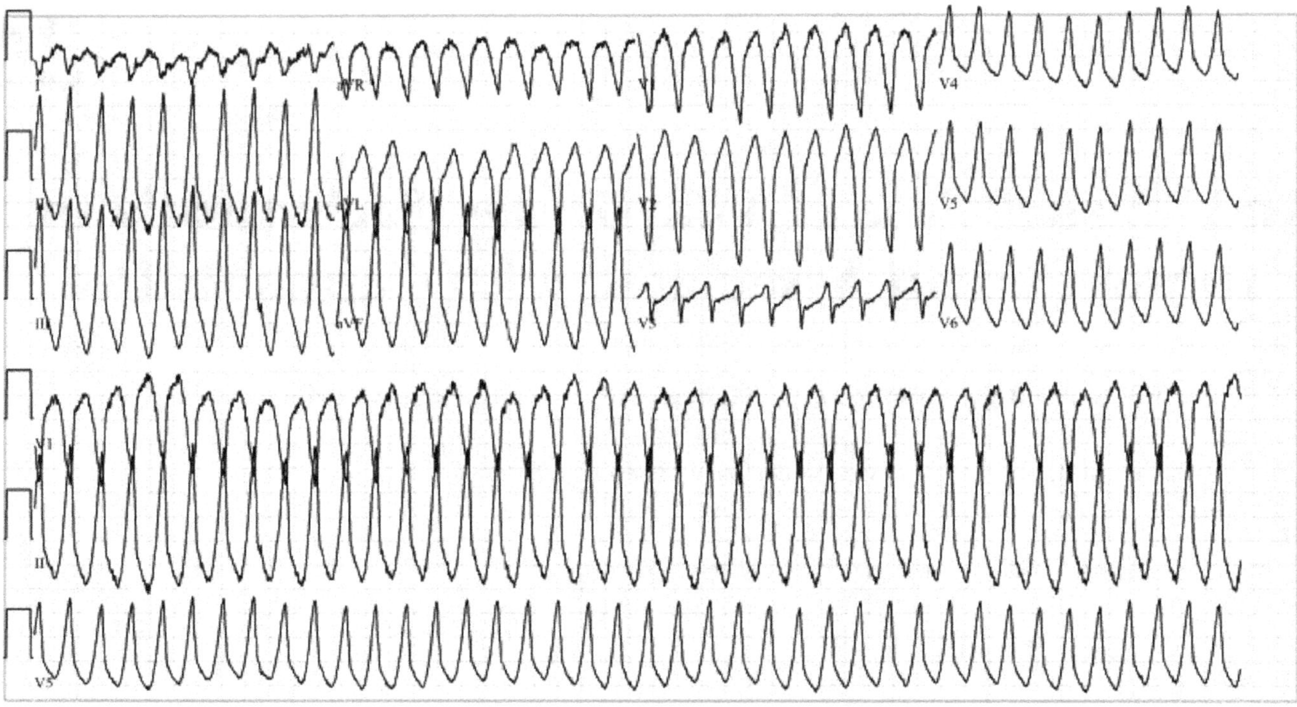

FIGURE 1: EKG showing right ventricular outflow tract ventricular tachycardia with left bundle branch pattern and inferior axis pattern.

a respiratory rate of 16. He was started on IV amiodarone 150 mg over 10 minutes and was continued on a drip with a rate on 1 mg/min, which resolved the arrhythmia after the initial bolus (Figure 2). He smokes 3 g marijuana daily. He denied the use of any drugs other than marijuana. He also denied any history of arrhythmia in the family.

An extensive workup was performed to find the cause of ventricular tachycardia. A urine toxicology report was significant only for cannabinoids in urine. Urine metanephrines and normetanephrines were within normal range. Serum magnesium was 1.7 mg/dL; potassium was 4.6 mmol/L at the time of admission. Troponin T levels were trended which remained negative for three occurrences. TSH was 0.903 IU/ml. Morning cortisol was 9.4 microgram/dL. Cardiac catheterization was performed to rule out ischemic causes of ventricular tachycardia, which showed normal coronaries. Echocardiogram obtained showed a left ventricular ejection fraction of 55-60% with normal valvular function, and no structural disease noted on echocardiogram. He was monitored on cardiac telemetry throughout his hospital course, and he was not found to have any further episodes of ventricular arrhythmias or ectopy.

With the consideration of ventricular tachycardia in a structurally normal heart and no coronary artery disease, he was started on metoprolol succinate 25 mg daily and was discharged with outpatient follow-up. He was provided education regarding marijuana cessation and was discussed.

He did undergo an electrophysiology study after discharge, which did not reveal any inducible ventricular or supraventricular tachycardia. A cardiac magnetic resonance imaging (MRI) was offered to the patient for further workup of arrhythmia; however, patient declined further workup. He has been continued on metoprolol succinate 25 mg and has remained asymptomatic since then.

3. Discussion

With workup largely negative, we believe that marijuana could have a potential role in the development of ventricular tachycardia in our patient.

Cannabis has over 400 active chemical entities with tetrahydrocannabinol (THC) being the most active chemical [15]. THC acts upon cannabinoid receptors CB_1 and CB_2 causing its effects on the heart. [2]

Mechanisms by which arrhythmias occur after use of marijuana remain unknown; however, multiple mechanisms have been proposed. The arrhythmogenic effects secondary to cannabis use may be related to its biphasic effects on the autonomic nervous system of the heart [16]. Lower doses cause sympathetic stimulation leading to tachycardia and increase in cardiac output, whereas higher doses cause parasympathetic stimulation [16]. Other likely mechanisms are increased myocardial oxygen demand, increased platelet activation, and coronary vasospasm leading to ischemic environment which can likely induce ischemia-induced arrhythmias even with the presence of nonobstructive coronary arteries [3]. Ischemia-induced arrhythmias can occur due to multiple mechanisms including damage to ion channels [17]. Decreased coronary flow has also been described in one care report associated with ventricular tachycardia and cannabis use [13].

With the increase in the use of marijuana, it is imperative to study the cardiovascular effects of marijuana. Even though our case does not show a causal effect of marijuana causing ventricular tachycardia, it is important to consider substance use when evaluating any type of arrhythmia. Screening of drug use by history and laboratory tests become essential in these situations.

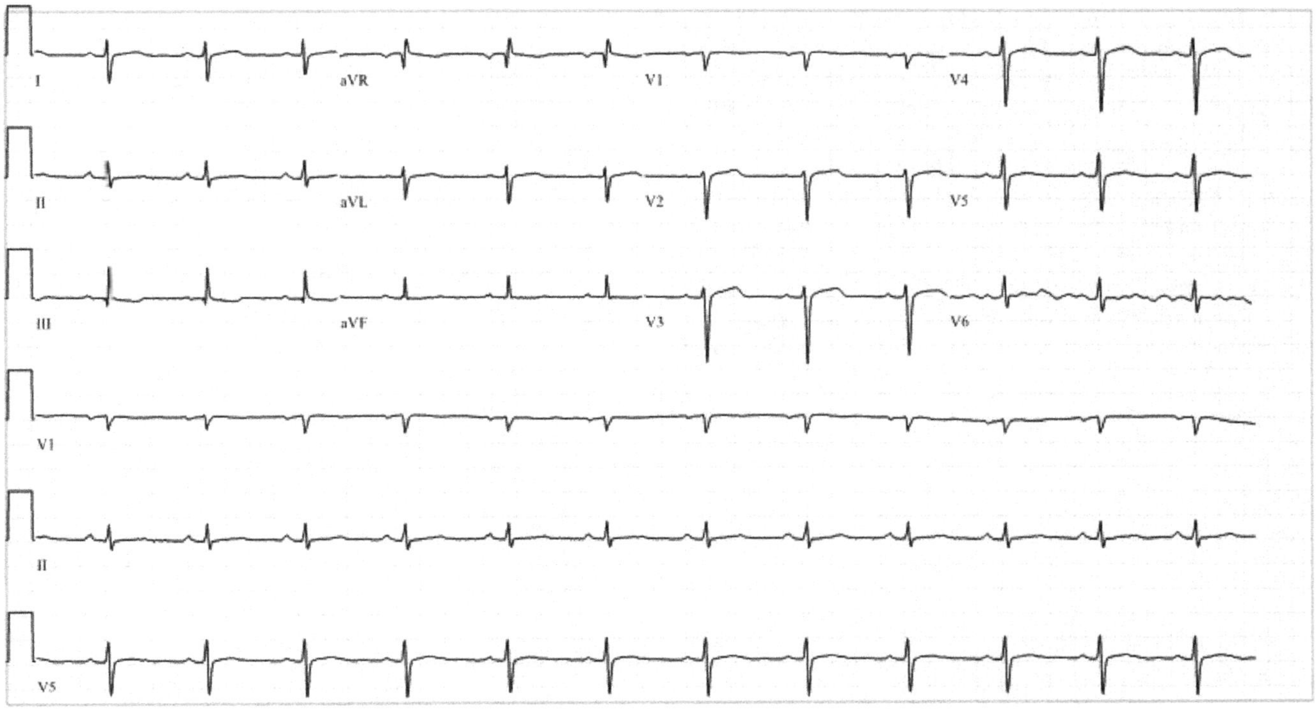

Figure 2: EKG showing normal sinus rhythm.

4. Conclusion

Given various association of marijuana with cardiovascular effects in literature, we conclude that a detailed social history with screening for cannabis use by history of laboratory tests including urine toxicology studies can be helpful in determining the etiology of a new onset arrhythmia. More studies are required to prove association of marijuana with ventricular tachycardia.

Authors' Contributions

Parth Sampat contributed to the conceptualizing and writing the original draft. Sana Riaz contributed to the writing the original draft. Maneesh Bisen contributed to the reviewing and editing. Robert Carhart contributed to the supervising and reviewing.

References

[1] R. N. Lipari, "Park-Lee E. Key substance use and mental health indicators in the United States: results from the 2018 National Survey on Drug Use and Health2019, May 7, 2020 https://www.samhsa gov/data/.

[2] P. Pacher, S. Bátkai, and G. Kunos, "Cardiovascular pharmacology of cannabinoids," *Handbook of Experimental Pharmacology*, vol. 168, pp. 599–625, 2005.

[3] P. T. Kariyanna, P. Wengrofsky, A. Jayarangaiah et al., "Marijuana and Cardiac Arrhythmias: A Scoping Study," *International Journal of Clinical Research & Trials*, vol. 4, no. 1, 2019.

[4] A. Goel, S. Kadavath, F. Habash, H. Paydak, and J. Mehta, "BURDEN and impact of arrhythmias in marijuana users across the UNITED STATES," *Journal of the American College of Cardiology*, vol. 73, no. 9, p. 467, 2019.

[5] R. Desai, U. Patel, A. Deshmukh, R. Sachdeva, and G. Kumar, "Burden of arrhythmia in recreational marijuana users," *International Journal of Cardiology*, vol. 264, pp. 91-92, 2018.

[6] J. Cardiol, C. Ther, T. Doctorian, and E. Chou, "Case report cannabis-induced Brugada syndrome presenting as cardiac arrest," May 11, 2020 https://juniperpublishers.com/online-submission.php.

[7] A. J. Romero-Puche, N. Trigueros-Ruiz, M. C. Cerdán-Sánchez, F. Pérez-Lorente, D. Roldán, and T. Vicente-Vera, "Patrón electrocardiográfico de Brugada inducido por cannabis," *Revista Española de Cardiología*, vol. 65, no. 9, pp. 856–858, 2012.

[8] J. V. Alonso, B. H.-Y. Teo, F. J. F. del Pozo, M. A. Aguayo, and A. Sanchez, "Brugada electrocardiogram pattern induced by cannabis; is cannabis safe? Am," *The American Journal of Emergency Medicine*, vol. 34, pp. 1738.e1–1738.e4, 2016.

[9] A. Akinlonu, R. Suri, P. Yerragorla et al., "Brugada Phenocopy Induced by Recreational Drug Use," *Case Reports in Cardiology*, vol. 2018, 4 pages, 2018.

[10] I. J. Sánchez Lázaro, L. Almenar Bonet, M. José Sancho-Tello, and L. Martínez-Dolz, "Taquicardia Ventricular por cannabis en trasplantado cardiaco," *Revista Española de Cardiología*, vol. 62, no. 4, pp. 459–461, 2009.

[11] S. T. Şengül, M. Erat, İ. Guliyev, V. O. Tanık, and M. Tulmaç, "Cannabis-Induced Ventricular Tachycardia Leading to Death in an Old Man," *The American Journal of Cardiology*, vol. 121, no. 8, p. e121, 2018.

[12] M. Diffley, P. Armenian, R. Gerona, O. Reinhartz, and K. Avasarala, "Catecholaminergic polymorphic ventricular tachycardia found in an adolescent after a methylenedioxymethamphetamine and marijuana-induced cardiac arrest," *Critical Care Medicine*, vol. 40, pp. 2223–2226, 2012.

[13] S. H. Rezkalla, P. Sharma, and R. A. Kloner, "Coronary no-flow and ventricular tachycardia associated with habitual marijuana use," *Annals of Emergency Medicine*, vol. 42, pp. 365–369, 2003.

[14] B. Hartung, S. Kauferstein, S. Ritz-Timme, and T. Daldrup, "Sudden unexpected death under acute influence of cannabis," *Forensic Science International*, vol. 237, pp. e11–e13, 2014.

[15] Z. Atakan, "Cannabis, a complex plant: different compounds and different effects on individuals," *Therapeutic Advances in Psychopharmacology*, vol. 2, no. 6, pp. 241–254, 2012.

[16] B. A. C. Fisher, A. Ghuran, V. Vadamalai, and T. F. Antonios, "Cardiovascular complications induced by cannabis smoking: a case report and review of the literature," *Emergency Medicine Journal*, vol. 22, no. 9, pp. 679-680, 2005.

[17] E. Carmeliet, "Cardiac ionic currents and acute ischemia: from channels to arrhythmias," *Physiological Reviews*, vol. 79, no. 3, pp. 917–1017, 1999.

32

Lactococcus garvieae: An Uncommon Human Pathogen Causing Infective Endocarditis in a Valve-in-Valve Transcatheter Aortic Valve Replacement

Diego H. González-Bravo,[1] Sergio Alegre-Boschetti,[1] Richard Silva-Cantillo,[1] Joshua Mercado-Maldonado,[1] Reyshley Ramos-Márquez,[2] Gabriel Torres-Rivera,[2] Carlos Cortés,[3] and Josue Mercado-Crespo[1]

[1]*Cardiovascular Division, Department of Medicine, VA Caribbean Healthcare System, San Juan, Puerto Rico*
[2]*Internal Medicine Division, Department of Medicine, VA Caribbean Healthcare System, San Juan, Puerto Rico*
[3]*Internal Medicine and Nephrology Division, Department of Medicine, VA Caribbean Healthcare System, San Juan, Puerto Rico*

Correspondence should be addressed to Diego H. González-Bravo; diego.gonzalez1@upr.edu

Academic Editor: Tong Liu

Lactococcus garvieae is a fish pathogen and an uncommon cause of human infections. There is a growing body of evidence showing its potential for causing endocarditis especially in those with prior valve surgery. In this case report, we present what we believe is the first case of endocarditis by *L. garvieae* affecting a valve-in-valve transcatheter aortic valve replacement that was successfully treated. Specific guidelines for the management of these patients are lacking. Our experience can contribute to the current knowledge regarding this life-threatening infection as well as to the future care of these patients. We aim to emphasize that despite not being recognized as a typical endocarditis microorganism by the Duke Criteria, the possibility of endocarditis needs to be highly entertained in patients with *L. garvieae* bacteremia, especially when prosthetic valves are present. Consequently, clinicians should pursue further this diagnosis with transesophageal echocardiogram and/or alternative imaging modalities (e.g., PET-CT scan and MRI) regardless of an initial negative transthoracic echocardiogram. Reaching a diagnosis of *L. garvieae* endocarditis led us to the decision of prolonging the antibiotic course for 6 weeks with successful results. Ultimately, surgery was not required owing to the absence of prosthetic aortic valve dysfunction and paravalvular extension of the infection.

1. Introduction

Lactococcus garvieae is a gram-positive coccus (Figure 1) and catalase-negative bacterium known for producing fish infection outbreaks in warm waters (rainbow trout) [1–3]. Its zoonotic potential was unknown until recently when multiple case reports have shown the spectrum of pathogenic capabilities of this bacterium, capable of causing urinary tract infections, liver abscess, and most importantly infective endocarditis (IE) [3–6].

Human consumption of raw seafood seems to be the main contamination source; nonetheless, infection from unpasteurized dairy products has also been described [2–4]. Other risk factors for infection are an immunosuppressed state, prior heart valve surgery, and the presence of gastrointestinal diseases that compromise the mucosal lining integrity (polyps, diverticulosis, peptic ulcers, and gastroesophageal reflux disease [GERD]) [2, 4].

We present a case that we believe is the first instance of *L. garvieae* endocarditis in a valve-in-valve transcatheter aortic valve replacement (TAVR). We aim to raise awareness about the potential for endocarditis of this blooming human pathogen as we discuss its diagnosis and our treatment experience.

2. Case Presentation

2.1. History of Present Illness. A 78-year-old man who presented with a one-day history of fever, chills, and altered

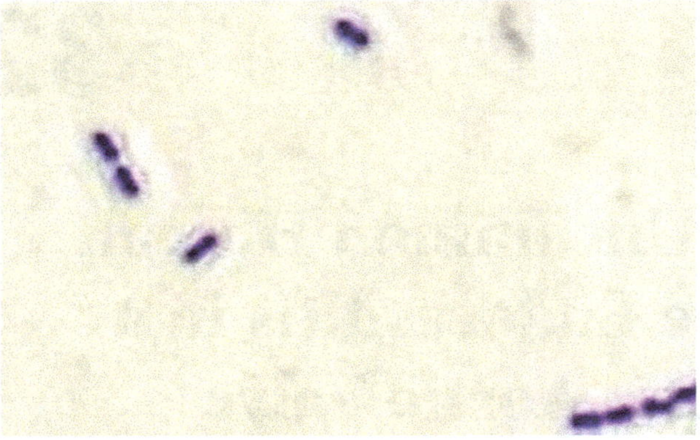

Figure 1: Microscopy. Gram-stain smear (1000× magnification) showing gram-positive (violet) cocci in chains consistent with *Lactococcus garvieae.*

mental status (AMS) preceded by 7 days of malaise and anorexia. At the emergency room (ER), he was found normotensive (107/67 mmHg), afebrile (37.1°C), not hypoxic (98%), and without tachypnea (19 rpm), yet tachycardia (131 bpm) was present. He was disoriented and lethargic but showed no focal neurological deficit nor signs of meningeal irritation. His heart rhythm was irregular, and a systolic ejection murmur (II/VI) was present at the right upper sternal border. Jugular venous distension was not evident, and his extremities were warm and without edema. His abdomen was nontender. Lungs were clear to auscultation, and no skin stigmata for endocarditis was appreciated (splinter hemorrhages, Osler, and Janeway lesions). Recent surgeries, new medications, travels, and toxic habits were all denied.

2.2. Past Medical History. His medical history was remarkable for essential hypertension, dyslipidemia, GERD, atrial fibrillation (afib) on chronic anticoagulation (apixaban 5 mg twice per day), and a bioprosthetic surgical aortic valve replacement (SAVR) in 2008 followed by valve-in-valve TAVR (2017) two years prior to presentation. Dietary habits included regular consumption of raw salmon.

2.3. Investigations. Initial electrocardiogram (Figure 2) showed afib with a fast ventricular response (FVR), without chest pain or new ST-segment changes compelling for an acute coronary syndrome. Chest X-ray (Figure 3) and head CT scan were negative for acute pathologies. However, mild leukocytosis ($11.3 \times 10^3/\mu L$) with neutrophilia, elevated ESR (72 mm/1Hr), CRP (214.7 mg/L), and procalcitonin levels (0.20 ng/mL) were present, all suggestive of an underlying bacterial infection. His toxicology, urinalysis, and HIV tests were unremarkable.

2.4. Differential Diagnosis and Management. His encephalopathy in the context of afib was worrisome for stroke; however, no focal neurological deficits were found, plus his head CT scan was negative, and he had been compliant with anticoagulation therapy. His laboratories and tachycardia suggested an underlying bacterial infection of unclear foci. At first, meningoencephalitis was contemplated although meningeal irritation signs were missing. A lumbar puncture was attempted but ultimately deferred as the patient became aggressive and uncooperative with the procedure. As per the sepsis protocol, the patient was pan-cultured, resuscitated with intravenous (IV) fluids, and started on broad-spectrum IV antibiotics (vancomycin and cefepime). Acyclovir was added given the possibility of herpetic meningoencephalitis.

Subsequently, blood cultures (4/4) grew *Lactococcus garvieae* (Figure 1). Transthoracic echocardiogram (TTE) revealed no prosthetic aortic valve dysfunction nor large vegetations (Figure 4). Nonetheless, a transesophageal echocardiogram (TEE) showed a pedunculated/oscillating echodense structure measuring 0.7 cm in its largest dimension attached to the right coronary cusp of the TAVR consistent with vegetation (Figure 5, Video 1). There were no cusp perforations, significant valvular insufficiencies, paravalvular abscess or leaks, nor evidence of valve thrombosis (normal valve hemodynamics by Doppler, plus valve was bioprosthetic and not mechanical, and patient was compliant with chronic anticoagulation).

3. Discussion

Prosthetic valve endocarditis (PVE) accounts for only 10-30% of all cases of infective endocarditis (IE) with an incidence of 1-6%, affecting the TAVR and SAVR population to a similar extent [7, 8]. It is believed to be the worst presentation of IE, a life-threatening infection of the lining of the heart (endocardium) that can lead to systemic embolization, valve destruction, heart failure, and death [9]. Most cases of PVE are caused by the typical endocarditis microorganisms: *Staphylococcus aureus* or coagulase-negative staphylococci. Nevertheless, in our patient, it was surprisingly caused instead by *Lactococcus garvieae*, a fish pathogen. Our patient's GERD and regular consumption of raw salmon were risk factors for infection.

Lactococcus garvieae is becoming a blooming human pathogen. Its potential for causing endocarditis has been unraveling for the last few years [5, 6]. There are less than 30 cases reported in the available literature, this one being the ninth case involving an aortic valve replacement (AVR), the sixth case reported in the USA, the first one documented in the island of Puerto Rico, and the first one affecting a valve-in-valve TAVR [6]. Multiple cases (20% = 5/25) have also been described in the Asian continent [6]. The incidence and prevalence remain unknown, plus it is believed to be underdiagnosed since misclassification of this pathogen as other gram-positive cocci (enterococci and streptococci) has been commonly described [5]. In our case, mass spectroscopy (MALDI-TOF MS) provided the identity of this unusual pathogen; however, 16 rRNA PCR has also been used successfully [1, 5].

Malek et al. evaluated 25 cases of *L. garvieae* IE and showed that infection affected more commonly older men (median age = 68 years) and most frequently presented as subacute fever with chills (median = 14 days) [5]. A history of valve replacement (8/25 aortic, 5/25 mitral) was identified in 52% of these patients, for which 54% (7/13) of them had evidence of vegetations associated to their prosthetic valves. The native mitral valve (64%) was the most infected valve,

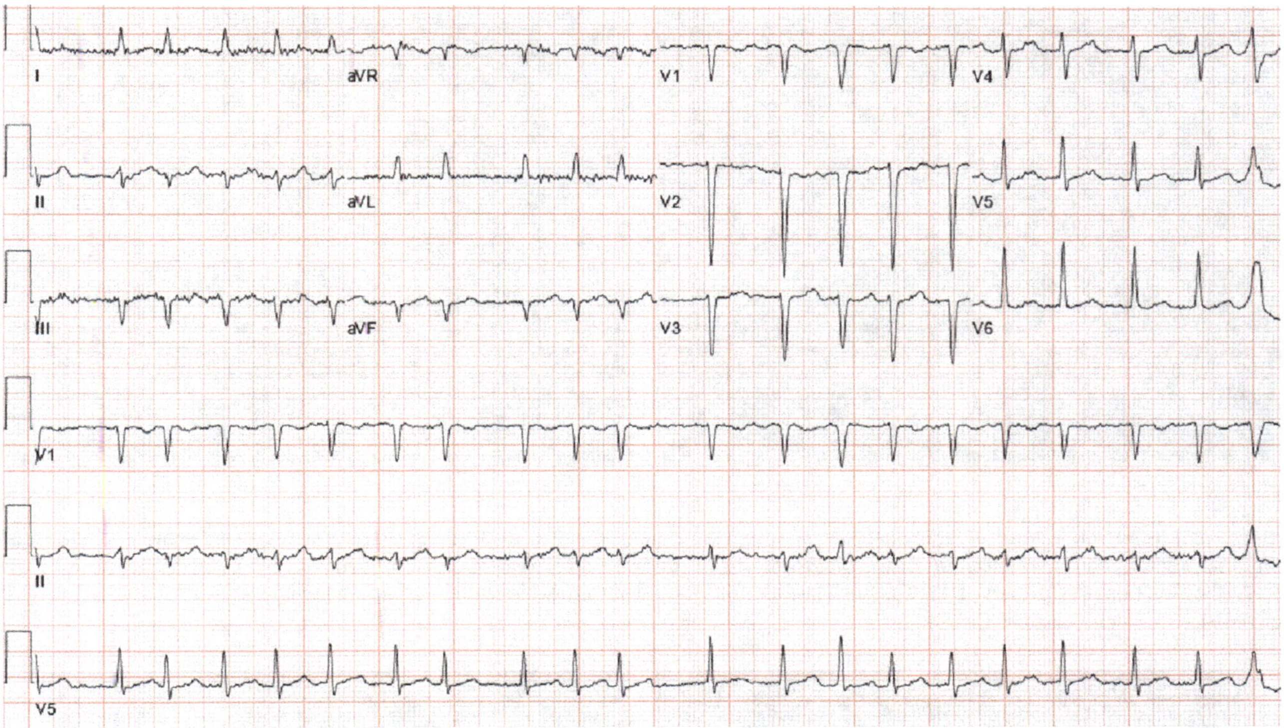

FIGURE 2: Electrocardiogram. Initial electrocardiogram revealing atrial fibrillation with fast ventricular response (126 bpm). There were no new ST-segment changes suggestive of acute ischemia.

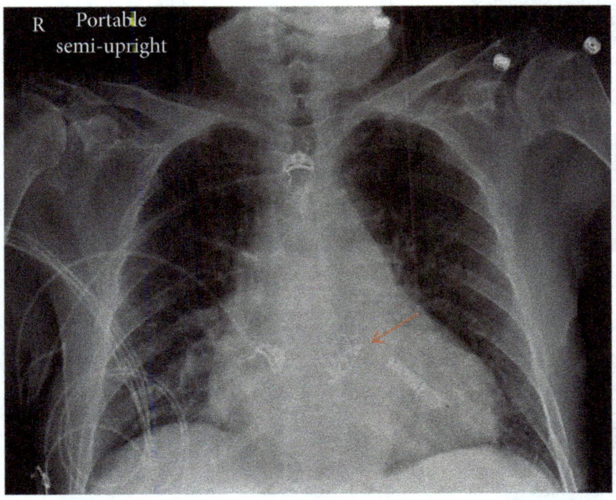

FIGURE 3: Chest X-ray (CXR): there are mildly increased interstitial markings (chronic in character), cardiomegaly, and no evidence of consolidation or pleural effusion. Loop monitor can be visualized in the CXR at the left lower chest wall as well as a valve-in-valve TAVR (red arrow).

even in cases where an AVR was present. Moreover, *L. garvieae* IE seems to have profound implications in terms of morbidity and mortality. The fatality rate was 16%, and half of the patients had complications such as valve dehiscence/rupture, septic emboli, heart failure, stroke, shock, or renal failure. Furthermore, 48% of cases required surgery.

An appropriate diagnosis of IE is done so by using the Duke Criteria (DC) that proposes a definite diagnosis in those with bacteremia and imaging evidence of valvular involvement (vegetations and paravalvular abscess) [9]. Initially, our patient had an unremarkable TTE and unfulfilled DC for definitive endocarditis (only 3 minor criteria were present: atypical microorganism, fever and predisposition/AVR). We were initially hesitant to perform a TEE as this was not a typical endocarditis microorganism (staphylococci and yeast) for which the probability of endocarditis is known to be high. Nevertheless, discovering the growing evidence of IE surrounding this pathogen pushed us to perform the TEE, which provided the major criteria that was missing in order to establish a definitive diagnosis of IE (1 major + 3 minor). Consequently, we want to emphasize that since the risk of endocarditis in these patients seems to be high, it is reasonable to pursue an in-depth evaluation with TEE or alternative imaging modalities (e.g., MRI and PET-CT) before ruling out such diagnosis after an initial negative TTE [9].

Arriving at this diagnosis changed drastically the management of our patient. First, by extending his antibiotic course to 6 weeks instead of providing him with only 2 weeks, as indicated for uncomplicated bacteremia, and second, it prompted cardiothoracic surgery evaluation.

There is no standardized treatment of *L. garvieae* endocarditis due to lack of randomized control trials (RCT), but it has been treated successfully with beta-lactams (ampicillin 2 g q4hrs or ceftriaxone 2 g q12-24 hrs), or vancomycin (30 mg/kg/day divided in 2-3 doses), with or without aminoglycosides (gentamycin 3 mg/kg/day) for 6 weeks [5, 6, 9]. Whether surgery is always required for the treatment of these patients remains elusive.

In general, indications for PVE surgical intervention follow the same principles as for native valve endocarditis [7].

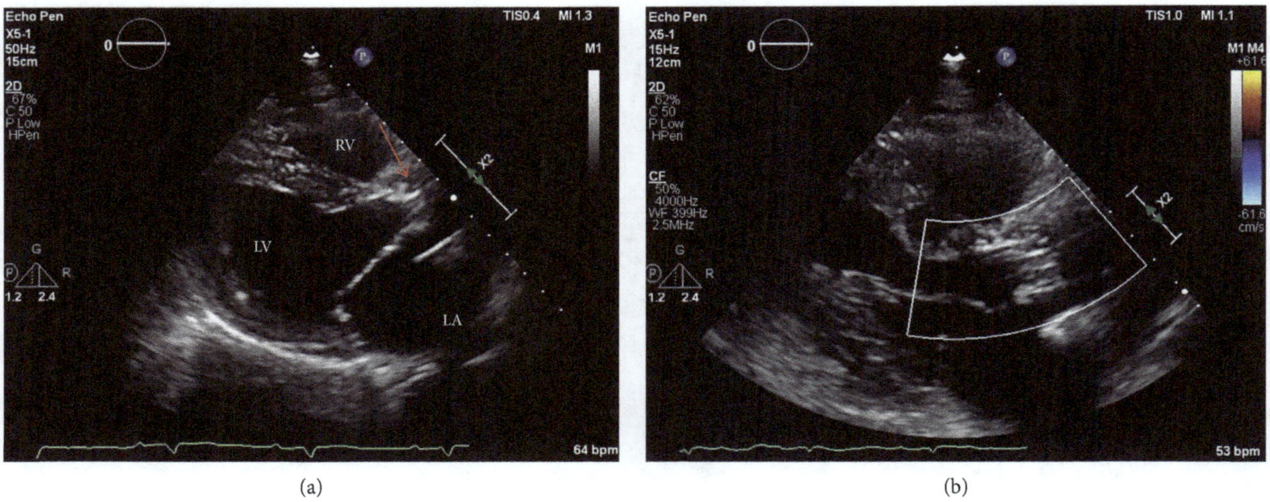

FIGURE 4: Transthoracic echocardiogram parasternal long-axis view. (a) Valve-in-valve TAVR (red arrow) with some artifacts causing suboptimal resolution and visualization of the bioprosthesis, yet no overt large vegetations were detected. No pericardial effusion present and systolic function was preserved (55%). (b) Diastolic frame showing no evidence of significant regurgitation by color Doppler. RV: right ventricle; LV: left ventricle; LA: left atrium.

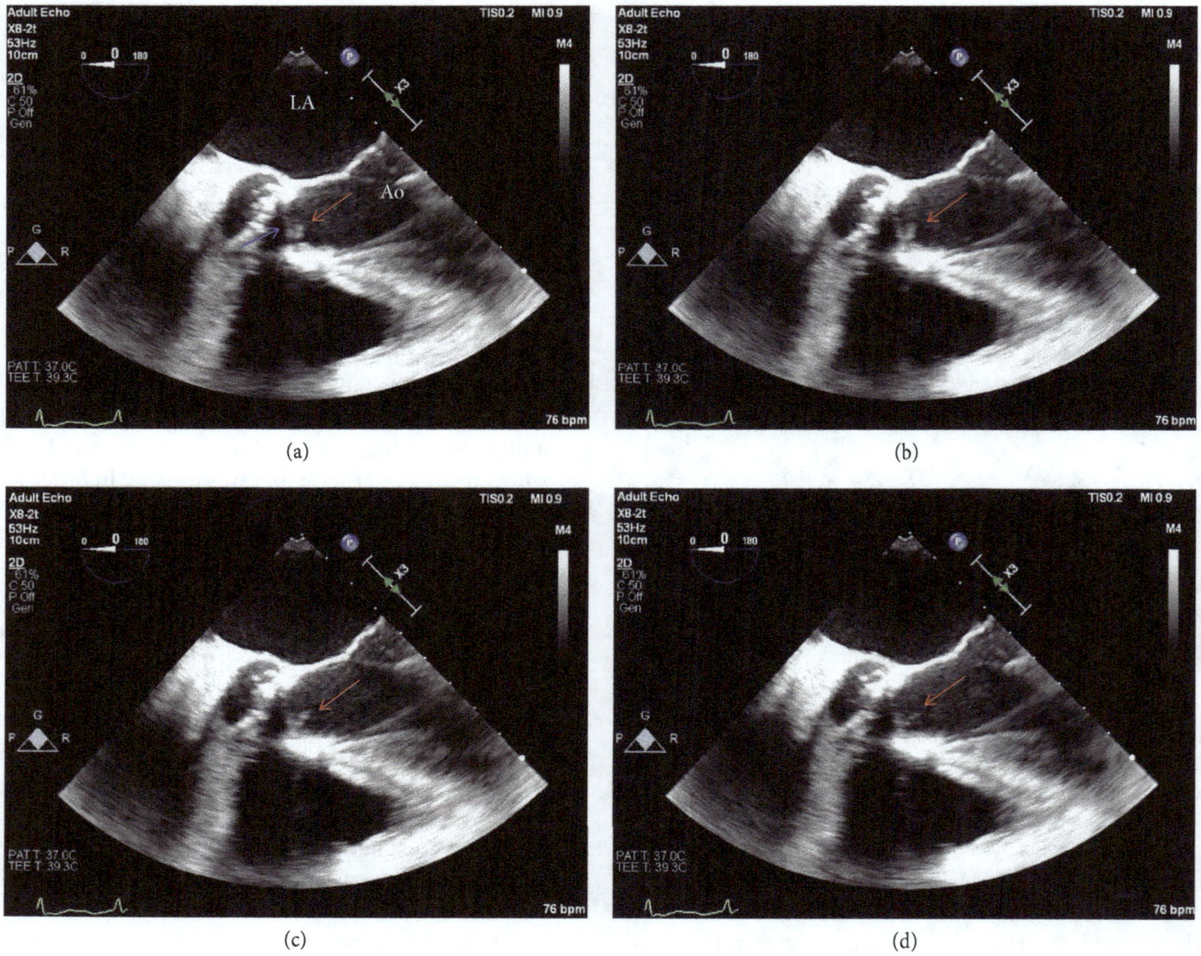

FIGURE 5: Transesophageal echocardiogram (TEE) midesophageal views (Video 1). Various frames of TEE images showing an elongated and oscillating echogenic structure (red arrow) attached to the right coronary cusp leaflet of the valve-in-valve TAVR (blue arrow) consistent with an infective endocarditis vegetation (measuring 0.7 cm). No significant insufficiency or paravalvular extension of infection was detected. No evidence in favor of valvular thrombosis. The other native valves (especially the mitral valve) had no vegetations. LA: left atrium; Ao: ascending aorta.

```
CULTURE RESULTS:  COCCUS, GRAM POSITIVE - Quantity: FROM SET OF BOTTLES
                        Comment: LACTOCOCCUS GARVIEAE
                                 CEFTRIAXONE MIC: 1 (S)
                                 LEVOFLOXACIN MIC: 1 (S)
                                 PENICILLIN MIC: 0.5 (I)


ANTIBIOTIC SUSCEPTIBILITY TEST RESULTS:

                                   COCCUS, GRAM POSITIVE
                                   :
                                   SUSC  INTP
VANCOMYCIN.......................  1     S
```

Figure 6: *Lactococcus garvieae* antimicrobial sensitivities.

Guidelines recommend a heart team-based approach to this decision. Patients who benefit the most from surgery are the ones with highly virulent pathogens (staphylococci or fungi), those with prosthetic valve dysfunction (severe regurgitation, paravalvular abscess/fistula, heart block, dehiscence, and perforation) causing heart failure, persistent bacteremia (after 5-7 days of antibiotics), recurrent embolic events, or vegetations larger than 1 cm [7, 9]. Our patient had none of these complications and since he responded positively to antibiotic therapy with rapid clearance of bacteremia plus subsequent TTE remain essentially unremarkable, the decision was taken in conjunction with a cardiothoracic surgeon to continue conservative management.

4. Follow-Up

Pathogen susceptibility (Figure 6) allowed for de-escalation of antibiotics to ceftriaxone (2 g q12 hrs) achieving sterile blood (hospitalization day #2) and resolution of tachycardia and AMS. He was discharged and completed 6 weeks of IV ceftriaxone at a skilled nursing facility without complications.

5. Conclusions

The possibility of endocarditis needs to be highly entertained when confronting patients with *L. garvieae* bacteremia, especially in the presence of prosthetic heart valves. Therefore, despite an initial negative TTE, the clinician should seek an in-depth evaluation with TEE and/or alternative imaging modalities (e.g., PET-CT, MRI) in view that these patients seem to have a high risk for endocarditis. A missed diagnosis could be fatal since about half of these patients can develop complications and require open-heart surgery. However, we presented a case of *L. garvieae* endocarditis, which we believe is the first one affecting a valve-in-valve TAVR that was successfully treated conservatively and did not develop complications that required surgery possibly due to early identification.

Abbreviations

Afib:	Atrial fibrillation
AMS:	Altered mental status
AVR:	Aortic valve replacement
FVR:	Fast ventricular response
GERD:	Gastroesophageal reflux disease
IE:	Infective endocarditis
MALDI-TOF MS:	Matrix-assisted laser desorption/ionization time-of-flight mass spectrometry
MRI:	Magnetic resonance imaging
PET-CT:	Positron emission tomography-computed tomography
PVE:	Prosthetic valve endocarditis
TAVR:	Transcatheter aortic valve replacement
TEE:	Transesophageal echocardiogram
TTE:	Transthoracic echocardiogram.

Disclosure

The authors have no relationship with the industry to disclose.

Acknowledgments

This material is the result of work supported with resources and the use of facilities at the Veterans Affairs, Caribbean Healthcare System San Juan, P.R. The contents of this publication do not represent the views of the Veterans Affairs Caribbean Healthcare System, the U.S. Department of Veterans Affairs, or the United States Government.

References

[1] M. E. Navas, G. Hall, and D. El Bejjani, "A case of endocarditis caused by Lactococcus garvieae and suggested methods for identification," *Journal of Clinical Microbiology*, vol. 51, no. 6, pp. 1990–1992, 2013.

[2] C. Y. Wang, H. S. Shie, S. C. Chen et al., "Lactococcus garvieae infections in humans: possible association with aquaculture outbreaks," *International Journal of Clinical Practice*, vol. 61, no. 1, pp. 68–73, 2007.

[3] E. F. Tariq, Y. Irshad, H. B. Khalil, A. S. Khakwani, and U. A. Khan, "Urinary tract infection caused by the novel pathogen, Lactococcus garvieae: a case report," *Cureus*, vol. 12, no. 7, article e9462, 2020.

[4] T. T. Choksi and F. Dadani, "Reviewing the emergence of Lactococcus garvieae: a case of catheter associated urinary tract infection caused by Lactococcus garvieae and Escherichia coli coinfection," *Case Reports in Infectious Diseases*, vol. 2017, Article ID 5921865, 4 pages, 2017.

[5] A. Malek, A. De la Hoz, S. I. Gomez-Villegas, C. Nowbakht, and C. A. Arias, "Lactococcus garvieae, an unusual pathogen in infective endocarditis: case report and review of the literature," *BMC Infectious Diseases*, vol. 19, no. 1, p. 301, 2019.

[6] R. M. Rösch, K. Buschmann, L. Brendel, T. Schwanz, and C. F. Vahl, "Lactococcus garvieae endocarditis in a prosthetic aortic valve: a case report and literature review," *Journal of Investigative Medicine High Impact Case Reports*, vol. 7, p. 232470961983205, 2019.

[7] G. Habib, P. Lancellotti, M. J. Antunes et al., "2015 ESC guidelines for the management of infective endocarditis: the task force for the management of infective endocarditis of the European Society of Cardiology (ESC). Endorsed by: European Association for Cardio-Thoracic Surgery (EACTS), the European Association of Nuclear Medicine (EANM)," *European Heart Journal*, vol. 36, no. 44, pp. 3075–3128, 2015.

[8] J. H. Butt, N. Ihlemann, O. de Backer et al., "Long-term risk of infective endocarditis after transcatheter aortic valve replacement," *Journal of the American College of Cardiology*, vol. 73, no. 13, pp. 1646–1655, 2019.

[9] L. M. Baddour, W. R. Wilson, A. S. Bayer et al., "Infective endocarditis in adults: diagnosis, antimicrobial therapy, and management of complications: a scientific statement for healthcare professionals from the American Heart Association," *Circulation*, vol. 132, no. 15, pp. 1435–1486, 2015.

33

Intravascular Lithotripsy for Underexpanded Stent in Heavily Calcified Coronary Artery Disease

Tejas Raxwal [1], **Cauvery Balhara** [2] **and Dipak Parekh** [1]

[1]Access Health Care Physicians, Hudson, Florida, USA
[2]Regional Medical Center Bayonet Point, Hudson, Florida, USA

Correspondence should be addressed to Tejas Raxwal; raxwal@yahoo.com

Academic Editor: Ertugurul Ercan

Objective. Can intravascular lithotripsy safely modify calcium in an underexpanded stent and result in optimal expansion and improved outcome? Coronary artery calcification results in difficulty with stent delivery and expansion and is associated with adverse outcomes. Intravascular lithotripsy (IVL) by delivering acoustic pressure waves modifies calcium plaque that improve vessel compliance resulting in optimizing stent deployment. *Results.* A 63-year-old patient presented with acute coronary syndrome with symptoms of unstable angina who underwent angiography that showed calcified right coronary artery which was treated with balloon angioplasty and stenting with drug eluting stent. However, after multiple inflations with noncompliant balloon, the patient was noted to have persistent residual in stent stenosis of 70%. Stenotic lesion in poorly expanded stent was treated with Shockwave C2 Coronary Intravascular Lithotripsy catheter resulting in 0% residual stenosis. The patient was followed for major adverse cardiovascular events at 30 days and 12 months. The patient remained MACE free at 30 days and 12 months. *Conclusions.* Coronary IVL safely and effectively facilitated stent expansion in severely calcified lesion in a poorly expanded stent with MACE free at 12-month follow-up.

1. Background

Severely calcified coronary arteries are known to portend lower procedural success rates and increased periprocedural complications. Lithotripsy technology is used for treatment of ureterorenal calculi, which has now been adapted as a new technique of intravascular lithotripsy (IVL) for heavily calcified lesions in coronary arteries [1].

IVL is a novel technique in which multiple lithotripsy emitters mounted on a traditional catheter platform deliver localized pulsatile sonic pressure waves to circumferentially modify vascular calcium by inducing calcium fractures. In the Disrupt CAD II study, the safety and effectiveness of IVL were reported for vessel preparation of severely calcified vessel in stenotic de novo coronary lesions before stent implantation [2].

Success and safety of the use of intravascular lithotripsy in a newly deployed underexpanded drug-eluting stent are unclear. Does it cause delamination of drug and polymer from stents and alter elution kinetics and drug delivery? Short- and long-term adverse cardiac events are unknown.

2. Case Report

63-year-old male has a history of diabetes, hyperlipidemia, HTN, and severe COPD and pulmonary HTN. The patient is a current smoker for over 50 years. Echocardiogram showed EF 60% with a PA pressure of 70 mmHg, and ECG showed sinus rhythm with occasional PVCs and incomplete RBBB. The patient had an episode of SVT with HR of 170 beats per minute. The patient had mildly elevated troponin of 0.15 ng/dl. Stress test showed an inferior-lateral perfusion defect in view of the fact that coronary angiography was performed.

Coronary angiogram showed the right coronary artery was severely diseased with 95% stenosis, so a decision was made to perform angioplasty (Figure 1). A coronary guidewire was crossed and placed in the distal PDA. A 2.5×12 mm compliant balloon was used to predilate the lesion. A 2.75×28 mm Xience DES was deployed distally, and an overlapping 3.0×18 mm Xience DES was deployed proximally. The stents

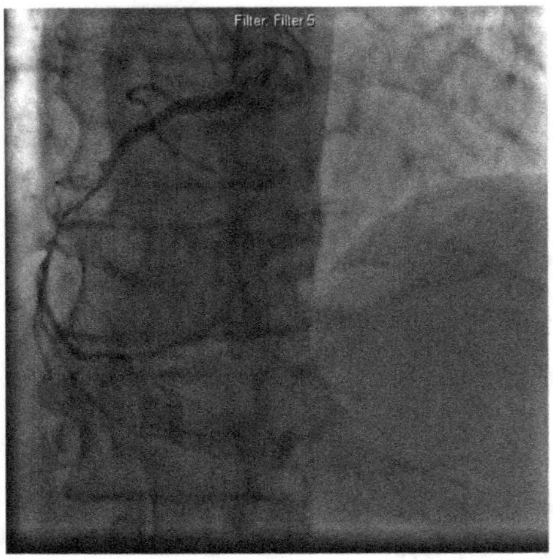

Figure 1: Right coronary artery with severe stenosis.

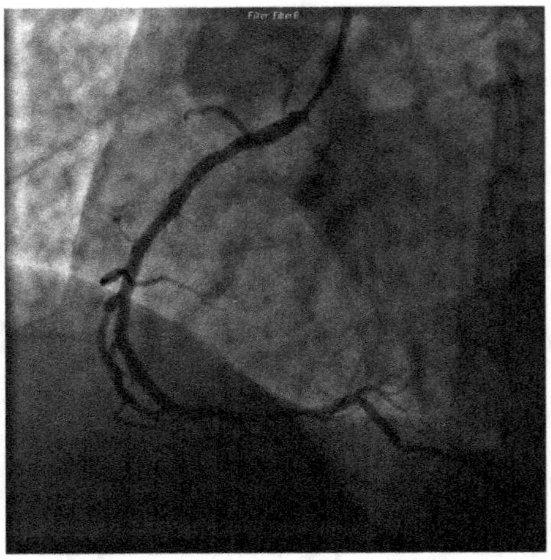

Figure 3: Right coronary artery after intravascular lithotripsy.

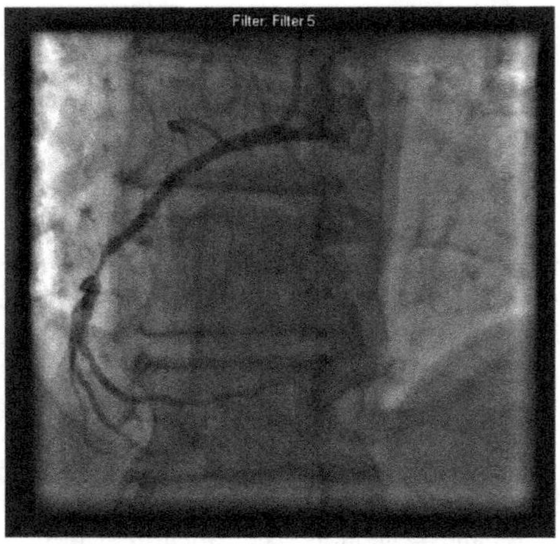

Figure 2: Right coronary artery with severe residual stenosis post balloon angioplasty and stenting.

were postdilated using a 3.5 × 12 noncompliant balloon. Repeat angiography despite multiple high pressure inflations showed the stent had a residual stenosis of approximately 70% (Figure 2). At this point, a decision was made to evaluate options of intravascular lithotripsy, laser versus coronary artery bypass surgery.

In discussion with the cardiac surgery team, it was decided attempting intravascular lithotripsy would be favorable in view of the patient having severe pulmonary HTN with severe COPD; his cardiac surgery risk would outweigh compared to attempting lithotripsy.

Patient was brought to the cardiac catheterization laboratory, and a Shockwave C2 Coronary Intravascular Lithotripsy catheter 3 mm × 12 mm balloon was inserted, and lithotripsy was done. Followed by lithotripsy, a 3.5 mm × 15 mm noncompliant balloon was inserted and balloon angioplasty was successfully performed which resulted in 0% residual stenosis (Figure 3).

The primary endpoint was in-hospital major adverse cardiac events (MACE) defined as cardiac death, MI, or target vessel revascularization. Secondary endpoints included angiographic success, defined as the ability of IVL to produce a residual diameter stenosis < 30% without serious angiographic complications (severe dissection impairing flow, perforation, abrupt closure, persistent slow flow, or no reflow). The patient had successful angioplasty with <10% residual stenosis facilitated by IVL with no MACE in-hospital, at 30 days and 12 months.

3. Discussion

Percutaneous coronary artery intervention of heavily calcified arteries remains a challenge. Specialty balloons like scoring, cutting, and ultrahigh pressure balloons have been used to pretreat these lesions. Rotational atherectomy is commonly used to facilitate PCI in calcified vessels; however, all techniques have significant limitations. Noncompliant balloon dilation, despite high pressures, may be of insufficient force to result in calcium fracture and thus artery expansion. In the presence of eccentric calcium, balloon dilation may be biased toward noncalcified segments of the artery, leading to dissection or perforation.

Rotational and orbital atherectomy, while highly effective for facilitating lesion crossing, may selectively ablate calcified segments of the artery resulting from guidewire bias, leaving significant calcium plaque unmodified within the lesion [3]. Periprocedural complications like slow-flow, periprocedural myocardial infarction, dissection, and perforation may result more often in atherectomy compared with balloon-based therapies.

Treatment of underexpanded stent still remains a challenge and poses an increased risk of early stent thrombosis and restenosis after PCI, while laser atherectomy has been used successfully in underexpanded stents using "explosion" technique [4]. However, it does have risk of dissection, perforation, and distal embolization.

In February 2021, the Shockwave C2 Coronary IVL Catheter was approved by the FDA for use before implanting a stent in heavily calcified coronary arteries. Intravascular lithotripsy is a novel technology, based on an established treatment strategy for renal calculi, delivered via a traditional catheter used to circumferentially modify vascular calcium.

The coronary IVL catheter contains multiple lithotripsy emitters enclosed in an integrated balloon. The emitters generate sonic pressure waves in the shape of a sphere, creating a field effect to treat vascular calcium. The generated sonic pressure waves selectively disrupt and fracture calcium in situ, altering vessel compliance while minimizing injury and maintaining the integrity of the fibroelastic components of the vessel wall.

Herein, we report safety and effectiveness of IVL for the modification of calcified plaque in an underexpanded stent. The IVL mechanism of action has been shown to be intraplaque calcium fracture, thereby modifying vascular compliance and facilitating stent expansion. IVL was safe with no dissection, perforation, abrupt closure, or slow flow/no reflow. There was no MACE reported at 30 days and 12 months. IVL is a feasible and safe frontline tool for calcified plaque modification, with the IVL catheter crossing the lesion and delivering therapy in complex cases including underexpanded stents.

In the Disrupt CAD study, the percentage of patients that underwent intravascular lithotripsy freedom from 30-day MACE was 92% [5, 6]. Thus, pending long-term results from the present case and additional studies, IVL may be a new, simple-to-use therapeutic option for patients with underexpanded stents as a bailout strategy to impact clinical outcomes of stent thrombosis, reduced restenosis, and reduced target lesion revascularization [7]. However, atherectomy remains the first-line therapy for optimal lesion preparation if there is difficulty in crossing the lesion with even contemporary low-profile balloon catheters.

In multicenter IVL-Dragon Registry, 62 consecutive patients with stent underexpansion were treated with IVL procedural success (72.6% of patients) [8]. Intravascular imaging confirmed increased stent expansion following IVL from 37.5% to 86% by optical coherence tomography and from 57% to 89% by intravascular ultrasound. One patient had cardiac death; however, there was no target lesion revascularization or target vessel myocardial infarction during the 30-day follow-up.

IVL is a potential bail-out treatment in nonexpanded stents with good safety and efficiency profile. On present review of data, IVL is an effective and safe method for facilitating stent expansion and increasing luminal gain.

References

[1] T. J. Brinton, Z. A. Ali, J. M. Hill et al., "Feasibility of shockwave coronary intravascular lithotripsy for the treatment of calcified coronary stenoses," *Circulation*, vol. 139, no. 6, pp. 834–836, 2019.

[2] Z. A. Ali, H. Nef, J. Escaned et al., "Safety and effectiveness of coronary intravascular lithotripsy for treatment of severely calcified coronary stenoses: the disrupt CAD II study," *Circulation: Cardiovascular Interventions*, vol. 12, no. 10, p. e008434, 2019.

[3] M. Abdel-Wahab, R. Toelg, R. A. Byrne et al., "High-speed rotational atherectomy versus modified balloons prior to drug-eluting stent implantation in severely calcified coronary lesions: the randomized prepare-CALC trial," *Circulation: Cardiovascular Interventions*, vol. 11, no. 10, p. e007415, 2018.

[4] T. Lee, R. A. Shlofmitz, L. Song et al., "The effectiveness of excimer laser angioplasty to treat coronary in-stent restenosis with peri-stent calcium as assessed by optical coherence tomography," *EuroIntervention*, vol. 15, no. 3, pp. e279–e288, 2019.

[5] S. Saito, S. Yamazaki, A. Takahashi et al., "Intravascular lithotripsy for vessel preparation in severely calcified coronary arteries prior to stent placement-primary outcomes from the Japanese Disrupt CAD IV Study," *Circulation Journal*, vol. 85, no. 6, pp. 826–833, 2021.

[6] D. J. Kereiakes, C. Di Mario, R. F. Riley et al., "Intravascular Lithotripsy for Treatment of Calcified Coronary Lesions: Patient-Level Pooled Analysis of the Disrupt CAD Studies," *JACC. Cardiovascular Interventions*, vol. 14, no. 12, pp. 1337–1348, 2021.

[7] M. Fedele, A. Iannone, D. Bartolini, and P. Rubartelli, "Shockwave intravascular lithotripsy in the treatment of underexpanded coronary stent: case series," *Clin Case Rep.*, vol. 9, no. 10, p. e04961, 2021.

[8] W. Wańha, M. Tomaniak, P. Wańczura et al., "Intravascular lithotripsy for the treatment of stent underexpansion: the Multicenter IVL-DRAGON Registry," *Journal of Clinical Medicine*, vol. 11, no. 7, p. 1779, 2022.

Flecainide-Associated Cardiogenic Shock in a Patient with Atrial Fibrillation

Erind Gjermeni, Andreas Bollmann, Gerhard Hindricks, and Andreas Müssigbrodt

Department of Electrophysiology, Heart Center University of Leipzig, Strümpellstraße 39, 04289 Leipzig, Germany

Correspondence should be addressed to Erind Gjermeni; erind_g@yahoo.com

Academic Editor: Christopher S. Snyder

Flecainide is a frequently used antiarrhythmic drug, recommended by current guidelines as a first-line treatment option for restoring and maintaining sinus rhythm in patients with atrial fibrillation and no significant structural heart disease. In overdose, it can induce severe cardiogenic shock. Cardiogenic shock after a therapeutic dose of flecainide in patients without contraindication has not yet been reported in literature. *Case Summary.* We report a case of flecainide-associated cardiogenic shock in a 52-year-old woman with paroxysmal atrial fibrillation after a therapeutic dose of flecainide. Pharmacological cardioversion of symptomatic tachyarrhythmic atrial fibrillation with flecainide was unsuccessful and shortly after, she developed cardiogenic shock with severely reduced LVEF. Electrical cardioversion was also unsuccessful. Coronarography was unremarkable, and the cardiac MRI showed no signs of inflammation or fibrosis. After amiodarone loading, she converted to SR. This rare but severe complication despite adequate treatment could be explained by increased susceptibility to negative inotropic effect of flecainide as a consequence of marked tachycardia. Therefore, cautious monitoring after new administration of flecainide or the administration of a higher dose is advisable.

1. Introduction

Flecainide is a class IC antiarrhythmic agent, frequently used for the management of atrial fibrillation (AF). Results from randomized clinical trials showed that flecainide is safe for patients with AF without significant structural heart disease [1] and is recommended as a first-line option for pharmacological conversion as well as the maintenance of SR [2]. Flecainide proved to be safe and effective as "pill-in-the-pocket" treatment strategy with a single oral dose of 200–300 mg for termination of recent-onset (<48 h) AF [3]. In the Cardiac Arrhythmia Suppression Trial (CAST) study on patients with myocardial infarction, flecainide showed a threefold increase of arrhythmic death compared to placebo [4]. In overdose, or in patients with significant heart disease, it can induce ventricular arrhythmias and severe cardiogenic shock [5–8]. Nevertheless, little is known about flecainide-induced cardiogenic shock at therapeutic doses.

2. Case Report

We report a case of a flecainide-induced cardiogenic shock in a 52-year-old (175 cm, 77 kg) woman with paroxysmal AF. She was previously effectively treated for one year with flecainide (200 mg) as PIP. The medication was well tolerated. Episodes of palpitations every 3-4 weeks disappeared typically after 1-2 hours after taking flecainide. Systolic function was normal in an echocardiography one year before the actual admission. She was otherwise fit and without any other known cardiovascular disease.

She presented one evening to the Emergency Department of a referring hospital with persisting palpitations. The symptoms had started the evening before, and the usual 200 mg flecainide had been ineffective.

Clinical examination showed a fast, irregular heartbeat and was otherwise unremarkable. Blood pressure (BP) was 136/87 mmHg and oxygen saturation (SpO_2) is 98% in room

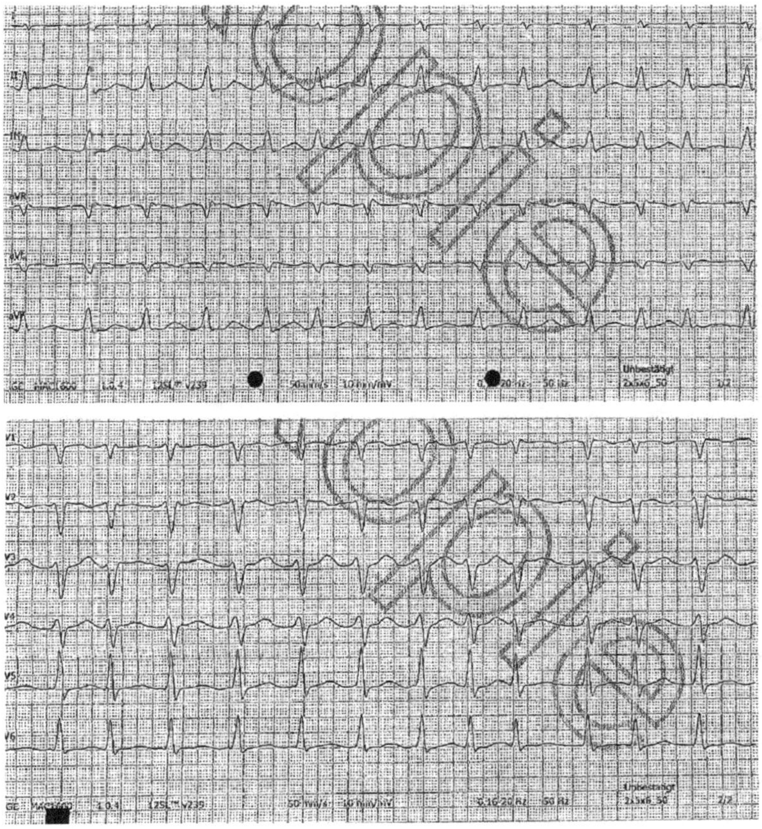

FIGURE 1: ECG on admission showing tachyarrhythmic atrial fibrillation with 158 bpm.

air. The electrocardiogram (ECG) showed tachyarrhythmic AF with 158 bpm (Figure 1).

The next day 300 mg flecainide p.o. (the recommended dose for patients with >70 kg) was given, and one hour later, the patient reported malaise and dyspnea, which rapidly worsened and she became tachypneic and severely hypotonic. Echocardiography revealed a severely reduced left ventricular ejection fraction (LVEF) of 30%. The patient was started on i.v. catecholamines and nasal oxygen and was urgently transferred to our center.

Upon arrival, the patient was dyspneic, SpO_2 96% with 2 l/min nasal oxygen, responsive and conscious, and BP was 100/48 mmHg under catecholamine support. ECG showed AF (120 bpm). Echocardiography revealed a severely reduced LVEF of only 18%. Chest X-ray showed pleural effusion and increased cardiothoracic ratio (Figure 2(a)).

As electrical cardioversion was unsuccessful, she was started on amiodarone. Bisoprolol was continued at 5 mg/day. Coronary angiography was unremarkable.

Heart rate decreased to around 100 bpm, and over the following 7 hours, catecholamines were fully weaned. Cardiac MRI on the fifth day after admission showed LVEF of 41%, without signs of inflammation or myocardial fibrosis. One day later, she converted into SR. An elective pulmonary vein isolation (PVI) was scheduled, and the patient was discharged with a full cardiovascular recovery (Figure 2(b)). At the time of this report, 4 months after the PVI and 5 months after the admission with cardiogenic shock, the patient negates any symptoms of AF recurrence or heart failure.

3. Discussion

Flecainide belongs to the class IC antiarrhythmic drugs that mainly act via potent and selective blockade of the cardiac fast inward sodium current. Its efficacy is use-dependent as it has a high affinity for open-state channels. Flecainide is safe and effective in preventing recurrent AF in patients without significant structural heart disease and is recommended as a first-line therapy by the current guidelines [1, 2, 9]. The PIP treatment strategy with flecainide in appropriately selected patients has been shown to be safe and effective and to significantly reduce hospitalizations [3]. Still, it is well known that its use may be associated with proarrhythmia [1, 10]. Moreover, flecainide has shown to exhibit mildly negative inotropic effects in healthy subjects, sometimes even causing dramatic but asymptomatic and reversible impairment of the systolic function [10].

Orally administered, its bioavailability is approximately 90%. Peak plasma concentration is reached within 1–3 hours and it has a half-life of 7–12 h. Cardiac manifestations appear after 30–120 minutes. The higher the dose, the shorter the delay [9]. Given the use-dependent properties of flecainide, its antiarrhythmic effect, but also the toxicity risk could rise significantly at higher heart rates [1].

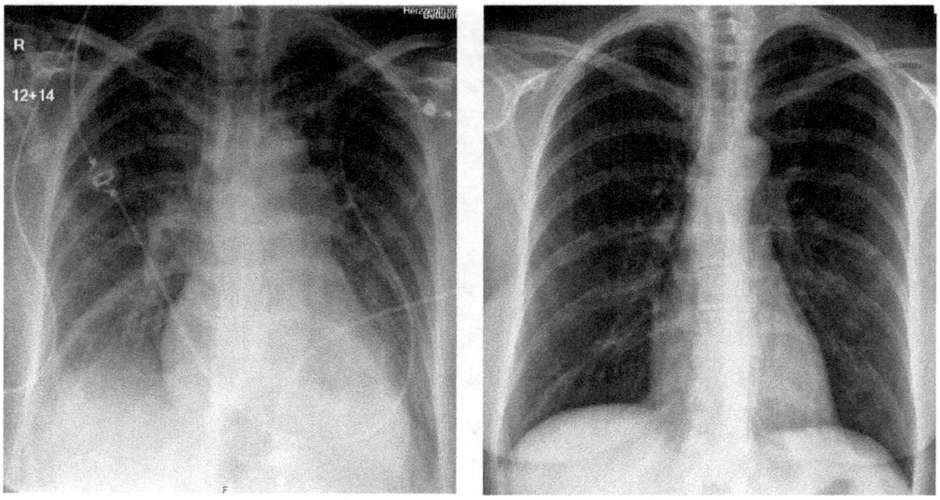

(a) (b)

Figure 2: Chest X-ray on admission (a) showing signs of heart enlargement and pleural effusion. Six days later before discharge (b), the heart size is normal again, and there is complete remission of pleural effusion.

There have been case reports of severe cardiogenic shock after large-dose ingestions, or at therapeutic levels in patients with clear contraindications (structural heart disease, before the publication of the CAST study) [5–8]. Cardiogenic shock after a therapeutic dose of flecainide in patients without contraindications has not yet been reported in literature.

This patient without known contraindications developed acute heart failure with severely reduced LVEF and cardiogenic shock after ingesting only the recommended dose of flecainide.

This severe complication despite adequate treatment based on extensive evidence could be explained by increased susceptibility to negative inotropic effect of flecainide as a consequence of marked tachycardia. As a differential diagnosis, tachycardia-induced cardiomyopathy or a combination of both could be considered.

Therefore, cautious monitoring after new administration of flecainide or after increasing the dose is advisable.

References

[1] E. Aliot, A. Capucci, H. J. Crijns, A. Goette, and J. Tamargo, "Twenty-five years in the making: flecainide is safe and effective for the management of atrial fibrillation," *Europace*, vol. 13, no. 2, pp. 161–173, 2011.

[2] P. Kirchhof, S. Benussi, D. Kotecha et al., "2016 ESC guidelines for the management of atrial fibrillation developed in collaboration with EACTS," *European Heart Journal*, vol. 37, no. 38, pp. 2893–2962, 2016.

[3] P. Alboni, G. L. Botto, N. Baldi et al., "Outpatient treatment of recent-onset atrial fibrillation with the "pill-in-the-pocket" approach," *The New England Journal of Medicine*, vol. 351, no. 23, pp. 2384–2391, 2004.

[4] D. S. Echt, P. R. Liebson, L. B. Mitchell et al., "Mortality and morbidity in patients receiving encainide, flecainide, or placebo. The cardiac arrhythmia suppression trial," *The New England Journal of Medicine*, vol. 324, no. 12, pp. 781–788, 1991.

[5] J. Buss, J. J. Lasserre, and D. L. Heene, "Asystole and cardiogenic shock due to combined treatment with verapamil and flecainide," *The Lancet*, vol. 340, no. 8818, p. 546, 1992.

[6] W. P. Forbes, T. T. Hee, S. M. Mohiuddin, and D. E. Hillman, "Flecainide-induced cardiogenic shock," *Chest*, vol. 94, no. 5, p. 1121, 1988.

[7] A. Ghannam, A. Tazi, A. Kettani, and M. Faroudy, "Non-accidental flecainide overdose-a case report," *International Journal of Medicine and Surgery*, vol. 1, no. 2, pp. 53–56, 2014.

[8] J. C. Reynolds and B. S. Judge, "Successful treatment of flecainide-induced cardiac arrest with extracorporeal membrane oxygenation in the ED," *The American Journal of Emergency Medicine*, vol. 33, no. 10, pp. 1542.e1–1542.e2, 2015.

[9] G. K. Andrikopoulos, S. Pastromas, and S. Tzeis, "Flecainide: current status and perspectives in arrhythmia management," *World Journal of Cardiology*, vol. 7, no. 2, pp. 76–85, 2015.

[10] V. Santinelli, M. Arnese, I. Oppo et al., "Effects of flecainide and propafenone on systolic performance in subjects with normal cardiac function," *Chest*, vol. 103, no. 4, pp. 1068–1073, 1993.

35

Atrial Septal Defect with Eisenmenger Syndrome: A Rare Presentation

Arnold Nongmoh Forlemu,[1] Muhammad Ajmal,[2] and Mehrdad Saririan[3]

[1]Creighton University School of Medicine-Phoenix/Maricopa Integrated Health System, Department of Internal Medicine-Cardiology, 2601 E Roosevelt St., Phoenix, AZ 85008, USA
[2]University of Arizona College of Medicine-Tucson, Sarver Heart Center, Department of Cardiology, 750 W Orange Grove Road, Tucson, AZ 85704, USA
[3]Creighton University School of Medicine-Phoenix/Maricopa Integrated Health System, Department of Cardiology, 2601 E Roosevelt St., Phoenix, AZ 85008, USA

Correspondence should be addressed to Arnold Nongmoh Forlemu; arnold.forlemu@ndus.edu

Academic Editor: Manabu Shirotani

Atrial septal defects (ASDs) are common congenital heart defects (CHD). The clinical course in patients without closure of the ASD is associated with significant morbidity and mortality in advanced age. A small percentage of patients may develop pulmonary arterial hypertension (PAH) due to left to right shunting that impacts morbidity and mortality. Advances in prenatal screening and fetal echocardiography have allowed timely interventions. Nonetheless, some patients still may be diagnosed with ASD in adulthood as an incidental finding or presenting with clinical symptoms such as shortness of breath from right heart failure. We report a case of an adult female presenting with shortness of breath due to ASD causing PAH with Eisenmenger physiology.

1. Introduction

Atrial septal defects (ASDs) are the second most common congenital heart defects (CHD) [1]. It accounts for about 13% of CHD cases with a 2 : 1 female to male ratio. The most common type of ASD is the secundum type that is located at the fossa ovalis [2]. ASDs may be benign, but occasionally left to right shunting can overload the right heart leading to right heart failure (RHF) and arrhythmias. In its advanced form, Eisenmenger syndrome (ES) with shunt reversal may develop, with a worse prognosis [2]. Shunt closure is indicated in the presence of severe shunting with signs of RHF with a pulmonary vascular resistance < 5 Wood units [3]. However, when irreversible pulmonary arterial hypertension (PAH) and ES develop, closure is contraindicated and medical management becomes the focus [3].

2. Case Report

A 44-year-old female with a history of heart murmur since age 15 and chronic dyspnea on exertion was admitted to the hospital with new-onset chest pain and shortness of breath. The pain was retrosternal, worse when lying flat, and improved with leaning forward. She was hypoxic on admission with an oxygen saturation of 86%. Physical examination revealed cyanosis, jugular venous distention, a right ventricular heave, and a loud pulmonic diastolic murmur. Blood work revealed a hemoglobin concentration of 14.2 g/dl, a normal troponin level < 0.012 ng/ml, serum creatinine of 0.51 mg/dl, negative antinuclear antibodies, negative HIV serology, and a negative pregnancy test. An electrocardiogram showed severe right ventricular hypertrophy (Figure 1).

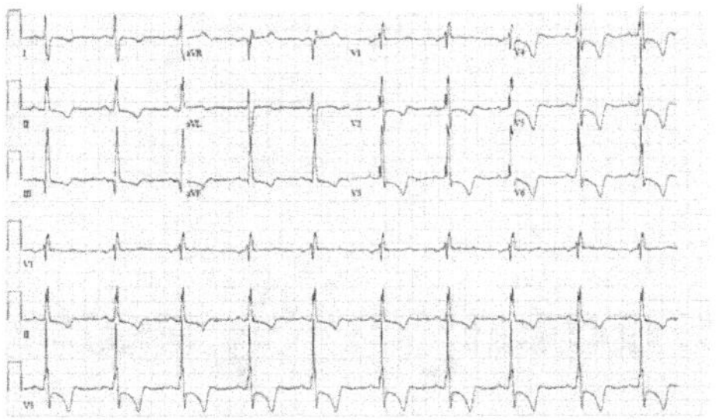

FIGURE 1: Electrocardiogram demonstrating Right Ventricular Hypertrophy Pattern.

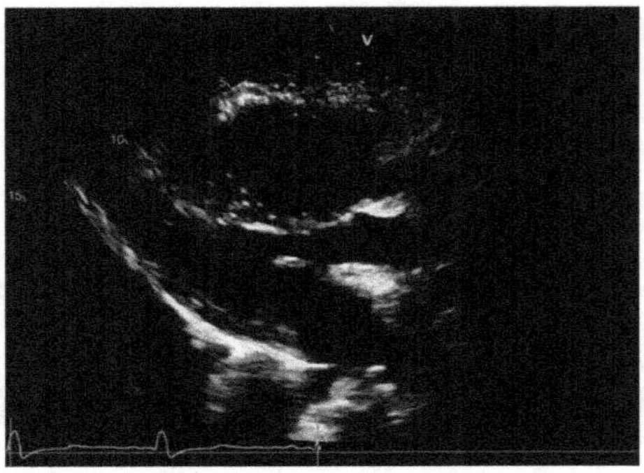

FIGURE 2: Transthoracic Echocardiogram Parasternal Long Axis View showing enlarged right ventricle from volume overload.

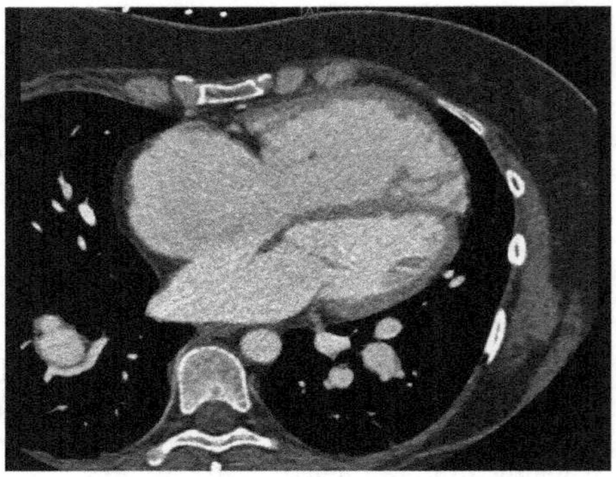

FIGURE 3: Cardiac CT showing large ASD.

Echocardiography revealed severe right atrial and right ventricular enlargement, severe pulmonary hypertension with right ventricular systolic pressure (RSVP) of 70 mmHg, and suspicion for a large ASD (Figure 2).

She underwent right heart catheterization (RHC) with a shunt run. This revealed 10% oxygen step-up from high superior vena cava to the right atrium, suggestive of ASD. Effective pulmonary blood flow to systemic blood flow (Qp/Qs) was 1, suggestive of equal bidirectional shunting and Eisenmenger physiology. RHC confirmed severe PAH (PVR = 8.7 Wood units) that did not respond to inhaled nitric oxide. The mean wedge pressure was 2 mmHg. She also underwent a computed tomography (CT) pulmonary angiogram that was negative for thromboembolic disease. A pulmonary function test (PFT) and diffusion lung capacity for carbon monoxide (DLCO) were normal.

To better delineate the anatomy of the atrial septum, she underwent cardiac CT which revealed a large (2.5 × 3.5 cm) secundum-type defect (Figure 3).

She had a six-minute walk test for prognostic purposes which revealed reduced walk distance of 300 meters or 50% of the predicted distance. She was classified as WHO class III functional status and started on combination therapy with Sildenafil 20 mg three times daily and Macitentan 10 mg once daily. She was also placed on two forms of contraception (barrier and nonestrogen contraceptives). Her shortness of breath and chest pain improved significantly, and she was scheduled for outpatient follow-up with a pulmonologist and cardiologist. At 30 days, the patient no longer felt short of breath with activities of daily living and her 6-minute walk test doubled to 600 meters.

3. Discussion

ASD is often encountered in the adult population, as many patients are symptom-free in the first few decades of life. Secundum-type ASDs are located at the fossa ovalis and represent about 70% of all ASDs [2]. To determine shunt direction during RHC, the superior vena cava sample (SVC) for venous oxygen saturation is best taken at high-level SVC to avoid contamination with mixed venous oxygen in the lower level SVC blood, owing to the latter being closer to the right atrium and the inferior vena cava that may underestimate left-right shunting.

PAH is characterized by a pulmonary capillary wedge pressure ≤ 15 mmHg and a pulmonary vascular resistance (PVR) > 3 Wood units (WU). Cardiac output and PVR are often measured by thermodilution. However, this technique may be inaccurate in patients with intracardiac shunts, low cardiac output states, or significant tricuspid regurgitation. In such situations, the Fick principle may be preferable to calculate cardiac output and thus PVR [4].

PAH in secundum-type ASD seems to be related to age, size of the defect, female sex, and nonclosed ASD status [5, 6]. ASD recognition and correction early after childbirth has helped reduce the incidence of PAH [5]. Unrecognized ASD often presents in the 4th decade of life (as it did with our patient) with dyspnea on exertion, chest pain, palpitations, and sometimes RHF [6]. Severe pulmonary vascular disease with ES is very rare (<5%) and may be seen in those with genetic predispositions, like in idiopathic PAH [6].

Whether ASD ES is secondary to severe PAH due to the ASD shunt size alone or the ES is related to idiopathic PAH with a standby ASD is still a subject of debate. Therrien et al. [7] demonstrated the absence of bone morphogenetic protein receptor 2 (BMPR2) gene mutation in patients with ASD ES, suggesting ASD size plays a major role in ES development. The BMPR2 gene mutation is found in 70% of patients with familial PAH and 25% of patients with idiopathic PAH. The BMPR2 gene mutation has been implicated in abnormal vascular smooth muscle cell proliferation and endothelial apoptosis [7]. Patients presenting in their teenage years with PAH and ASD with BMPR2 mutation may have abnormal cell signaling from the mutation coupled with hemodynamic overload from the ASD promoting rapid progression of pulmonary vascular lesions resulting in severe

PAH [7]. Although the BMPR2 gene mutation was absent in the above study, patients with ASD may still carry an unknown genetic mutation predisposing them to PAH ES, which may become clinically apparent when triggered by an external stimulus such as high flow through large shunt size. This may explain why ASD patients rarely develop ES, as the genetic predisposition, if any, likely occurs rarely in the population or has a low penetrance in society.

In the study by Therrien et al. [7], patients with ASD ES also had significantly larger ASDs than the control patients (3.7 ± 1.2 cm versus 1.9 ± 0.7 cm). The patient in our case presented in her 4th decade with PAH ES and a large ASD (2.5×3.5 cm) suggesting that the magnitude of the ASD likely played a major hemodynamic role leading to shunt reversal and ES.

It is worth noting that other conditions can cause precapillary PH, with the most common being left heart diseases such as diastolic heart failure [8]. Also, precapillary PH in the presence of an ASD can be caused by obstructive lung disease, pulmonary fibrosis, and thromboembolism [8]. The patient in our case had a normal wedge pressure, normal PFT and DLCO, and a step-up of oxygen saturation from high superior vena cavae to the right heart chambers with bidirectional ASD shunting, all pointing towards an ASD as being the primary cause of the PAH.

4. Management

Secundum ASDs can be closed either surgically or percutaneously, and repair is indicated when there is evidence of RV compromise with or without symptoms [6]. Left to right shunt with $Qp : Qs \geq 1.5$ and $PVR < 2.3$ Wood units (or $PVRi < 4\,WU/m^2$) is safe for ASD closure. Closure of the defect and pregnancy are not recommended if the PVR is >4.6 WU ($PVRi > 8\,WU/m^2$), even when an Eisenmenger-type phenomenon has not been reached. For patients with PVR between 2.3 and 4.6 WU, the decision to close the ASD is made on a case-by-case basis. Once the shunt has reversed from right to left ($Qp : Qs < 1$) or is bidirectional ($Qp : Qs = 1$), PAH is often irreversible and ASD closure is contraindicated due to worsening RHF [6, 8]. This is because closing the shunt in such instances may sacrifice the right-sided pressure relief role that the ASD may be providing. Preserving right ventricular function by upfront combination therapy or by escalating pulmonary vasodilators can significantly improve patient outcomes when ES develops. As such, phosphodiesterase-type 5 inhibitors, endothelin receptor antagonists, prostacyclin analogues, and receptor agonists, either with upfront combination therapy or with sequential escalation of monotherapy, are recommended [9, 10]. The "treat and repair" strategy in which PVR is lowered enough by medications to allow for shunt closure remains controversial. Some authors have reported successful shunt closure without complications in patients with significant PVR after lowering the PVR to <4-6.5 WU with medical management [9, 11]. However, this approach is not currently supported by guidelines and could be potentially fatal.

Pregnancy is contraindicated in all forms of PAH due to risk of cardiac, fetal, and obstetric complications [10, 12]. Women of childbearing age found to have PAH should be placed on two different forms of contraceptive (excluding estrogen-containing products due to increased thromboembolism risk) before starting medical management, including a barrier method and nonestrogen contraceptives [10, 12].

5. Conclusion

ASDs are not commonly associated with Eisenmenger physiology. The morbidity and mortality in ASD-related PAH are due to cardiac complications including heart failure and arrhythmias. Once ES develops, ASD closure is contraindicated. Medical management and avoidance of situations that can alter hemodynamic balance (such as pregnancy) to reduce right-sided pressures are paramount to the patient's survival.

Additional Points

Learning Objective. ASDs are not commonly associated with Eisenmenger physiology, mostly owing to volume rather than pressure loading on the pulmonary circulation as well as early recognition and closure of ASD. Once ES develops, timely medical management with vasodilators, postponing closure, and avoidance of situations that alter hemodynamic balance (e.g., pregnancy) become paramount to the patient's survival.

References

[1] D. van der Linde, E. E. Konings, M. A. Slager et al., "Birth prevalence of congenital heart disease worldwide: a systematic review and meta-analysis," *Journal of the American College of Cardiology*, vol. 58, no. 21, pp. 2241–2247, 2011.

[2] S. Goetschmann, S. Dibernardo, H. Steinmann, M. Pavlovic, N. Sekarski, and J. P. Pfammatter, "Frequency of Severe Pulmonary Hypertension Complicating "Isolated" Atrial Septal Defect in Infancy," *The American Journal of Cardiology*, vol. 102, no. 3, pp. 340–342, 2008.

[3] M. C. van de Veerdonk, T. Kind, J. T. Marcus et al., "Progressive right ventricular dysfunction in patients with pulmonary arterial hypertension responding to therapy," *Journal of the American College of Cardiology*, vol. 58, no. 24, pp. 2511–2519, 2011.

[4] R. A. Nishimura and B. A. Carabello, "Hemodynamics in the cardiac catheterization laboratory of the 21st century," *Circulation*, vol. 125, no. 17, pp. 2138–2150, 2012.

[5] M. Vogel, F. Berger, A. Kramer, V. Alexi-Meshkishvili, and P. E. Lange, "Incidence of secondary pulmonary hypertension in adults with atrial septal or sinus venosus defects," *Heart*, vol. 82, no. 1, pp. 30–33, 1999.

[6] H. Baumgartner, P. Bonhoeffer, N. M. de Groot et al., "ESC guidelines for the management of grown-up congenital heart disease (new version 2010)," *European Heart Journal*, vol. 31, no. 23, pp. 2915–2957, 2010.

[7] J. Therrien, S. Rambihar, B. Newman et al., "Le syndrome d'Eisenmenger et les communications interauriculaires : Inne ou acquis?," *Canadian Journal of Cardiology*, vol. 22, no. 13, pp. 1133–1136, 2006.

[8] H. Nashat, C. Montanaro, W. Li et al., "Atrial septal defects and pulmonary arterial hypertension," *Journal of Thoracic Disease*, vol. 10, no. S24, pp. S2953–S2965, 2018.

[9] Y. Kijima, T. Akagi, Y. Takaya et al., "Treat and repair strategy in patients with atrial septal defect and significant pulmonary arterial hypertension," *Circulation Journal*, vol. 80, no. 1, pp. 227–234, 2016.

[10] N. Galiè, M. Humbert, J. L. Vachiery et al., "2015 ESC/ERS guidelines for the diagnosis and treatment of pulmonary hypertension: the joint task force for the diagnosis and treatment of pulmonary hypertension of the European Society of Cardiology (ESC) and the European Respiratory Society (ERS) endorsed by: Association for European Paediatric and Congenital Cardiology (AEPC), International Society for Heart and Lung Transplantation (ISHLT)," *European Respiratory Journal*, vol. 46, no. 4, pp. 903–975, 2015.

[11] E. A. Bradley, N. Ammash, S. C. Martinez et al., ""Treat-to-close": non-repairable ASD-PAH in the adult: results from the North American ASD-PAH (NAAP) multicenter registry," *International Journal of Cardiology*, vol. 291, pp. 127–133, 2019.

[12] M. Ladouceur, L. Benoit, J. Radojevic et al., "Pregnancy outcomes in patients with pulmonary arterial hypertension associated with congenital heart disease," *Heart*, vol. 103, no. 4, pp. 287–292, 2017.

Masked Hypotension due to Elevated Venous Pressure in a Patient with Complex Adult Congenital Heart Disease

Wytch Rigger,[1] **Sean P. Javaheri,**[2] **Gyanendra K. Sharma,**[2] **Norris Stanley Nahman Jr.,**[3] **Mark Sheynshteyn,**[4] **and Neal L. Weintraub**[2]

[1]*Department of Medicine, Medical College of Georgia at Augusta University, Augusta, GA, USA*
[2]*Division of Cardiology, Medical College of Georgia at Augusta University, Augusta, GA, USA*
[3]*Division of Nephrology, Medical College of Georgia at Augusta University, Augusta, GA, USA*
[4]*Division of Endocrinology, Diabetes and Metabolism, Medical College of Georgia at Augusta University, Augusta, GA, USA*

Correspondence should be addressed to Neal L. Weintraub; nweintraub@augusta.edu

Academic Editor: Kathleen Ngu

An adult with surgically corrected Tetralogy of Fallot presented with profoundly elevated central venous pressure (CVP) and acute renal dysfunction thought secondary to acute on chronic right heart failure. Treatment with dopamine promoted diuresis and a stabilization of renal function. Repeated attempts to wean the patient from dopamine were associated with hypotension and worsening renal failure. Invasive hemodynamic assessment unexpectedly demonstrated high cardiac output with low systemic vascular resistance (SVR). In retrospect, the markedly elevated CVP had concealed the impact of reduced SVR on blood pressure. After reversible causes of low SVR state were excluded, the patient was successfully managed with oral alpha-adrenergic agents. While typically negligible under physiologic conditions, elevated CVP can artificially increase mean arterial pressure. We have coined the term "masked hypotension" to describe this unique pathophysiological phenomenon.

1. Introduction

Due to advances in surgical techniques, the population of adults with congenital heart disease is growing [1]. As these patients age, understanding the interplay between their congenital heart disease and acquired diseases is imperative to providing comprehensive care. We report the case of an adult with Tetralogy of Fallot who presented with what appeared to be right-sided heart failure, only to discover that the patient was actually in a high cardiac output state. Management required an acute understanding of his unique hemodynamic physiology and the different determinants of tissue perfusion pressure.

2. Case

A 61-year-old male with a history of surgically corrected Tetralogy of Fallot presented with fatigue, edema, weight gain, and worsening renal insufficiency. He exhibited marked jugular venous distension, ascites, and edema on examination. Historically, he had undergone complete surgical repair at age 11, a right ventricular outflow tract reconstruction and pulmonary valve replacement at age 47, and a percutaneous pulmonary valve replacement at age 59. In the months prior to admission, the patient exhibited worsening signs and symptoms of volume overload requiring escalating diuretic doses. Prior to admission, a cardiac MRI demonstrated marked biatrial enlargement, right ventricular dilation and dysfunction, and moderate pulmonary and tricuspid regurgitation (Supplemental Figure 1). An echocardiogram on admission demonstrated right ventricular dilation with an estimated right ventricular systolic pressure of 54 mmHg, moderate tricuspid regurgitation, and mild pulmonary conduit stenosis. Electrocardiogram at the time of admission demonstrated sinus rhythm with a stable right bundle branch block (Figure 1).

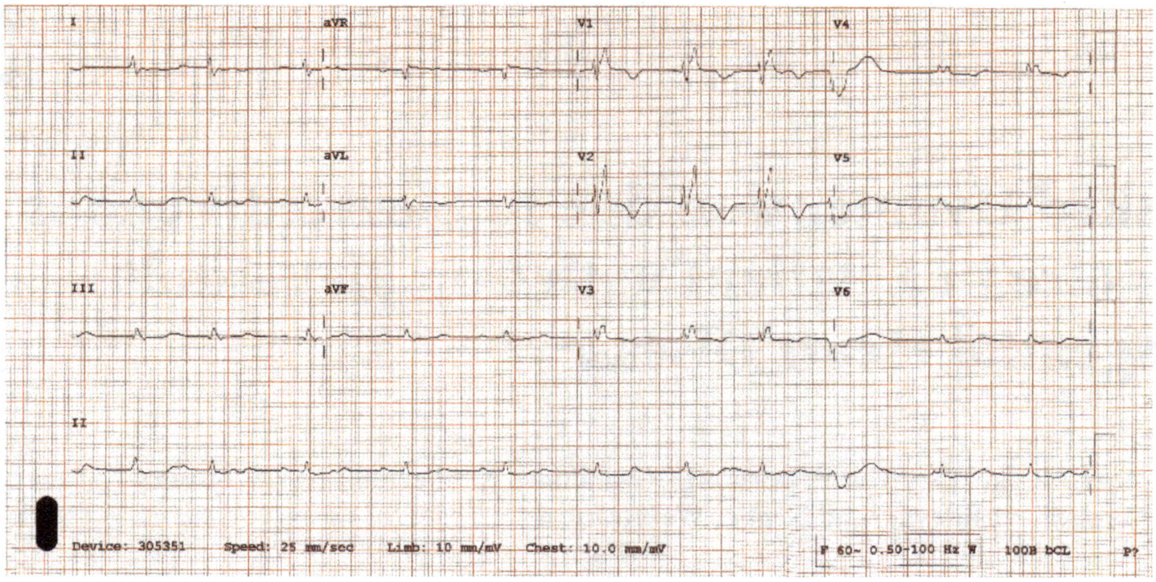

FIGURE 1: Electrocardiogram on presentation. The patient was noted to be in sinus rhythm with a first-degree AV block with a prolonged PR interval of 223 msec and a stable right bundle branch block that had been present for many years.

The patient was admitted for treatment of presumed decompensated right heart failure. MAP was 64 mmHg, and CVP was markedly elevated at 27 mmHg. He was started on intravenous diuretics and dopamine and successfully diuresed over 12 days to a negative fluid balance of 16.5 L with an improvement in renal function (Figure 2).

Three days after discharge, the patient was readmitted with frank hypotension, hyperkalemia, and oliguric renal failure. Dopamine infusion was resumed with improvement in renal function and urine output. Repeated attempts to wean the dopamine were associated with dramatic drops in blood pressure and oliguric renal failure (Figure 2). Simultaneous right and left heart catheterization performed off dopamine surprisingly demonstrated elevated CO and low SVR consistent with distributive shock (Table 1). Additionally, the patient was noted to have concordance of ventricular pressures that suggested of restrictive physiology (Figure 3). The pulmonary artery catheter was left in place, and subsequent measurements were made once the patient was placed back on dopamine (Table 1).

Potential reversible causes, including adrenal insufficiency and sepsis, were excluded. After a failed trial of dopamine weaning, a phenylephrine infusion was started. He was subsequently converted to oral phenylephrine and midodrine with stable hemodynamics, urine output, and renal function. Three weeks after discharge, he reported good exercise tolerance and urine output, with a stable creatinine.

On outpatient follow-up assessments, the patient remained stable on this medication regimen for several months until he suffered a mechanical fall at home and eventually died of complications related to this event.

3. Discussion

Initially, this patient's history and clinical features suggested a diagnosis of decompensated right heart failure, a common problem in adults with complex congenital heart disease. Therapy was initiated with diuretics and dopamine leading to improved symptoms and renal function, lending further credence to this diagnosis. After dopamine was withdrawn and he abruptly decompensated with hypotension and renal failure, a pulmonary artery catheterization led to the unexpected finding of high-output cardiac failure, low SVR, and a diagnosis of distributive shock. In retrospect, the markedly elevated CVP on presentation not only contributed to poor renal perfusion but also impeded the diagnosis of distributive shock in this patient. We have thus coined the term "masked hypotension" to describe this phenomenon.

Chronic high-output cardiac failure, characterized by an elevated CO and central venous congestion, is most often caused by anemia, thyrotoxicosis, obesity, hepatic disease, shunts, and COPD [2]. The cause of distributive shock was never fully explained in this case and was likely multifactorial. The patient was obese and had evidence of cirrhosis (not shown), although he did not exhibit signs or symptoms of advanced hepatic disease. Interestingly, his bilirubin level fell with dopamine infusion and diuresis (not shown), suggesting that liver dysfunction may have been a consequence, rather than a cause, of the high-output failure. Shunts are common in patients with adult congenital heart disease, but none was detected on catheterization (not shown). Other causes of distributive shock, including adrenal insufficiency, thyrotoxicosis, and sepsis, were excluded in this patient. Notably, patients with adult congenital heart disease were reported to exhibit elevated levels of endotoxin, which potentially could have contributed to low SVR in this patient [3].

Increased venous return from an elevated cardiac output alongside volume retention due to decreased renal perfusion pressure led to a dramatically elevated CVP. Under normal physiologic conditions, the contribution of CVP to MAP is negligible. However, markedly elevated CVP can

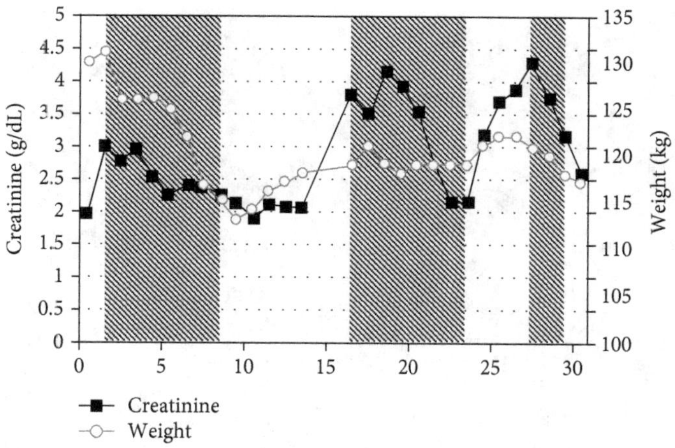

FIGURE 2: Plot of serum creatinine and weight over the 30 days after initial presentation. Shaded areas represent time periods where the patient received treatment with intravenous vasopressor agents. Dopamine was used as the vasopressor on days 1-8 and 16-23 while intravenous phenylephrine was used on days 27-29 with the patient being transitioned to oral phenylephrine thereafter. Note that despite correction of volume status by day 10, and the relative stability of weight thereafter, the patient still developed renal failure (second shaded area) supporting a pathophysiologic role for distributive shock in the face of high-output cardiac failure.

TABLE 1: Hemodynamic data obtained during right heart catheterization and bedside pulmonary artery catheter measurements.

	Without dopamine	With dopamine at 9 mcg/kg/min
MAP (mmHg)	45	94
CVP (mmHg)	14	20
Cardiac output (L/min)*	9.05	7.46
CI (L/min/m^2)	3.85	3.12
SVR (DS/cm^5)	256	793
PAP (mmHg)	33/11 (21)	40/19 (27)
PCWP (mmHg)	16	20
PVR (DS/cm^5)	35	75
RAP (mmHg)	12	n/a#
RVP (mmHg)	42/4 (12)	n/a#
LVP (mmHg)	113/-3 (16)	n/a#

*Cardiac output calculated using Fick's formula. #Direct measurements of right atrial pressure, right ventricular pressure, and left ventricular pressure were unable to be obtained using the bedside pulmonary artery catheter. CI = cardiac index; CVP = central venous pressure; MAP = mean arterial pressure; PAP = pulmonary artery pressure; PCWP = pulmonary capillary wedge pressure; SVR = systemic vascular resistance; RAP = right atrial pressure; RVP = right ventricular pressure; LVP = left ventricular pressure.

significantly contribute to MAP [MAP = (SVR × CO) + CVP] and potentially "mask" arterial hypotension. Only after diuresis was it apparent that this patient was profoundly hypotensive and dependent on vasopressor agents to maintain MAP. It is not known if this phenomenon is unique to high-output failure. However, given that SVR is a fixed value and CO is maximally elevated at baseline, it would appear that CVP would be a greater determinant of MAP in high-output failure compared to other physiologic states.

In this patient, the profoundly elevated CVP hampered recognition of the low SVR state while contributing to impaired renal perfusion. While volume retention is an appropriate response to inadequate arterial filling pressures, the maladaptive increase in CVP contributed to the patient's development of cardiorenal syndrome. Elevated CVP has been shown to decrease GFR via multiple mechanisms, including a decrease in the transrenal arterial-venous pressure gradient as well as an increase in hydrostatic pressure within the renal capsule [4].

Dopamine was chosen initially in this case for several reasons. First, dopamine was reported to preserve renal function in some patients with acute heart failure exacerbation, although results have been mixed [5]. Second, the patient was presumed to have right heart failure, and dopamine has been suggested to improve right ventricular contractility without increasing pulmonary vascular resistance [6]. Third, the patient had marginally low MAP, so inotropes associated with vasodilatory properties (i.e., dobutamine and milrinone) were less desirable. In retrospect, it appears that the benefit derived from dopamine therapy was related solely to peripheral vasoconstriction mediated through alpha-adrenergic stimulation (Table 1), as validated by the patient's clinical response to oral phenylephrine.

The unique physiology of our patient highlights the challenge in managing adults with congenital heart disease; the prevalence of which is expected to grow due to increased survival from surgical advances [1]. In addition to cardiac disease, these patients have significantly elevated rates of extracardiac organ dysfunction compared to the general population [7]. Thus, understanding the altered physiology in adult congenital heart patients is paramount to proper diagnosis and management.

4. Conclusion

In summary, we present a case of distributive shock that was concealed by markedly elevated CVP in a patient with complex adult congenital heart disease. We have coined the term

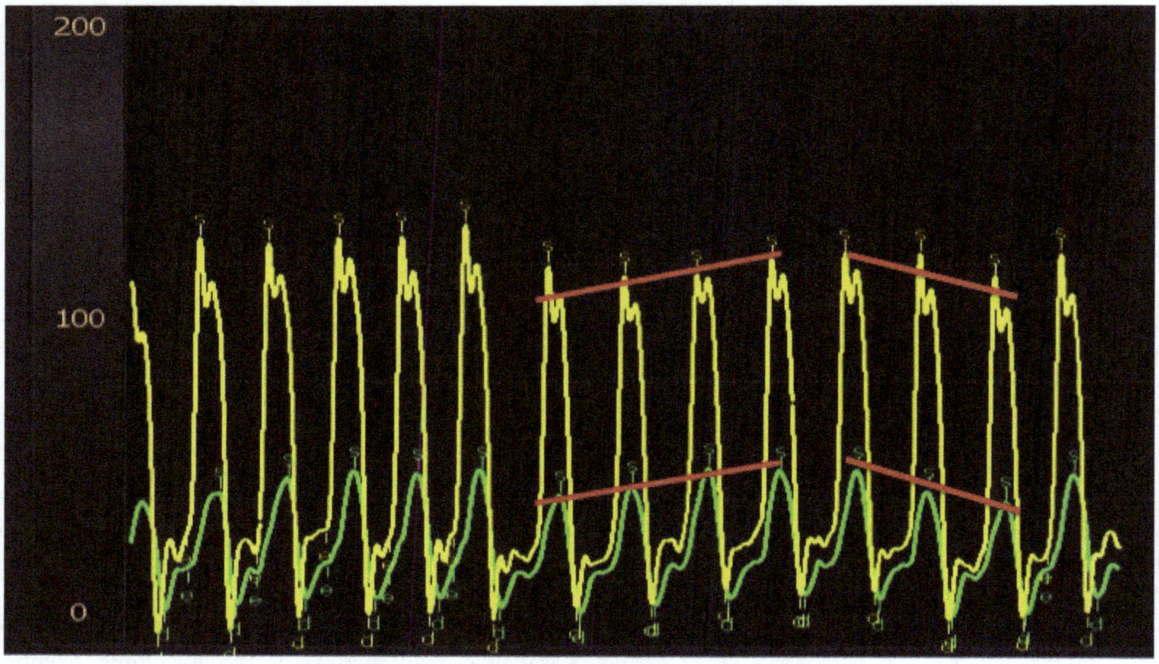

FIGURE 3: Simultaneous left and right ventricle hemodynamic monitoring with left ventricular pressure shown in yellow and right ventricular pressure shown in green. Red lines added to highlight the concordance between right ventricular and left ventricular pressure with respiration. Concordance between right ventricular and left ventricular pressures with respiration is suggestive of restrictive physiology.

"masked hypotension" to describe this phenomenon. Proper diagnosis led to treatment with alpha-adrenergic agents, which stabilized his hemodynamic state and renal function.

Abbreviations

MAP: Mean arterial pressure
CVP: Central venous pressure
CO: Cardiac output
SVR: Systemic vascular resistance
GFR: Glomerular filtration rate.

Acknowledgments

Dr. Weintraub is supported by grants HL126949, HL142097, HL134354, and AR070029 from the National Institutes of Health.

References

[1] C. P. Benziger, K. Stout, E. Zaragoza-Macias, A. Bertozzi-Villa, and A. D. Flaxman, "Projected growth of the adult congenital heart disease population in the United States to 2050: an integrative systems modeling approach," *Population Health Metrics*, vol. 13, no. 1, pp. 1–8, 2015.

[2] Y. N. V. Reddy, V. Melenovsky, M. M. Redfield, R. A. Nishimura, and B. A. Borlaug, "High-output heart failure: a 15-year experience," *Journal of the American College of Cardiology*, vol. 68, no. 5, pp. 473–482, 2016.

[3] R. Sharma, A. P. Bolger, W. Li et al., "Elevated circulating levels of inflammatory cytokines and bacterial endotoxin in adults with congenital heart disease," *The American Journal of Cardiology*, vol. 92, no. 2, pp. 188–193, 2003.

[4] B. Raam, W. A. Cupples, J. A. Joles, and C. Gaillard, "Systemic arterial and venous determinants of renal hemodynamics in congestive heart failure," *Heart Failure Reviews*, vol. 17, no. 2, pp. 161–175, 2012.

[5] H. H. Chen, K. J. Anstrom, M. M. Givertz et al., "Low-dose dopamine or low-dose nesiritide in acute heart failure with renal dysfunction the ROSE acute heart failure randomized trial," *Journal of the American Medical Association*, vol. 310, no. 23, pp. 2533–2543, 2013.

[6] C. E. Ventetuolo and J. R. Klinger, "Management of acute right ventricular failure in the intensive care unit," *Annals of the American Thoracic Society*, vol. 11, no. 5, pp. 811–822, 2014.

[7] K. Dimopoulos, G. P. Diller, E. Koltsida et al., "Prevalence, predictors, and prognostic value of renal dysfunction in adults with congenital heart disease," *Circulation*, vol. 117, no. 18, pp. 2320–2328, 2008.

37

Recurrent Multivalvular *Staphylococcus Lugdunensis* Endocarditis Causing Complete Heart Block after TAVR

Preeti Singhal,[1,2] **Somsupha Kanjanauthai**,[2,3] **and Wilson Kwan**[2,3]

[1]*Department of Internal Medicine, Keck School of Medicine of USC, Los Angeles, CA, USA*
[2]*Los Angeles County + University of Southern California Medical Center, Los Angeles, CA, USA*
[3]*Department of Cardiovascular Medicine, Keck School of Medicine of USC, Los Angeles, CA, USA*

Correspondence should be addressed to Preeti Singhal; preeti.singhal015@gmail.com

Academic Editor: Ertugurul Ercan

Prosthetic valve endocarditis after transcatheter aortic valve replacement (PVE after TAVR) is a feared complication most often observed during the early postprocedural period. We report a case of severe, multivalvular PVE after TAVR with complete heart block caused by an uncommon organism. A 78-year-old female with prior *Streptococcus agalactiae* mitral valve endocarditis treated with antibiotics presented one year later with severe, symptomatic aortic insufficiency. She subsequently underwent TAVR given high surgical risk. Six weeks post-TAVR, she presented with syncope, fever, and complete heart block. Transthoracic echocardiogram was not demonstrative of vegetation. Blood cultures were positive for *Staphylococcus lugdunensis*. Transesophageal echocardiogram (TEE) demonstrated vegetations of the aortic, mitral, and tricuspid valves and aorto-mitral continuity. While awaiting surgery, the patient developed cardiac arrest; she was resuscitated and taken to surgery emergently. The patient underwent TAVR explantation, bovine pericardial tissue aortic and porcine bioprosthetic mitral valve replacements, and tricuspid valve repair. Additionally, left main coronary artery endarterectomy was performed due to presence of infectious vegetative material. *Staphylococcus lugdunensis* is an unusual but virulent organism that may damage both native and prosthetic valves. Early surgery is recommended for PVE after TAVR, especially in cases with perivalvular disease causing conduction abnormalities. *Learning Objectives.* TAVR has revolutionized the management of severe aortic stenosis and has even been successfully utilized in select cases of aortic regurgitation. Unfortunately, there are a number of associated complications that can be difficult to diagnose, such as prosthetic valve endocarditis (PVE). We emphasize maintaining a high clinical suspicion for PVE after TAVR in patients presenting with conduction abnormalities and highlight the importance of early surgical management in cases complicated by heart block, abscesses, or destructive penetrating lesions.

1. Introduction

Transcatheter aortic valve replacement (TAVR) has become the treatment of choice for those with severe aortic stenosis and can be an effective option for patients with severe aortic regurgitation and high surgical risk. However, with the increasing rate of TAVRs being performed comes a need to better understand TAVR-associated complications such as prosthetic valve endocarditis (PVE), leaflet thrombosis, and paravalvular regurgitation. Here, we emphasize having a high clinical suspicion for PVE after TAVR in patients presenting with nonspecific symptoms and conduction abnormalities, an uncommon sequela. We highlight the importance of early surgical intervention in patients with PVE after TAVR whose clinical courses are complicated by heart block, paravalvular abscesses, and destructive penetrating lesions.

2. Case Report

A 78-year-old woman with past medical history significant for hypertension, type 2 diabetes mellitus, May-Thurner syndrome managed with iliac vein stenting, lower extremity lymphedema status post lymphovenous bypass, *Streptococcus agalactiae* endocarditis of the mitral valve treated with a six-week course of antibiotics with posttreatment TEE showing resolution of infection, and severe, symptomatic,

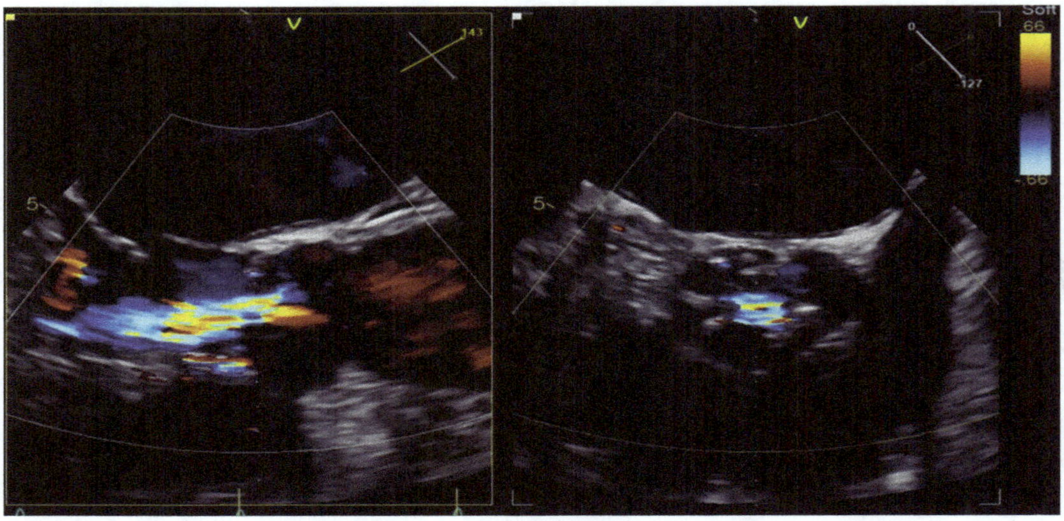

FIGURE 1: Transesophageal echocardiography image acquired prior to TAVR demonstrating thickened aortic valve with significant central aortic regurgitation without evidence of vegetation or perforation.

degenerative aortic regurgitation (Figure 1) status post uncomplicated TAVR (Edwards Lifesciences, Irvine, CA) given high surgical risk with postprocedure TTE showing peak and mean gradients of 27 mmHg and 12 mmHg, respectively, across the valve and no perivalvular regurgitation, presented six weeks post-TAVR after a syncopal episode. The patient reported several days of nausea, fevers, dizziness, and malaise.

On examination, her temperature was 38.7°C, heart rate 40/min, respiratory rate 19/minute, blood pressure 100/52 mmHg, and oxygen saturation 95% on room air. The patient was oriented but uncomfortable and lethargic appearing. Cardiovascular examination revealed an audible S1/S2 with a grade III/VI systolic ejection murmur. She also had bilateral lower extremity edema and crackles in bilateral lung bases. Electrocardiogram demonstrated new complete heart block. Transvenous pacing was initiated in the emergency department.

Laboratory studies revealed a leukocyte count of 7.0 K/cumm (reference range: 4.5-10), platelet count 18 K/cumm (reference range: 160-360), blood glucose 446 mg/dL, alkaline phosphatase 254 U/L (reference range: 35-104), and pro-BNP 3886 pg/mL (reference range: <450). Troponin-T, lactate, and TSH were within normal limits. A rapid SARS-CoV-2 assay was negative. Chest radiography demonstrated an enlarged cardiomediastinal silhouette with pulmonary vascular congestion. TTE showed a LVEF of 55%, normal right ventricular systolic function, and a well-seated bioprosthetic aortic valve with trace intravalvular aortic regurgitation without paravalvular leak (peak velocity 3.3 m/s, mean gradient 26 mmHg, and effective orifice area 1.2 cm^2). No vegetations or abscesses were visualized. Blood cultures were positive for *Staphylococcus lugdunensis*.

The patient was initiated on broad-spectrum antibiotics with vancomycin and piperacillin/tazobactam. Blood cultures remained positive for *Staphylococcus lugdunensis* for three consecutive days. Given persistent bacteremia and strong clinical suspicion for PVE following TAVR, antibiotic therapy was transitioned to vancomycin, gentamycin, and rifampin. TEE was performed on hospital day 3 and demonstrated bulky vegetative material extending from the aortic root to the atrial surface of the anterior mitral leaflet measuring 2.0 × 0.07 cm, as well as small discrete vegetative lesions measuring 0.5 × 0.3 cm and 0.5 × 0.3 cm on the atrial side of the anterior mitral leaflet and ventricular side of the aortic valve, respectively (Figure 2(a)–2(c) and Figure 3), moderate mitral regurgitation, trivial bioprosthetic aortic valve regurgitation, mild bioprosthetic aortic valve stenosis (peak velocity: 3.3 m/s) with moderately thickened leaflets along all three coaptation lines suggestive of vegetations, and mild tricuspid regurgitation. Antibiotics were narrowed to gentamycin, oxacillin, and rifampin based on blood culture susceptibilities. Surgical evaluation was initiated, and the patient was transferred to an outside hospital for further medical management and operative planning.

On hospital day 10, the patient developed ventricular tachycardia with cardiac arrest and was successfully resuscitated after one round of cardiopulmonary resuscitation. She was taken for emergent surgery, undergoing TAVR valve explantation (Figure 4), bovine pericardial tissue aortic and porcine bioprosthetic mitral valve replacement, tricuspid valve repair with anterior septal commissuroplasty, ventricular septal defect closure with a bovine pericardial patch, and right ventricular free wall perforation repair, likely a complication from transvenous pacemaker placement versus secondary to recent infarct from septic emboli. Additionally, ostial left main coronary artery endarterectomy was performed given intraoperative findings of near-total occlusion of the artery with clot and vegetative material, the likely etiology for the patient's cardiac arrest. A postintervention intraoperative transesophageal echocardiogram showed a well-seated and properly functioning bioprosthetic aortic valve with no obvious intra- or perivalvular regurgitation, a well-seated and properly functioning bioprosthetic mitral valve with trace intravalvular regurgitation and no definitive evidence of a perivalvular leak, mild tricuspid regurgitation, no evidence of residual VSD, and an ejection fraction preserved to prebypass baseline. Final surgical pathology report

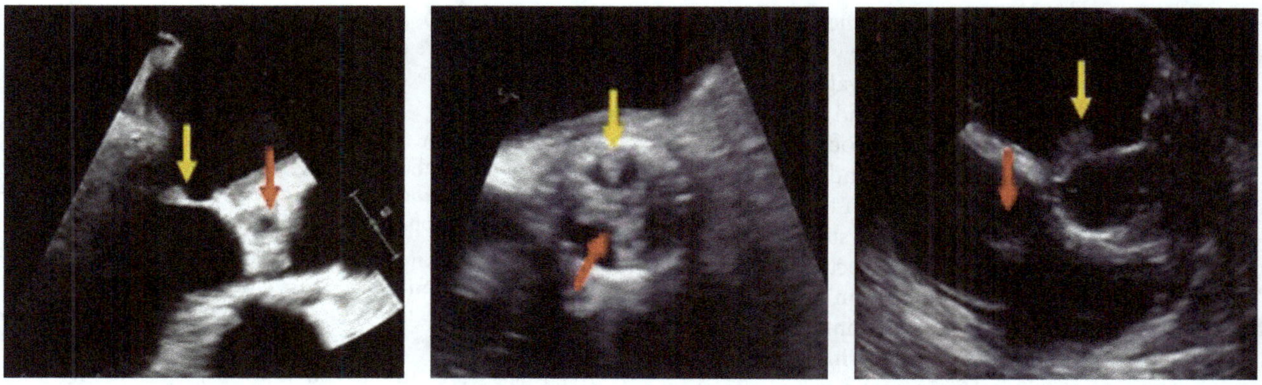

(a) (b) (c)

Figure 2: Transesophageal echocardiography of infected TAVR. (a) Thickened TAVR leaflets (red arrow) and vegetation of the mitral valve (yellow arrow). (b) Thickened TAVR leaflets (red arrow) and vegetation of the aortic cusp (yellow arrow). (c) Vegetations of the tricuspid valve (red arrow) and aortomitral continuity (yellow arrow).

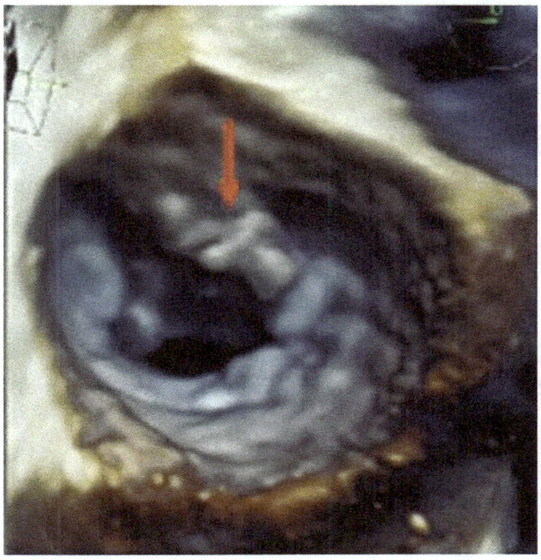

Figure 3: 3D transesophageal echocardiography of infected TAVR showing bulky vegetation on the anterior mitral valve leaflet (arrow).

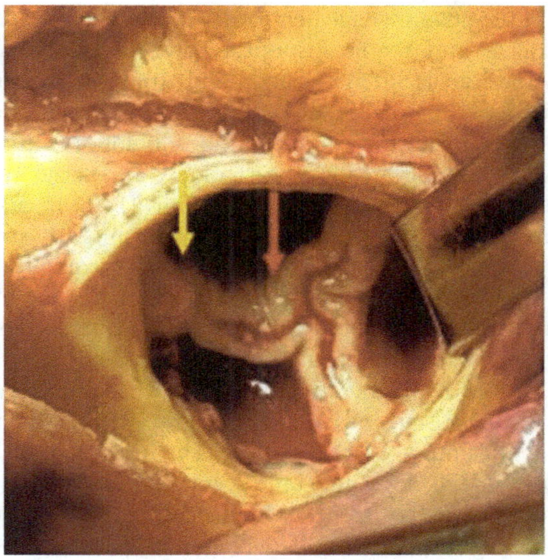

Figure 4: Intraoperative view of TAVR showing thickened TAVR leaflets (red arrow) and vegetative material (yellow arrow).

of the tissue from the aortic valve prosthesis, mitral valve, and left main endarterectomy showed organizing fibrin and prominent acute inflammation with gram stain negative for bacteria.

The patient's postoperative course was complicated by acute on chronic biventricular failure requiring inotropic and mechanical circulatory support, vasodilatory shock, and renal failure requiring continuous renal replacement therapy. After extensive discussions with the patient's family, a decision was made to change her code status to do not resuscitate. She passed seven days postoperatively from multiorgan failure.

3. Discussion

TAVR has become the treatment of choice for patients with severe aortic stenosis and can be an option for those with severe aortic regurgitation who are deemed high surgical risk. TAVR is associated with a unique set of complications [1, 2]. Albeit uncommon (incidence: 1-3%), PVE following TAVR is associated with an in-hospital mortality rate of 36% and a 2-year mortality of 67% according to a large 250 case registry [1, 3]. The risk of PVE is highest in the first year after TAVR; the most common organisms implicated overall are *Streptococcus spp.* (28.9%), followed by *Enterococcus spp.* (26.2%), and *Staphylococcus aureus* (21.5%) [2]. *Staphylococcus lugdunensis* is a relatively uncommon but highly virulent coagulase negative staphylococcus that is notable for its production of and adherence to biofilm, enabling growth on bioprosthetic materials and native tissues [4, 5].

Conduction disturbances occur in 4-10% of patients with IE. Those with aortic valve involvement are at higher risk of developing heart block due to the proximity of the His-Purkinje system to the aortic valve [6]. Recurrent IE is relatively uncommon; in a multicenter study of 1874 patients with IE, 91 (4.8%) had a documented episode of repeat IE, of which 74 (81%) involved a new bacterial species [7]. 16 cases (18%) involved a prosthetic valve; the causative organism was different between initial and recurrent infections in all 16 cases [7]. Repeat IE was associated with intravenous drug use and hemodialysis dependence, neither of which were characteristic of the patient in the case [7].

Although TTE and TEE are the cornerstones for diagnosis of endocarditis, echocardiographic detection of PVE after TAVR can be challenging in comparison to native valve endocarditis or PVE after SAVR [1]. Contributing factors include the absence of a surgical sewing ring or decalcification area, remnant native calcified aortic valve, and valve struts, all of which may cause significant echocardiographic artifacts and obscure visualization of the prosthetic valve [1]. Additionally, free space between the transcatheter and native aortic valve also presents a challenge for the diagnosis of vegetation or abscess by TEE [1].

Conservative management of PVE after TAVR is often inadequate and requires surgical valve replacement. [8] The American Heart Association and American College of Cardiology recommends early surgery during initial hospitalization prior to the completion of antibiotics in patients with PVE complicated by heart block, annular or aortic abscess, or destructive/penetrating lesions [1, 9]. In cases of uncomplicated PVE with a sensitive organism, early surgery is not required but should be considered if complications arise [1]. Our patient's significant conduction disease, multivalvular and aortic root involvement, and acute decompensation necessitated aggressive surgical management.

This case highlights the importance of prompt recognition of clinical signs of PVE, particularly when echocardiographic diagnosis is challenging. The presentation with complete heart block and intraoperative findings of widespread tissue involvement and left main coronary obstruction by vegetative material highlight the pathogenicity of *Staphylococcus lugdunensis*—an uncommon but virulent organism. Although we suspected PVE given the patient's history of prior *Streptococcus agalactiae* endocarditis and TAVR, we were surprised to find a different causative organism. It remains unclear how the patient acquired *S. lugdunensis* bacteremia. Early surgical intervention is recommended for PVE after TAVR when complicated by heart block, abscesses, or penetrating lesions given the propensity for acute decompensation.

Abbreviations

TAVR: Transcatheter aortic valve replacement
TEE: Transesophageal echocardiogram
TTE: Transthoracic echocardiogram
PVE: Prosthetic valve endocarditis
LVEF: Left ventricular ejection fraction.

References

[1] G. Habib, "Infective endocarditis after transcatheter aortic valve replacement: the worst that can happen," *Journal of the American Heart Association*, vol. 7, no. 17, 2018.

[2] S. Stortecky, D. Heg, D. Tueller et al., "Infective endocarditis after transcatheter aortic valve replacement," *Journal of the American College of Cardiology*, vol. 75, no. 24, pp. 3020–3030, 2020.

[3] M. S. Rawala, A. S. Ahmed, S. B. Rizvi, and A. Nanjundappa, "A case of transcatheter prosthetic aortic valve endocarditis," *Journal of Community Hospital Internal Medicine Perspectives*, vol. 10, no. 3, pp. 279–282, 2020.

[4] C. Ishiekwene, M. Ghitan, M. Kuhn-Basti, E. Chapnick, and Y. S. Lin, "*Staphylococcus lugdunensis* endocarditis with destruction of the ventricular septum and multiple native valves," *IDCases*, vol. 7, pp. 14-15, 2017.

[5] I. Anguera, A. Del Rio, J. M. Miro et al., "*Staphylococcus lugdunensis* infective endocarditis: description of 10 cases and analysis of native valve, prosthetic valve, and pacemaker lead endocarditis clinical profiles," *Heart*, vol. 91, no. 2, p. e10, 2005.

[6] M. Arai, K. Nagashima, M. Kato et al., "Complete atrioventricular block complicating mitral infective endocarditis caused by streptococcus Agalactiae," *American Journal of Case Reports*, vol. 17, pp. 650–654, 2016.

[7] L. Alagna, L. P. Park, B. P. Nicholson et al., "Repeat endocarditis: analysis of risk factors based on the International Collaboration on Endocarditis - Prospective Cohort Study," *Clinical Microbiology and Infection*, vol. 20, no. 6, pp. 566–575, 2014.

[8] S. Attaran, A. Chukwuemeka, P. P. Punjabi, and J. Anderson, "Do all patients with prosthetic valve endocarditis need surgery?," *Interactive Cardiovascular and Thoracic Surgery*, vol. 15, no. 6, pp. 1057–1061, 2012.

[9] R. A. Nishimura, C. M. Otto, R. O. Bonow et al., "2017 AHA/ACC focused update of the 2014 AHA/ACC guideline for the management of patients with valvular heart disease: a report of the American College of Cardiology/American Heart Association task force on clinical practice guidelines," *Journal of the American College of Cardiology*, vol. 70, no. 2, pp. 252–289, 2017.

38

Acute Myopericarditis after COVID-19 Vaccine in Teenagers

Shashikanth Ambati[1] **Michael Colon,**[2] **Maya Mihic,**[3] **Javier Sanchez,**[1] **and Adnan Bakar**[1]

[1]*Division of Pediatric Critical Care, Department of Pediatrics, Bernard & Millie Duker Children's Hospital, Albany, New York, USA*
[2]*Pediatric Cardiology, Capital District Pediatric Cardiology Associates, Albany, New York, USA*
[3]*Department of Pediatrics, Bernard & Millie Duker Children's Hospital, Albany, New York, USA*

Correspondence should be addressed to Shashikanth Ambati; ambatis@amc.edu

Academic Editor: Luigi Sciarra

Background. There have been an increasing number of reports of myocarditis and pericarditis in adolescents and young adults after coronavirus disease 19 vaccinations. The pathophysiology of myocarditis after this vaccination is indeterminate currently. The problem is a relatively new phenomenon, and so there are no current guidelines on how to manage these cases of myopericarditis. We intend to describe our management in these two cases so that it can help guide pediatricians, intensivists, and cardiologists taking care of similar cases. *Case Summaries.* The first case is a young adolescent who presented with chest pain after receiving his second dose of coronavirus disease 19 vaccination with no other symptoms. His troponin was found to be 40 ng/mL. He had a normal echocardiogram and chest CT angiogram. His troponins trended down with symptomatic pain management after 3 days. The second case is another adolescent who presented with fever, fatigue, headache, and chest pain 3 days after receiving his second dose of coronavirus vaccine. His troponin was elevated to 5 ng/mL, electrocardiogram with ST segment elevations, and mildly decreased systolic function on echocardiogram. His troponins and electrocardiogram were normalized in 3 days at the time of his discharge. *Conclusion.* The clinical course of vaccine-associated myocarditis appears favorable as both our patients have responded well to medications and rest with prompt improvement in symptoms with full recovery. The experience remains limited at this time regarding the investigations, management, and follow-up of this novel clinical entity. It is vital for all the health care providers taking care of adolescents to have knowledge about this phenomenon and make correct diagnosis in those presenting with chest pain after COVID-19 vaccine and in preventing unnecessary invasive procedures such as coronary angiogram to rule out acute coronary syndromes.

1. Introduction

There have been increased reported cases of myocarditis and pericarditis after the mRNA COVID-19 vaccines (Pfizer-BioNTech and Moderna) particularly in adolescent and young adults since April 2021 [1]. The Advisory Committee on Immunization Practices (ACIP) issued the recommendation for use of Pfizer-BioNTech COVID-19 vaccine in adolescents aged 12-15 years under the Food and Drug Administration's (FDA) Emergency Use Authorization (EUA) on May 12, 2021 [2]. More than 20 million adolescents and young adults have been vaccinated in the United States so far. Recently, the Center for Disease Control (CDC) confirmed 226 cases of myocarditis or pericarditis in people younger than 30 years of age who have received an mRNA COVID-19 vaccine [3]. Although rare, the case rates per million doses after second dose of the vaccine are higher than the expected for this age group. The numbers above were reported to vaccine adverse event reporting system (VAERS), and there are another 250 more reports that federal health officials are investigating. It is not yet clear whether these cases represent true myocarditis or pericarditis. The true incidence of myocarditis/pericarditis after COVID-19 vaccine may not be known as every case may not be reported.

Marshall et al. [4] recently published a case series of seven adolescents with myocarditis following Pfizer-BioNTech COVID-19 vaccine. Currently, there is no definite causal relationship of myocarditis with the COVID-19 vaccine. The pathophysiology of myocarditis after COVID-19 vaccine is indeterminate at this time. However, there have been multiple reports of myopericarditis associated with active COVID-19 infection, as a delayed complication in COVID-19 adult survivors, and as a part of multi-inflammatory syndrome in children (MIS-C) [5]. The pathogenesis of myocarditis or pericarditis associated with COVID-19 infection is thought to be the combination of direct viral injury or the host's immune response resulting in myocardial damage [6].

The problem is a relatively new phenomenon, and there are no current guidelines on how to manage these cases of myopericarditis. Here, we describe two adolescents who developed myopericarditis after receiving the second dose of Pfizer-BioNTech COVID-19 vaccine requiring intensive care unit admission followed by full recovery. At this time, there are not many case reports published about this condition in adolescents other than the reports to VAERS and some anecdotal reports. Hence, we intend to describe our management in these two cases so that it can help guide pediatricians, intensivists, and cardiologists taking care of similar cases.

2. Case 1

A 16-year-old male with history of Von Willebrand disease, anxiety disorder, and Lennox-Gastaut syndrome on multiple seizure medications and vagal nerve stimulator presented to the emergency department (ED) with chest pain 2 days after receiving his second dose of Pfizer-BioNTech COVID-19 vaccine. There was no associated shortness of breath, palpitations, or syncope. The chest pain was described as stabbing in nature, localized to the substernal area, and worsened with respirations. He also reported to have couple episodes of emesis the morning of presentation but denied any fevers, abdominal pain, diarrhea, or any breakthrough seizures. There was no known exposure or history of COVID-19 in the past. He initially presented to a local urgent care after his chest pain got worsened. His electrocardiogram (ECG) demonstrated diffuse ST segment elevations and elevated troponin I to 38 ng/mL with a normal B Type Natriuretic Peptide (BNP). On arrival to our ED, his repeat troponin was found to be 40 ng/mL. He had normal biventricular systolic function with normal coronary origins and size on transthoracic echocardiogram. He was admitted to the pediatric intensive care unit (PICU) for close monitoring due to severely elevated troponin and ECG changes. He was monitored with serial troponins every six hours and symptomatic management with nonsteroidal anti-inflammatory agents. His respiratory viral panel was negative for all the viruses. Due to the possibility of MIS-C, labs such as ferritin 128 ng/mL (normal), CRP 86.5 mg/L (elevated), d-dimers 0.75 mg/L (slightly elevated), and ESR 4 mm/hr (normal) were performed. His chest pain completely resolved, ST segment elevations improved, and troponins trended down within 24 hours to 11 ng/mL. Cardiac magnetic resonance imaging was planned to confirm the diagnosis of myocarditis but deferred due to the presence of vagal nerve stimulator in proximity to the heart.

Although his chest pain improved, the troponins plateaued between 11 and 13 ng/mL for another 24 hours with some diffuse T wave inversions on EKG. Computerized Tomographic Angiography (CTA) of the coronary arteries demonstrated a normal appearance of the coronary arteries without anomaly, stenosis, or occlusion. On PICU day #3, his troponins trended down to 4 ng/mL and he remained without chest pain. He was discharged home on ibuprofen with close follow-up with cardiology. He was evaluated in the outpatient cardiology office a week after discharge from PICU, where his repeat echocardiogram was normal and troponin I level of 0.17 ng/mL. He has planned follow-up in 6 weeks.

3. Case 2

A 17-year-old male with history of attention deficit hyperactivity disorder and mild intermittent asthma presented to a local urgent care center with chest pain. He received his second dose of Pfizer-BioNTech COVID-19 vaccine 3 days prior to presentation. Starting the day, he received his vaccine, he experienced fatigue, generalized body aches, headache, and fever of 101 F. He denied any cough, congestion, nausea, emesis, abdominal pain, or diarrhea. There was no known exposure or history of COVID-19 in the past. He described his chest pain as sharp, nonradiating, and constant pain localized to the sternum. It was exacerbated by deep inspiration but no change with movement or palpation. Additionally, he complained of shortness of breath with the chest pain. His labs showed an elevated troponin I of 5 ng/mL and ST segment elevations on the ECG concerning for myocarditis which prompted the transfer to our ED for cardiology evaluation. Echocardiogram showed mildly decreased left ventricular systolic function. He was admitted to the PICU for close monitoring due to his EKG changes and elevated troponin I. He also had negative viral respiratory panel, and his MIS-C labs included a normal ferritin and d-dimer with BNP of 121 pg/mL (mildly elevated) and CRP 95 mg/L (elevated), ESR 43 mm/hr (elevated), and negative SARS-CoV-2 IgG antibody. He was managed with serial troponins and supportive management with ibuprofen and narcotics for chest pain. He was transferred out of the PICU to the floor at hospital day 2 and then discharged home on day 3. His troponin level at the time of discharge is 0.55 ng/mL, and EKG showed normal ST segments. Follow-up is planned in 2-3 weeks.

4. Discussion

As per a report from Centers for Disease Control and Prevention, a total of 789 cases of myocarditis or pericarditis across all ages have been reported since April 2021 after the Pfizer/BioNTech and Moderna vaccines, most commonly after the second dose. After the FDA authorized the use of Pfizer-BioNTech COVID-19 vaccine in young people between ages 12 and 15 years of age in May 2021, federal agencies began receiving more reports about cases of chest pain or palpitations or other signs consistent with myocarditis or pericarditis in young adolescents. There were nearly

226 reports of myocarditis or pericarditis under age 30 years among which had been confirmed, and other 250 reports are still being investigated [3]. In those ages 16 to 17 years, there were 79 cases of myocarditis/pericarditis following 2.3 million administered second dose mRNA vaccinations [3]. The annual incidence of myocarditis from other causes in children and adolescents in United States is estimated to be 1-2 per 100,000 [7]. The number of these cases exceeds the cases expected in general unvaccinated children.

The cases that were reported to the vaccine adverse event reporting system (VAERS) have been predominantly males with a median age of 24 years following the second dose of the vaccine. The most common symptoms reported included chest pain, elevated cardiac enzymes, ST or T wave changes on ECG, dyspnea, and abnormal echocardiography/imaging. Both our patients presented with chest pain with elevated cardiac enzymes and ST segment changes on ECG. The echocardiograms in our patients appeared grossly normal with good biventricular systolic function. We ruled out acute COVID-19 infection as part of workup for the etiology of myocarditis in both our patients as there are many reports of acute myocarditis or pericarditis from COVID-19 infection both in the acute phase and delayed complication [7, 8]. Though children and young adolescents had been relatively spared from COVID-19 pulmonary manifestations, some of them succumbed to inflammatory syndrome called MIS-C proposed to be mediated by cytokine activation after several weeks of COVID-19 infection. Both our patients had reported no history of COVID-19 infection or known exposure to someone with COVID-19. The role of SARS-CoV-2 IgG antibodies in ruling out prior exposure in these cases is unknown due to vaccine-induced immunogenicity. Vaccines trigger antibodies to specific viral protein targets and currently authorized COVID-19 mRNA vaccines induce antibodies to the spike protein. If the patient had natural infection from COVID-19, the antibodies are produced to the nucleocapsid and spike proteins of the virus and at this time our SARS-CoV-2 antibody testing cannot differentiate the antibodies from either one making it difficult to differentiate the immunogenicity from vaccine or prior infection in our patients. Both our patients were ruled out for MIS-C due to low ferritin, d-dimer, fibrinogen, and no other clinical signs of multisystem involvement.

All patients presenting with chest pain, palpitations, shortness of breath, or syncope within 7 days from COVID-19 vaccination should get an ECG and troponin level to rule out postvaccine myocarditis. Patients with elevated troponins or ECG changes consistent with pericarditis or myocarditis should be admitted to the hospital with telemetry. These patients should be followed with serial troponin levels and ECGs. Echocardiogram should be obtained on admission to evaluate ventricular function, pericardial effusion, chamber enlargement, or valvular abnormalities. It should be repeated if there are any new arrhythmias or clinical deterioration. Elevated levels of cardiac enzymes such as cardiac troponin I can be seen in most patients with myocarditis, but the degree of elevation does not consistently correlate with disease severity as some patients with only mild ventricular dysfunction can have higher levels of troponin I than patients with moderate to severe ventricular dysfunction [9]. The highest level of troponin I that was reported by Marshall et al. [4] recently in their case series of seven adolescents with myocarditis after COVID-19 vaccine was 22 ng/mL. Our patient (case 1) had a level of 40 ng/mL which rapidly decreased to 11 ng/mL within 24 hours. Although troponin I is very specific marker for myocardial injury, there have been reports of troponin I elevation after a seizure [10, 11]. Since our patient has history of Lennox-Gastaut syndrome, he might have had some seizures contributing to such an elevation. It remains to be determined if the presence of copathologies in both our patients favored the increase in the troponin.

Extensive diagnostic evaluation for other infectious myocarditis etiologies should be performed in these patients. Infectious, particularly viral, etiologies are most common in children. The most common causes of viral myocarditis are enterovirus (coxsackie group B), adenovirus, parvovirus B19, Epstein-Barr virus, cytomegalovirus, and human herpes 6 [12]. These patients should be tested for SARS-CoV-2 PCR to rule out active COVID-19 infection. If the antibody testing can differentiate the vaccine-induced antibodies and infection-induced antibodies, then SARS-CoV-2 antibody testing is helpful to rule out prior infection as there are several reports of myocarditis or pericarditis as a part of MIS-C in children and young adolescents. Labs such as CRP, d-dimer, ferritin, and ESR should be sent in these patients to rule out MIS-C [13].

Endomyocardial biopsy (EMB) is considered the gold standard to confirm a clinical diagnosis of myocarditis but it has a fairly low sensitivity and is associated with considerable risk as it requires cardiac catheterization [14]. For these reasons, cardiac magnetic resonance imaging (CMRI) is increasingly used to diagnose myocarditis in children. CMRI can show myocardial edema, late gadolinium enhancement consistent with necrosis, or scarring and regional wall motion abnormalities [15]. Recent publication by Rosner et al. reported multifocal subepicardial late gadolinium enhancement in all their patients with myocarditis after COVID-19 vaccine and myocardial edema in 3 out of 7 patients [16]. CMRI was not performed in either of our patients as one of our patients (case 1) had a vagal nerve stimulator situated close to the heart and other patient (case 2) had resolving troponin leak within 24 hours. CMRI may be considered in patients with myocarditis from COVID-19 vaccine if the troponins are increasing and there is ventricular dysfunction on the echocardiogram to confirm the diagnosis of myocarditis.

The symptoms of vaccine-induced myocarditis mimic acute coronary syndromes. The incidence of acute coronary syndromes in children and young adolescents is very rare compared to middle-aged and elderly patients [17]. There have been multiple case reports of acute coronary syndrome associated with COVID-19 in adults who required invasive coronary angiography but no reports of coronary involvement in any patients who received COVID-19 vaccine so far [18]. Rosner et al. [16] performed coronary angiography in 3 out of 7 middle-aged patients with COVID-19 vaccine-associated myocarditis, and none of them revealed any obstructive coronary disease, and all of them were early or middle-aged patients. Marshall et al. [4] reported none of their adolescents required any coronary angiography in their case series. The role of cardiac catheterization in these adolescent patients with postvaccine myocarditis to rule out acute coronary syndrome is unclear at this time but considering the prevalence of acute coronary syndromes in this age group makes it of little or no benefit considering the risks associated.

In most cases that were reported, the clinical course of vaccine-associated myocarditis appears favorable as most of the patients have responded well to medications and rest with prompt improvement in symptoms with full recovery. Though the risk of myocarditis from vaccine seems higher than the general population, the benefit of COVID-19 vaccines clearly outweighs the risks given the potential morbidity of COVID-19 or any type of viral myocarditis. This problem is relatively new, and the CDC and its partners are actively monitoring reports and reviewing data and medical records to see if there is any association between the COVID-19 vaccine and myocarditis. The experience remains limited at this time regarding the investigations, management, and follow-up of this novel clinical entity. It is critical to report all these events to VAERS, and further studies are needed to explain the pathophysiological mechanism of this phenomenon so that these patients can be identified and treated appropriately. It is vital for all the health care providers taking care of adolescents to have knowledge about this phenomenon and make correct diagnosis in those presenting with chest pain after COVID-19 vaccine and in preventing unnecessary invasive procedures such as coronary angiogram to rule out acute coronary syndromes.

5. Patient Perspective

One of the patients shared that he was glad that the damage to the heart is temporary, and he was happy that he was able to go home in few days. He said that he did not regret taking the vaccine.

Consent

No written consent has been obtained from the patients as there is no patient identifiable data included in this case report/series.

Disclosure

This research was performed as part of employment of the authors under Albany Medical Center.

References

[1] National Center for Immunization and Respiratory Diseases (NCIRD), "Division of Viral Diseases," *Myocarditis and pericarditis following mRNA COVID-19 vaccination*, 2021, https://www.cdc.gov/coronavirus/2019-ncov/vaccines/safety/myocarditis.html.

[2] Pfizer-BioNTech, *Full Emergency Use Authorization (EUA) Prescribing Information*, 2021, http://labeling.pfizer.com/ShowLabeling.aspx?id=14471&format=pdf&&page=13.

[3] M. Jenco, *CDC confirms 226 cases of myocarditis after COVID-19 vaccination in people 30 and under*, 2021, https://www.aappublications.org/news/2021/06/10/covid-vaccine-myocarditis-rates-061021.

[4] M. Marshall, I. D. Ferguson, P. Lewis et al., "Symptomatic acute myocarditis in 7 adolescents After Pfizer-BioNTech COVID-19 vaccination," *Pediatrics*, vol. 148, no. 3, article e2021052478, 2021.

[5] I. Valverde, Y. Singh, J. Sanchez-de-Toledo et al., "Acute cardiovascular manifestations in 286 children with multisystem inflammatory syndrome associated with COVID-19 infection in Europe," *Circulation*, vol. 143, no. 1, pp. 21–32, 2021.

[6] B. Siripanthong, S. Nazarian, D. Muser et al., "Recognizing COVID-19-related myocarditis: the possible pathophysiology and proposed guideline for diagnosis and management," *Heart Rhythm*, vol. 17, no. 9, pp. 1463–1471, 2020.

[7] S. E. Lipshultz, L. A. Sleeper, J. A. Towbin et al., "The incidence of pediatric cardiomyopathy in two regions of the United States," *New England Journal of Medicine*, vol. 348, no. 17, pp. 1647–1655, 2003.

[8] R. Bajaj, H. C. Sinclair, K. Patel et al., "Delayed-onset myocarditis following COVID-19," *The Lancet Respiratory Medicine.*, vol. 9, no. 4, pp. e32–e34, 2021.

[9] R. J. Butts, G. J. Boyle, S. R. Deshpande et al., "Characteristics of clinically diagnosed pediatric myocarditis in a contemporary multi-center cohort," *Pediatric cardiology.*, vol. 38, no. 6, pp. 1175–1182, 2017.

[10] Y. Ghandi, F. Sharitmadari, D. Habibi, and S. Sadrnia, "Evaluation of cardiac troponin level following generalized tonic-clonic seizure in children; cross-sectional study," *Shiraz E-Medical Journal*, vol. 22, no. 7, 2021.

[11] A. Brobbey and K. Ravakhah, "Elevated serum cardiac troponin I level in a patient after a grand mal seizure and with no evidence of cardiac disease," *The American journal of the medical sciences.*, vol. 328, pp. 189–191, 2004.

[12] C. E. Canter and K. E. Simpson, "Diagnosis and treatment of myocarditis in children in the current era," *Circulation*, vol. 129, no. 1, pp. 115–128, 2014.

[13] J. C. McMurray, J. W. May, M. W. Cunningham, and O. Y. Jones, "Multisystem inflammatory syndrome in children (MIS-C), a post-viral myocarditis and systemic vasculitis-a critical review of its pathogenesis and treatment," *Frontiers in Pediatrics*, vol. 8, p. 626182, 2020.

[14] M. Brighenti, A. Donti, M. Giulia Gagliardi et al., "Endomyocardial biopsy safety and clinical yield in pediatric myocarditis: an Italian perspective," *Catheterization and cardiovascular interventions: official journal of the Society for Cardiac Angiography & Interventions.*, vol. 87, no. 4, pp. 762–767, 2016.

[15] P. Banka, J. D. Robinson, S. C. Uppu et al., "Cardiovascular magnetic resonance techniques and findings in children with myocarditis: a multicenter retrospective study," *Journal of cardiovascular magnetic resonance: official journal of the Society for Cardiovascular Magnetic Resonance.*, vol. 17, no. 1, 2015.

[16] C. M. Rosner, L. Genovese, B. N. Tehrani et al., "Myocarditis temporally associated with COVID-19 vaccination," *Circulation*, vol. 144, no. 6, pp. 502–505, 2021.

[17] S. Puricel, C. Lehner, M. Oberhänsli et al., "Acute coronary syndrome in patients younger than 30 years – aetiologies, baseline characteristics and long-term clinical outcome," *Swiss medical weekly.*, vol. 143, 2013.

A Case of Systemic Lupus Erythematosus in a Patient Presenting with Libman-Sacks Endocarditis

Mariann Al-Jehani,[1] Faisal Al-Husayni,[2,3] Ahmed Almaqati,[3] Jomanah Shahbaz,[1] Saad Albugami,[1,2,4] and Wail Alameen[4]

[1]*King Saud bin Abdulaziz University for Health Sciences, Jeddah, Saudi Arabia*
[2]*King Abdullah International Medical Research Center, Jeddah, Saudi Arabia*
[3]*Department of Internal Medicine, National Guard Hospital, Jeddah, Saudi Arabia*
[4]*Department of Cardiac Sciences, King Faisal Cardiac Center, National Guard Hospital, Jeddah, Saudi Arabia*

Correspondence should be addressed to Saad Albugami; sbugami@gmail.com

Academic Editor: Christopher S. Snyder

Background. Libman-Sacks endocarditis (LSE) is a rare cardiovascular manifestation of systemic lupus erythematosus/antiphospholipid syndrome that is described as a sterile verrucous nonbacterial vegetative lesion. These lesions can cause progressive damage to the heart valves leading to valve surgery. The most common valves to be affected are the aortic and mitral valves. Libman-Sacks endocarditis is associated with malignancies, other systemic diseases like systemic lupus erythematosus (SLE) and antiphospholipid antibody syndrome (APS). The majority of LSE patients are usually asymptomatic. *Case Summary*. We describe a 39-year-old male patient who presented with increasing shortness of breath and pulmonary congestion. He was found to have severe mitral valve regurgitation and mitral stenosis. Transesophageal echocardiogram confirmed the diagnosis of Libman-Sacks endocarditis with thickened mitral valve leaflets with symmetrical mass-like structure causing a restriction in the valve function during both cardiac phases later diagnosed with systemic lupus erythematosus by immunology. The patient was started on diuretics, anticoagulants, angiotensin inhibitors, beta-blockers, and hydroxychloroquine. He underwent successful mechanical mitral valve replacement with a 27 mm St. Jude valve. The mitral valve was found to be grossly thickened with friable tissue and complete amalgamation of the leaflets with subvalvular apparatus. The patient suffered some warfarin adverse effects a year later but did well otherwise. *Conclusion*. This case demonstrates that Libman-Sacks endocarditis can be the first manifestation of systemic lupus erythematosus. Early and prompt diagnosis of LSE can prevent and lessen the many side effects associated with thromboembolism. Additionally, addressing the underlying disease is key to successful treatment.

1. Introduction

Libman-Sacks endocarditis (LSE) is noninfectious endocarditis that is sometimes referred to as nonbacterial thrombotic endocarditis (NBTE), marantic endocarditis, or verrucous endocarditis. It is characterized by deposition of thrombi mainly on aortic and mitral valves; involvement of other valves is less common. It was first described by Emanuel Libman and Benjamin Sacks in 1924 [1]. LSE was mostly associated with malignancies, for example, patients with pancreatic adenocarcinoma were found to have a higher risk of developing LSE with systemic embolization being the leading cause of morbidity [2]. Additionally, LSE is linked to other systemic diseases like systemic lupus erythematosus (SLE) and antiphospholipid antibody syndrome (APS). LSE is encountered among 10% of patients with SLE; it correlates with the disease activity, duration, anticardiolipin antibodies, and APS manifestations. SLE patients with LSE frequently have evidence of valvular affection and lesion progression as shown by Moyssakis et al. [1].

The majority of LSE patients are usually asymptomatic, while if the patient was symptomatic it is usually due to embolic infarctions either as cerebrovascular or systemic thromboembolism. SLE and APS patients may present with signs and symptoms of their underlying diseases, such as malar rash and recurrent miscarriages.

The prognosis of LSE has not been well defined; it is usually considered poor, especially if those patients develop recurrent thromboembolism [3].

We are describing an adult patient who presented with LSE as the first manifestation of SLE.

2. Case Presentation

A 39-year-old male, who was medically free prior to this, presented complaining of a three-month history of exertional dyspnea classified as New York Heart Association (NYHA) Class III, associated with cough and palpitation. The patient suffered from five ill-defined syncopal attacks during the past year. He reported a three-month history of lethargy, loss of appetite, and weight loss. The patient denied any personal history of fever, joint pain, or drug abuse. Family history was unremarkable for malignancies or cardiac conditions. Upon admission, the patient was vitally stable with normal saturation on ambient air. Chest examination revealed decreased breath sounds in the right lower zone with bilateral basal crackles, soft first heart sound, normal second heart sound, loud pansystolic murmur, and a soft diastolic rumble at the mitral area. His initial blood work is shown in Table 1. ECG revealed T-wave inversion in leads II, III, and AVF (Figure 1).

Chest imaging revealed cardiomegaly and right pleural effusion with right lower lobe consolidations (Figure 2). Echocardiogram showed a dilated right ventricle with mild to moderate tricuspid regurgitation and severe rheumatic mitral stenosis with moderate to severe mitral regurgitation (Figure 3). The patient was then commenced on diuretics, anticoagulants, angiotensin inhibitors, and beta-blockers. Transesophageal echocardiogram showed thickened mitral valve leaflets with symmetrical mass-like structure on the ventricular surface involving the tips of both leaflets extending to the body, causing a restriction in the valve function during both cardiac phases (Figure 4). Later, the patient underwent a diagnostic angiography, which showed normal coronary arteries. The immunology test came back confirming the diagnosis of SLE (Table 2). Following cardiac team discussion, the patient underwent mitral valve replacement surgery. During the operation, the mitral valve was found to be grossly thickened with friable tissue and complete amalgamation of the leaflets with subvalvular apparatus (Figure 5). The valve was replaced with a 27 mm St. Jude valve. Postop echocardiogram was performed; thus, the surgery was deemed successful and his hospital stay was uneventful. Tissue biopsy showed degenerative changes, myxoid areas with hemorrhage admixed with acute and chronic inflammatory cell infiltrate. In addition, fibroid necrosis was present without calcification. The diagnosis of LSE was confirmed with SLE as underlying disease. The patient was started on hydroxychloroquine 400 mg daily, warfarin, and aspirin. At one-year follow-up, he had an increased intraocular pressure, hyphema, total vitreous hemorrhage, and choroidal hemorrhage. The patient was admitted and underwent hyphema drainage and trabeculectomy. Otherwise, the patient was doing well.

Table 1: Initial laboratory data for the patient at presentation.

Labs	Results	Reference range
White blood count	5.5×10^9/L	$4.0 - 11.0 \times 10^9$/L
Hemoglobin	11.9 g/dL	11.5–16.5 g/dL
Platelet	111×10^9/L	$150 - 450 \times 10^9$/L
Neutrophil count	3.14×10^9/L	$2 - 7.5 \times 10^9$/L
Lymphocyte count	1.08×10^9/L	$1.5 - 4 \times 10^9$/L
Blood urea nitrogen	8.1 mmol/L	2.1–7.1 mmol/L
Creatinine	150 μmol/L	62–106 μmol/L
Brain natriuretic peptide	1585 pg/mL	<100 pg/mL
High-sensitivity troponin	>0.03 ng/mL	>0.03 ng/mL

3. Discussion

Cardiac involvement in SLE is common. It is estimated that more than 50% of SLE/APS patients have cardiovascular manifestations in the form of pericarditis, myocarditis, LSE, pulmonary arterial hypertension, conduction disease, and coronary artery disease. Left-sided heart valves are by far the most affected. It has previously been reported to have cardiac involvement as the main reason for presentation; however, this is extremely rare [1–8].

Multivalvular involvement often occurs, but typically, the most frequently affected valve is the mitral valve with the vegetations occurring near the edge of the valve or on both of its surfaces. Involvement of the atrial or ventricular endocardium or the chordae tendineae and papillary muscles is rare.

The approach to diagnose LSE might not be simple as some SLE or APS patients are asymptomatic. Echocardiography is the best first modality to diagnose LSE, but transesophageal echocardiography is more sensitive and specific than transthoracic echocardiography [9, 10]. Doppler echocardiography detects between 18% and 50% of valve diseases [1–10], while transesophageal echocardiography detects up to 74% [9, 10]. LSE on imaging is described as irregular heterogeneous echo density with the absence of independent motion of the verrucous vegetations on the cardiac valves and endocardium [9, 10]. The mitral and aortic valves are most affected by leaflet thickening and regurgitation. Although the origin of valvular lesions in SLE is closely linked to the presence of antiphospholipid antibodies [10], negative test results have been described in literature in other patients with SLE and LSE [8] or even in nonbacterial thrombotic endocarditis without underlying disease.

The LSE diagnosis is difficult to be confirmed by laboratory tests; however, patients who are suspected of having LSE must have complete blood count, comprehensive metabolic workup, blood cultures, autoimmune profile, and hypercoagulable workup [1–9].

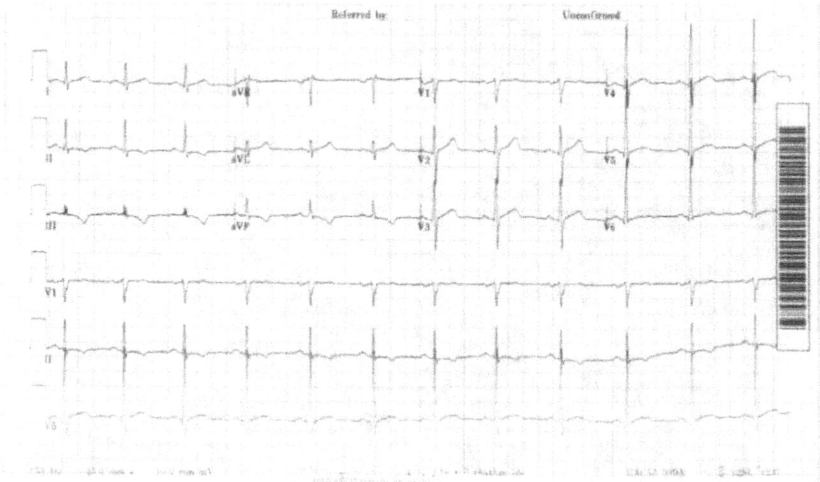

FIGURE 1: Patient's electrocardiogram showing inverted T-wave in leads II, III, and AVF.

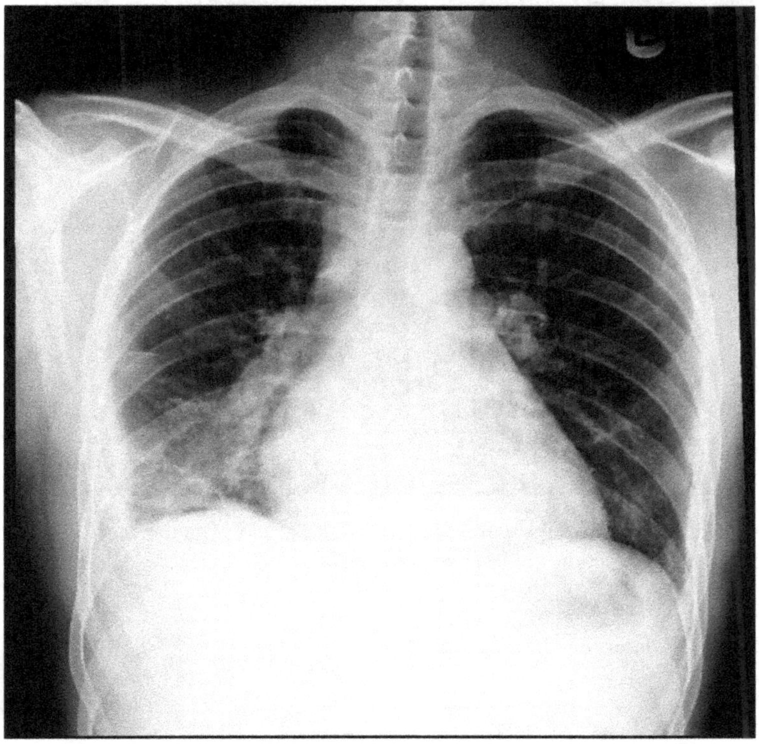

FIGURE 2: Patient's chest X-ray demonstrating cardiomegaly and right lower lobe consolidations with pleural effusion.

When treating LSE, the underlying disease, either SLE or APS, must be addressed. Hydroxychloroquine (HCQ), an antimalarial drug, has been an effective option for managing SLE, especially in the early stages [1–10]. Its effectiveness has been established in the mild form of SLE, while not as effective in preventing severe SLE manifestations such as glomerulonephritis and central nervous system involvement [11].

Corticosteroids are considered a treatment option to reduce the inflammatory reaction caused by LSE; however, they can lead to tissue scarring and fibrosis, predisposing to further valvular damage [11, 12]. Anticoagulation should be considered in SLE/APS patients as secondary prevention for thromboembolic events, especially those who have had previous thromboembolic events [11–15].

Surgical valve replacement is recommended for symptomatic and severe cases of LSE. Mechanical valve replacement in females of reproductive age is not preferable as they would require to be put on an anticoagulation regime with increased fetal and maternal side effects. Nonetheless, it is still recommended as many authors believe that SLE/APS patients will eventually end up on anticoagulants for the disease-associated thromboembolism [14, 15].

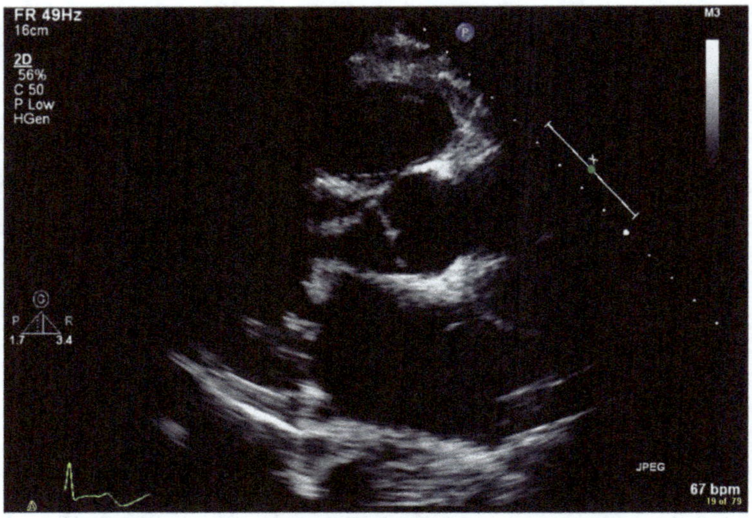

Figure 3: Parasternal long axis view revealing a diffused leaflet thickening of the mitral valve.

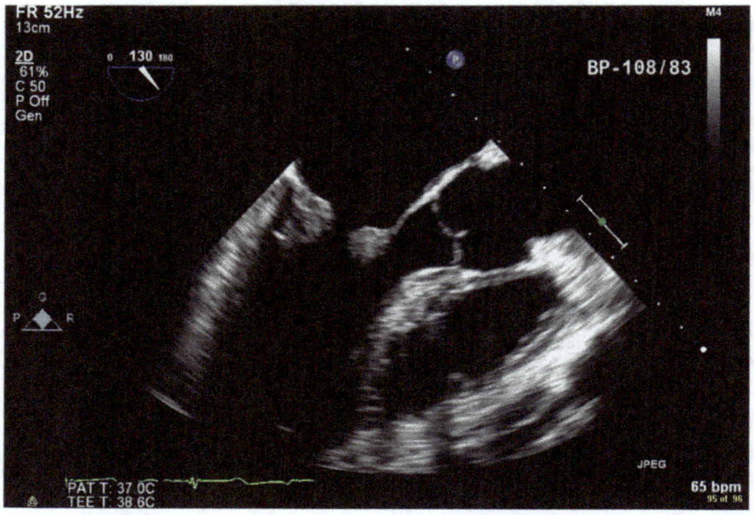

Figure 4: Transesophageal echocardiogram showing a symmetrical mass-like structure on the ventricular surface involving the tips of both leaflets extending to the body, causing a restriction in the valve function.

Table 2: Autoimmune laboratory tests concerning the diagnosis of systemic lupus erythematosus.

Labs	Results	Reference range
Antinuclear antibody	Positive	Negative
Anti-double-stranded DNA	355.7	<68.6 is negative 68.6–229 is moderately positive >229 is strongly positive
Ribonucleoprotein antibody	472.5	<20 is negative 20–39 is weakly positive 40–80 is moderately positive >80 is strongly positive
Anti-Smith antibody	114.71	<20 is negative 20–39 is weakly positive 40–80 is moderately positive >80 is strongly positive
C3 complement	0.8 g/dL	0.9–1.9 g/dL
C4 complement	>0.06	0.1–0.4 g/dL

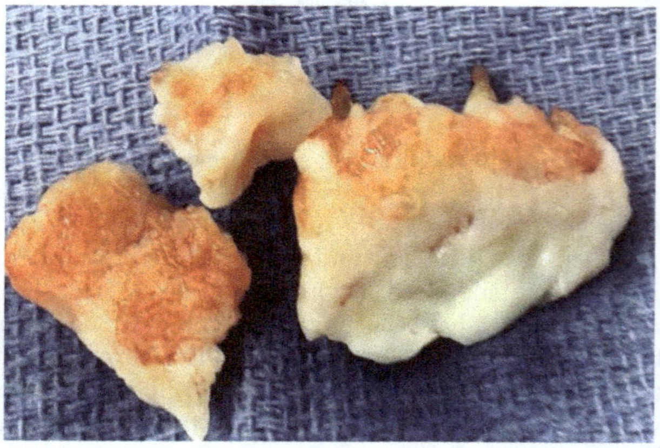

Figure 5: Gross anatomy of the mitral valve leaflets in keeping with Libman-Sacks endocarditis.

4. Conclusion

LSE is rare as the first manifestation of SLE/APS. We presented a 39-year-old male with LSE as the initial manifestation of SLE. It was successfully diagnosed by echocardiography and treated with mitral valve replacement surgery. The case highlights SLE as a differential diagnosis when encountering a healthy individual with new-onset valve disease. Early and prompt diagnosis of LSE can prevent and lessen the many side effects associated with thromboembolism.

References

[1] I. Moyssakis, M. G. Tektonidou, V. A. Vasilliou, M. Samarkos, V. Votteas, and H. M. Moutsopoulos, "Libman-Sacks endocarditis in systemic lupus erythematosus: prevalence, associations, and evolution," *The American Journal of Medicine*, vol. 120, no. 7, pp. 636–642, 2007.

[2] A. González Quintela, M. J. Candela, C. Vidal, J. Román, and P. Aramburo, "Non-bacterial thrombotic endocarditis in cancer patients," *Acta Cardiologica*, vol. 46, no. 1, pp. 1–9, 1991.

[3] C. A. Roldan, W. L. Sibbitt, C. R. Qualls et al., "Libman-Sacks endocarditis and embolic cerebrovascular disease," *JACC: Cardiovascular Imaging*, vol. 6, no. 9, pp. 973–983, 2013.

[4] N. E. Doherty and R. J. Siegel, "Cardiovascular manifestations of systemic lupus erythematosus," *American Heart Journal*, vol. 110, no. 6, pp. 1257–1265, 1985.

[5] M. Foroughi, M. Hekmat, M. Ghorbani, H. Ghaderi, M. Majidi, and M. Beheshti, "Mitral valve surgery in patients with systemic lupus erythematosus," *The Scientific World Journal*, vol. 2014, Article ID 216291, 9 pages, 2014.

[6] M. F. de Godoy, C. M. de Oliveira, V. A. Fabri et al., "Long-term cardiac changes in patients with systemic lupus erythematosus," *BMC Research Notes*, vol. 6, no. 1, 2013.

[7] J. Sharma, Z. Lasic, A. Bornstein, R. Cooper, and J. Chen, "Libman-Sacks endocarditis as the first manifestation of systemic lupus erythematosus in an adolescent, with a review of the literature," *Cardiology in the Young*, vol. 23, no. 1, pp. 1–6, 2013.

[8] S. Chen, B. Smith, M. Ilina, C. Bowen, and N. Martin, "PReS-FINAL-2307: Libman-Sacks endocarditis as a presentation for systemic lupus erythematous in an adolescent with isolated mitrial regurgitation and Noonan syndrome," *Pediatric Rheumatology*, vol. 11, Supplement 2, 2013.

[9] H. Gouya, L. Cabanes, L. Mouthon, A. Pavie, P. Legmann, and O. Vignaux, "Severe mitral stenosis as the first manifestation of systemic lupus erythematosus in a 20-year-old woman: the value of magnetic resonance imaging in the diagnosis of Libman-Sacks endocarditis," *The International Journal of Cardiovascular Imaging*, vol. 30, no. 5, pp. 959-960, 2014.

[10] C. A. Roldan, B. K. Shively, C. C. Lau, F. T. Gurule, E. A. Smith, and M. H. Crawford, "Systemic lupus erythematosus valve disease by transesophageal echocardiography and the role of antiphospholipid antibodies," *Journal of the American College of Cardiology*, vol. 20, no. 5, pp. 1127–1134, 1992.

[11] U. P. Dandekar, R. Watkin, N. Chandra et al., "Aortic valve replacement for Libman-Sacks endocarditis," *The Annals of Thoracic Surgery*, vol. 88, no. 2, pp. 669–671, 2009.

[12] A. Akhlaq, T. A. Ali, and S. H. Fatimi, "Mitral valve replacement in systemic lupus erythematosus associated Libman-Sacks endocarditis," *Journal of the Saudi Heart Association*, vol. 28, no. 2, pp. 124–126, 2016.

[13] A. M. Ibrahim and M. S. Siddique, "Libman Sacks endocarditis," in *Stat Pearls*, Stat Pearls Publishing, Treasure Island FL, 2020.

[14] A. Doria, M. Zen, M. Canova et al., "SLE diagnosis and treatment: when early is early," *Autoimmunity Reviews*, vol. 10, no. 1, pp. 55–60, 2010.

[15] M. Hojnik, J. George, L. Ziporen, and Y. Shoenfeld, "Heart valve involvement (Libman-Sacks endocarditis) in the antiphospholipid syndrome," *Circulation*, vol. 93, no. 8, pp. 1579–1587, 1996.

A Rare Case of Multivessel SCAD Successfully Treated with Conservative Medical Management

Lance Alquran[1] **Ankita Patel,**[1] **Lucy Safi,**[2] **and Ankitkumar Patel**[1,2]

[1]*Department of Internal Medicine, Hackensack Meridian Health Mountainside Medical Center, Montclair, New Jersey 07028, USA*
[2]*Department of Cardiology, Hackensack University Medical Center, Hackensack, New Jersey 07601, USA*

Correspondence should be addressed to Lance Alquran; dr.alquran@gmail.com

Academic Editor: Man-Hong Jim

A female patient presented with severe, symptomatic multivessel spontaneous coronary artery dissection (SCAD) with no known medical history or risk factors. The affected vessels were left anterior descending artery (LAD), right coronary artery (RCA), and the ramus. She was treated with conservative medical management. Two months later, repeat coronary angiogram to evaluate for any residual disease was performed which showed near-complete resolution of all involved vessels.

1. Case History

A 51-year-old African American female with no known past medical history presented to the emergency department with substernal chest pain, after being found in the field with frequent nonsustained ventricular tachycardia. The patient described the pain as pressure-like, moderate in intensity, which has been bothering her for the past twelve hours, alleviated by rest, and aggravated by exertion. On physical examination, she appeared anxious, well nourished, and in no acute distress. Initial vital signs showed she was hypertensive with a blood pressure of 165/94 and a regular heart rate of 89. Her neck was supple, jugular venous pressure normal, and trachea was midline. Cardiac examination revealed no abnormalities in point of maximal impulse or carotid bruits. There were no murmurs, rubs, or gallops, with normal S1/S2 components. The examination of other systems was unremarkable. In the context of substernal chest pain, the patient initially received an electrocardiogram that showed normal sinus rhythm with old anterior and inferior lateral wall myocardial infarction (Figure 1). The initial troponin upon arrival to the emergency department was 8.5 ng/mL. She was brought for an emergent coronary catheterization, for ongoing ischemic symptoms, and was found to have multivessel SCAD involving the LAD, ramus, and RCA (Figures 2–4). Echocardiogram revealed mildly depressed systolic function and regional wall motion abnormalities. Given her anatomical features, percutaneous coronary intervention (PCI) was deemed of elevated risk. Optimal medical therapy began with dual antiplatelet therapy aspirin and clopidogrel. Nitroglycerin infusion was started for symptomatic relief, as well as heparin drip for the non-ST-segment myocardial infarction. The patient developed symptom relief. Her hospital course was uncomplicated and with conservative therapy she has done well. After receiving conservative medical management, repeat coronary angiogram was preformed to access for residual disease, to see if the dissections have resolved. The repeat angiogram showed near-complete resolution of the LAD, RCA, and ramus (Figures 5–7). Repeat electrocardiogram two weeks after PCI showed no acute ST-T changes. Her New York Heart Association (NYHA) functional class was class I; she had no signs or symptoms of heart failure post-procedure. Taking into account the patient's functional status with only minor deficits on initial echocardiogram, there was no repeat scan

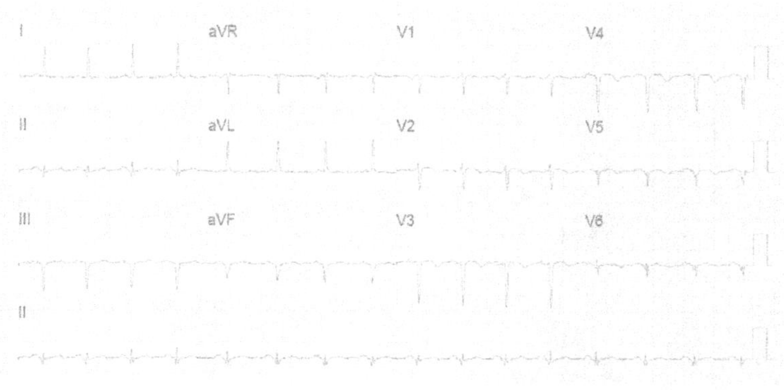

FIGURE 1: Normal sinus rhythm with an old anterior and inferolateral wall myocardial infarct.

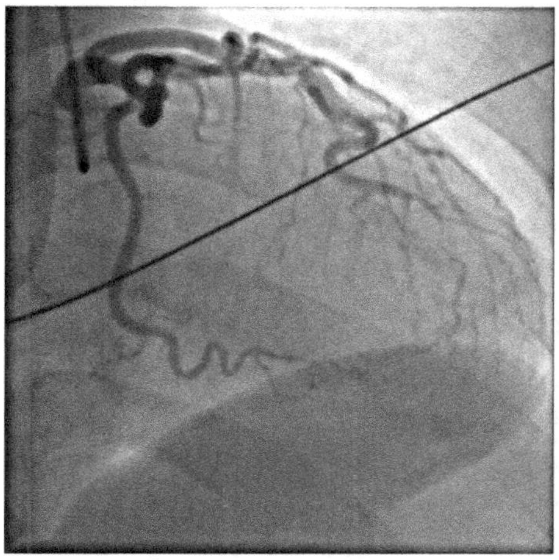

FIGURE 2: LAD with a normal caliber type 3 tortuous vessel and distal 80% long dissected section with normal apical vessel.

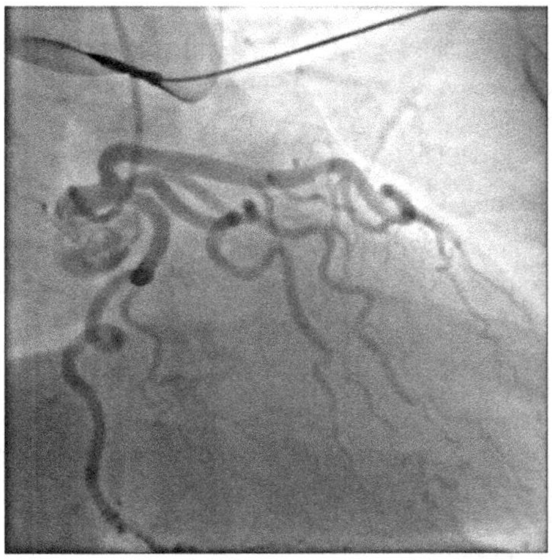

FIGURE 3: Ramus with a normal caliber tortuous vessel and distal 80% long dissected section.

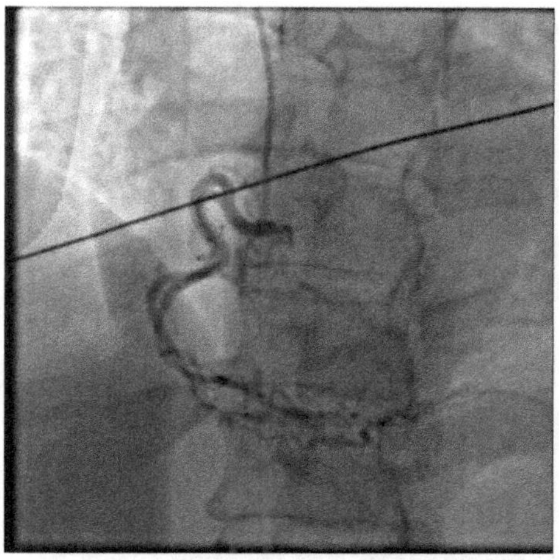

FIGURE 4: RCA with a normal caliber dominant vessel, early bifurcation, and extreme tortuosity distal area of dissection.

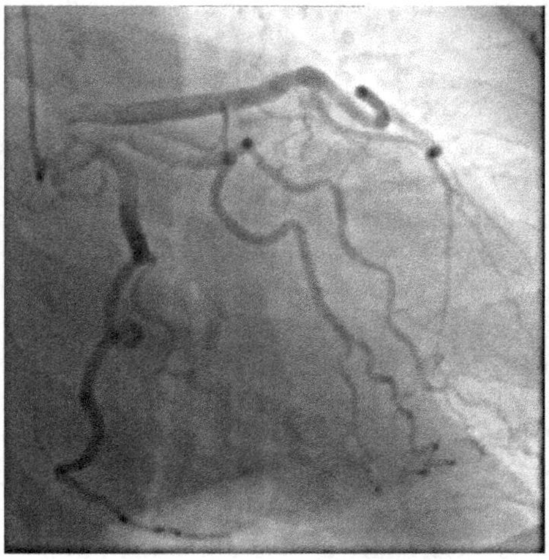

FIGURE 5: LAD with normal caliber type 3 vessel with 20% midstenosis and distal nearly completely healed SCAD long segment.

preformed. At post-procedure, she did not have exertional angina, making her class 0 on the Canadian Cardiovascular Society grading of angina pectoris.

2. Discussion

SCAD is a relatively rare cause of myocardial infarction, being diagnosed in approximately 0.07-0.2% of all angiograms [1]. It is thought that the true incidence remains

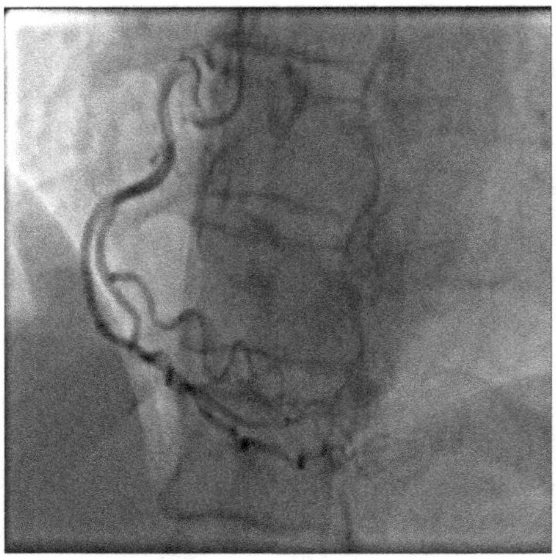

Figure 6: RCA with normal caliber codominant vessel with tortuosity.

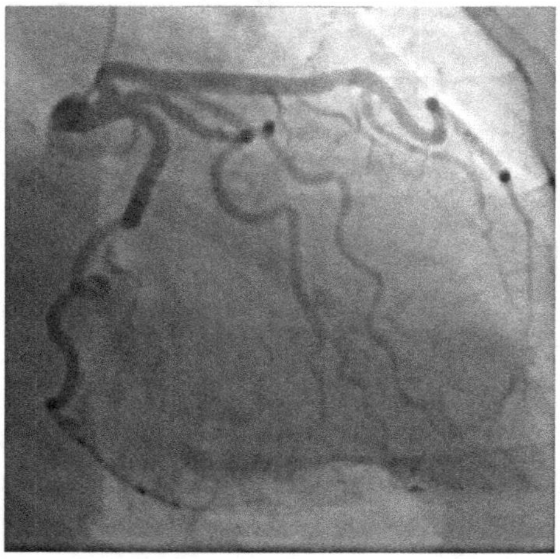

Figure 7: Ramus with normal caliber vessel with healed distal SCAD segments.

unclear because of the cases which go underdiagnosed [2, 3]. There has been an increased rate of diagnosis in recent years, likely secondary to increased use of coronary angiograms, and application of high-resolution intracoronary imaging [4]. Multivessel SCAD is much more rare and occurs in 9-23% of described cases [5]. Patients who are correctly diagnosed usually present with acute coronary syndrome positive biomarkers [2]. Ventricular arrhythmias have been associated with 2.8-10% cases [2, 6–8]. Patients usually present with the same signs and symptoms of acute coronary syndrome, with chest pain being the most common complaint [5]. Coronary angiogram is the first-line method used to diagnose SCAD if suspected [5]. There have been no dedicated studies regarding the role of coronary computed tomography angiography (CCTA) in the setting of acute SCAD [5]. CCTA is generally contradicted in patients with a high likelihood of acute coronary syndrome and is not recommended as a first-line investigation [5]. Also, normal findings on CCTA cannot exclude SCAD [5]. Traditionally, SCAD is described as multiple radiolucent lumens with extraluminal contrast staining that can show intraluminal filling defects or spiral dissections [9]. When treating SCAD, the goals of care are to provide symptomatic relief, prevent reoccurrence, and improve short/long-term outcomes [5]. Some experts recommend dual-antiplatelet therapy for a minimum of 1 year after diagnosis of SCAD, as well as lifetime aspirin therapy [10]. There is no clear evidence supporting the use of dual-antiplatelet therapy in patients with SCAD who did not receive coronary intervention [5]. The theoretical benefit of early dual-antiplatelet therapy is protection from subsequent thrombus formation [5]. No studies have been performed to compare the short- and long-term outcomes, as well as risk of bleeding, in patients treated with dual-antiplatelet therapy and aspirin alone [5]. Studies have shown PCI therapy to cause high rates of technical failure and does not protect against reoccurrence or vessel revascularization [6]. Conservative management with close observation can be preferred [6]. There have been no comprehensive prospective studies that performed angiographic restudy after the diagnosis of SCAD [5]. However, there is observational data that indicates angiographic healing of SCAD in (70-97%) of patients who were restudied weeks to months after being conservatively managed [5].

3. Conclusion

Multivessel SCAD is a rare but serious cause of ACS that requires prompt diagnosis and treatment. We describe a case of multivessel SCAD, which was treated conservatively. The repeat coronary angiogram to evaluate for any residual disease was performed two months after initial diagnosis and showed near-complete resolution of all involved vessels.

References

[1] G. Vanzetto, E. Berger-Coz, G. Barone-Rochette et al., "Prevalence, therapeutic management and medium-term prognosis of spontaneous coronary artery dissection: results from a database of 11,605 patients," *European Journal of Cardio-Thoracic Surgery*, vol. 35, no. 2, pp. 250–254, 2009.

[2] D. Adlam, F. Alfonso, A. Maas et al., "European Society of Cardiology, Acute Cardiovascular Care Association, SCAD study group: a position paper on spontaneous coronary artery dissection," *European Heart Journal*, vol. 39, no. 36, pp. 3353–3368, 2018.

[3] J. Saw, K. Humphries, E. Aymong et al., "Spontaneous coronary artery dissection: clinical outcomes and risk of recurrence," *Journal of the American College of Cardiology*, vol. 70, no. 9, pp. 1148–1158, 2017.

[4] J. Saw, G. B. J. Mancini, and K. H. Humphries, "Contemporary review on spontaneous coronary artery dissection," *Journal of the American College of Cardiology*, vol. 68, no. 3, pp. 297–312, 2016.

[5] S. N. Hayes, C. E. S. H. Kim, J. Saw et al., "Spontaneous coronary artery dissection: current state of the science: a

scientific statement from the American Heart Association," *Circulation*, vol. 137, no. 19, pp. e523–e557, 2018.

[6] M. S. Tweet, M. F. Eleid, P. J. M. Best et al., "Spontaneous coronary artery dissection: revascularization versus conservative therapy," *Circulation Cardiovascular Interventions*, vol. 7, no. 6, pp. 777–786, 2014.

[7] J. Saw, E. Aymong, T. Sedlak et al., "Spontaneous coronary artery dissection," *Circulation. Cardiovascular Interventions*, vol. 7, no. 5, pp. 645–655, 2014.

[8] C. Lettieri, D. Zavalloni, R. Rossini et al., "Management and long-term prognosis of spontaneous coronary artery dissection," *The American Journal of Cardiology*, vol. 116, no. 1, pp. 66–73, 2015.

[9] J. H. Rogers and J. M. Lasala, "Coronary artery dissection and perforation complicating percutaneous coronary intervention," *The Journal of Invasive Cardiology*, vol. 16, no. 9, pp. 493–499, 2004.

[10] E. A. Amsterdam, N. K. Wenger, R. G. Brindis et al., "2014 AHA/ACC guideline for the management of patients with non–ST-elevation acute coronary syndromes: executive summary," *Circulation*, vol. 130, no. 25, pp. 2354–2394, 2014.

Surgery for Bacterial Endocarditis Complicated by Diffuse Alveolar Hemorrhage

Kazuhiro Kurisu, Hiroshi Mitsuo, and Yasutaka Ueno

Department of Cardiovascular Surgery, Shimonoseki City Hospital, Shimonoseki, Japan

Correspondence should be addressed to Kazuhiro Kurisu; kazukurisu@outlook.jp

Academic Editor: Hajime Kataoka

Diffuse alveolar hemorrhage is a very rare but potentially lethal condition resulting from various disorders. We report the case of a patient who suffered diffuse alveolar hemorrhage subsequent to bacterial endocarditis and survived aortic valve replacement, which was applied after improvement in respiratory distress. We believe that the strategy of respiratory functional recovery by aggressive rehabilitation is essential for the achievement of a successful surgical outcome in patients with alveolar hemorrhage.

1. Introduction

Diffuse alveolar hemorrhage (DAH) is a very rare but potentially fatal condition [1–3]. Its etiology is wide and includes, *inter alia*, autoimmune vasculitis, infection, drug toxicities, and organ transplantation [1–3]. As this condition is caused by bleeding into the alveoli resulting from the disruption of the alveolar-capillary basement membrane, respiratory distress is frequently a serious concern [1–3]. Cardiac valve surgery should be avoided in this situation because it may lead to further bleeding and exacerbated respiratory failure. We describe a patient who suffered DAH following bacterial endocarditis and survived aortic valve replacement after improvement in respiratory distress syndrome.

2. Case Presentation

A 45-year-old woman, on a regimen of steroids for a diagnosis of Behçet's disease or systemic lupus erythematosus, was admitted with pyrexia, cough, and worsening dyspnea of a week's duration. She had a history of small bowel resection for intestinal necrosis and had been on parenteral nutrition since then. She presented a fever of 39.1°C, tachycardia of 116/min, and hypoxia with oxygen saturation of 94% in nasal oxygen cannula. A grade 3/6 regurgitant diastolic murmur was heard in the left third intercostal space on auscultation. She soon fell into respiratory failure and was immediately supported by mechanical ventilation. The ratio of the arterial oxygen pressure and the fraction of inspired oxygen (PaO_2/-FiO_2) was initially calculated as 105. Chest radiography and computed tomography revealed diffuse extensive consolidation in bilateral fields corresponding with DAH (Figure 1). This diagnosis was confirmed by bronchoalveolar lavage with increasing bloody secretion in three consecutive aliquots. In a peripheral blood examination, the white blood cell count was 11,540/mm^3, hemoglobin 6.6 g/dL, and platelet count 132,000/mm^3. Aspartate aminotransferase, alanine aminotransferase, and lactate dehydrogenase were 18, 16, and 164 IU/L, respectively. Renal function was slightly affected, with a creatinine level of 1.5 mg/dL. C-reactive protein was elevated to 12.3 mg/dL. Blood cultures afterward grew *Staphylococcus warneri*. Echocardiography showed aortic regurgitation and a mobile vegetation of 15×9 mm in size on the commissure between the left and right coronary cusps. Left ventricular function was preserved with an ejection fraction of 62%. The patient was diagnosed with bacterial endocarditis [4] complicated with respiratory distress related to the DAH.

At this point, she was judged not to tolerate cardiac surgery because of the exacerbating bleeding and respiratory failure related to heparinized extracorporeal circulation. The management plan was as follows: (1) antibiotic and inotropic therapies with diuretics for the bacterial endocarditis

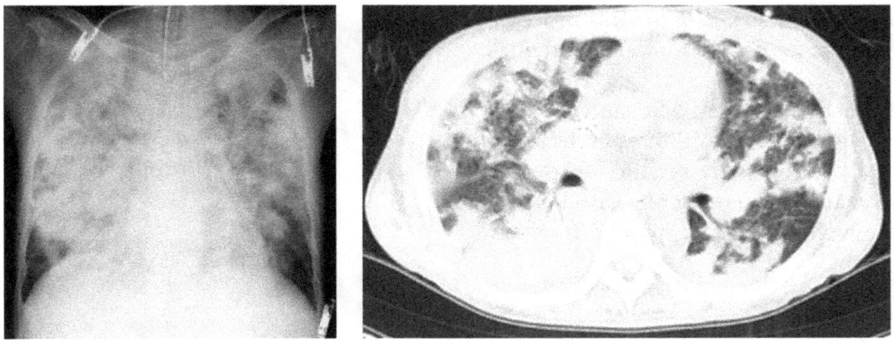

(a) (b)

FIGURE 1: Preoperative chest radiography (a) and computed tomography (b) showing bilateral diffuse consolidation.

and heart failure, (2) steroid pulse and hemostatic drug therapies for DAH, and (3) postponement of cardiac surgery until sufficient improvement in respiratory function unless circulation collapses. Nevertheless, the respiratory function initially made little improvement despite adequate cardiac condition. Because the clot in the alveolar space could not be excreted in the usual supine position, a tracheotomy followed by aggressive positional changes to include an abdominal position was planned. The tracheotomy was performed on hospital day 12. Thereafter, respiratory function gradually improved although mechanical ventilation was still needed, and the PaO_2/FiO_2 ratio reached 356 on hospital day 31. Methylprednisolone was then adjusted to a maintenance dose of 40 mg/day, and daptomycin was administered at 210 mg/day. The white blood cell count was 8,210/mm^3 with a shift to the left, and C-reactive protein was 10.2 mg/dL. Repeated echocardiography revealed worsening aortic regurgitation suggesting the disruption of the commissure between the left and right coronary cusps and the mildly enlarged vegetation. We decided to perform the valve surgery in this timing when the respiratory distress improved.

J shaped partial sternotomy was performed between the second intercostal space and the xiphoid process. A cardiopulmonary bypass was equipped with right femoral artery perfusion and right atrial drainage. A 19 mm St. Jude Medical mechanical prosthesis (St. Jude Medical, St. Paul, MN, USA) was inserted with subannular reinforcement [5] using a rifampicin-soaked woven Dacron graft (Vascutek, Terumo, Inchinnan, UK) to prevent valve detachment associated with Behçet's disease. Respiratory function was well maintained, and mechanical ventilation support was discontinued on the seventh postoperative day. The control of infection was satisfactory. The patient was discharged home following closure of the tracheotomy. Methylprednisolone therapy was continued at the maintenance dose of 40 mg/day during the operative and postoperative days. Daptomycin was also used at the same dose of 210 mg/day, and ampicillin sodium/sulbactam sodium was added only on the day of operation.

3. Discussion

DAH is a potentially fatal condition because the respiratory function is seriously impaired by bleeding into the alveoli resulting from the disruption of the alveolar-capillary basement membrane [1–3]. Its etiology is wide and includes autoimmune vasculitis, infection, drug toxicities, and organ transplantation [1–3]. In this particular case, we speculate the autoimmune vasculitis resulted from inflammation provoked by the bacterial infection and caused the disruption of the alveolar-capillary basement membrane and further alveolar hemorrhage. Systemic lupus erythematosus probably participated in the mechanism of this illness. DAH resulting from bacterial endocarditis is extremely rare, and this combination has been reported only once, by Wu et al. [6], who treated their patient with intravenous antibiotic therapy but not surgically. To our knowledge, the present patient is the first to survive surgery for infective endocarditis complicated with DAH.

The reported in-hospital mortality of DAH ranged from roughly 25% to 50% [1–3]. Quadrelli et al. reported that mortality is higher in patients who require dialysis and/or mechanical ventilation and SaO_2 under 90% at admission [1]. Zamora et al. showed that the factors associated with increased mortality include mechanical ventilation, infection, and cyclophosphamide therapy [2]. Kohashi et al. proposed that factors for poor prognosis are a lactate dehydrogenase level over 230 IU/L, PaO_2/FiO_2 ratio under 300, and consolidation shadows on computed tomography [3]. The condition of our patient, with respiratory distress requiring mechanical ventilation support, active infective endocarditis, and consolidation shadows on images, was presumed to be very serious. Although surgical intervention was considered indispensable for the treatment of this endocarditis, we concluded that the patient would be unable to tolerate the surgery at first. We surmised that a procedure for respiratory functional improvement by excreting the clot from the alveolar space would be essential to obtain a successful surgical outcome in this situation. Although initially not sufficient, remarkable improvement in respiratory distress was achieved by aggressive respiratory rehabilitation with frequent positional change following the tracheotomy. The patient consequently underwent aortic valve replacement without any respiratory and infectious complications.

We adopted subannular reinforcement [5] using a woven Dacron graft in aortic valve replacement to prevent valve detachment. Although other surgeons consider the technique troublesome and time-consuming, this procedure might an effective adjunct for pathology with a potentially fragile annulus.

In conclusion, we describe a patient who survived aortic valve replacement for bacterial endocarditis complicated by DAH. We believe that improving respiratory distress by aggressive respiratory rehabilitation to excrete any clots from alveoli is essential for successful cardiac surgery in patients with DAH.

References

[1] S. Quadrelli, D. Dubinsky, M. Solis et al., "Immune diffuse alveolar hemorrhage: clinical presentation and outcome," *Respiratory Medicine*, vol. 129, pp. 59–62, 2017.

[2] M. R. Zamora, M. L. Warner, R. Tuder, and M. I. Schwarz, "Diffuse alveolar hemorrhage and systemic lupus erythematosus: clinical presentation, histology, survival, and outcome," *Medicine*, vol. 76, no. 3, pp. 192–202, 1997.

[3] Y. Kohashi, Y. Saito, Y. Totani et al., "The relationships between initial clinical features and prognosis in 14 cases of diffuse alveolar hemorrhage syndrome," *Annals of the Japanese Respiratory Society*, vol. 47, no. 4, pp. 265–270, 2009.

[4] J. S. Li, D. J. Sexton, N. Mick et al., "Proposed modifications to the Duke criteria for the diagnosis of infective endocarditis," *Clinical Infectious Diseases*, vol. 30, no. 4, pp. 633–638, 2000.

[5] T. Azuma, K. Yamazaki, S. Saito, and H. Kurosawa, "Aortic valve replacement in Behcet's disease: surgical modification to prevent valve detachment," *European Journal of Cardio-Thoracic Surgery*, vol. 36, no. 4, pp. 771-772, 2009.

[6] H. C. Wu, Y. K. Wen, M. L. Chen, and C. S. Fan, "Pulmonary-renal syndrome in a patient with bacterial endocarditis," *Journal of the Formosan Medical Association*, vol. 104, no. 8, pp. 588–592, 2005.

A Case of Acute Massive Bioprosthetic Mitral Valve Thrombosis Leading to Fulminant Heart Failure

Zeid Nesheiwat,[1] Pinang Shastri,[1] Rohit Vyas,[1] Cameron Burmeister,[1] Robert Grande,[2] and Hazem Malas[2]

[1]*Department of Internal Medicine, The University of Toledo College of Medicine, 3000 Arlington Avenue, Toledo, Ohio 43614, USA*
[2]*Division of Cardiovascular Medicine, Toledo Hospital, 2142 N Cove Boulevard, Toledo, Ohio 43606, USA*

Correspondence should be addressed to Zeid Nesheiwat; nesheiwatzeid@gmail.com

Academic Editor: Alfredo E. Rodriguez

Bioprosthetic valve thrombosis has been considered to be extremely unlikely, typically freeing patients from the potential complications of long-term anticoagulation. However, there have been several documented cases of bioprosthetic valve thrombosis and there are concerns that its incidence may be underreported. Experience with diagnosis and management of this condition is limited. Here, we present a case of acute massive bioprosthetic mitral thrombosis manifesting as fulminant heart failure.

1. Introduction

Over 150,000 valve replacements are performed annually in the United States and over 80% of these procedures utilize bioprosthetic valves [1]. The large shift from mechanical valves to BPVs is related to the growing high-risk population that require valve replacement, the appeal of short-term anticoagulation therapy, and options for minimally invasive procedures making them a good option for patients who are poor surgical candidates or have an increased risk of bleeding. BPV replacements are relatively safe procedures with a minimal rate of serious complications, typically 2-3%, which include thromboembolic events, structural valve dysfunction, endocarditis, and hemolysis [2]. Current guidelines support short-term oral anticoagulation with or without aspirin as well as dual antiplatelet therapy following transcatheter aortic valve replacement [1].

Valve thrombosis is a rare and life-threatening complication of valve replacement surgery. While more common in mechanical valves, valve thrombosis can occur in bioprosthetic valves with severe consequences. The diagnosis remains challenging mainly due to a general lack of awareness of its existence [2]. Typically, bioprosthetic valve thrombosis occurs within 1-2 years of implantation with some studies showing as early at 6 months postimplantation [1, 3]. Treatment options include surgical excision and reimplantation, fibrinolysis, and anticoagulation. Here, we present a case of acute bioprosthetic mitral valve thrombosis with fulminant heart failure requiring emergent invasive cardiac surgery.

2. Case Presentation

A 65-year-old male with a past medical history significant for hypertension, asthma, and minimally invasive bioprosthetic mitral valve replacement with a 33 mm mosaic mitral porcine valve one year prior presented with severe respiratory distress requiring emergent intubation. Initial electrocardiogram (EKG) revealed sinus rhythm with left anterior fascicular block, right bundle branch block, and evidence of left atrial enlargement. Initial troponin was normal at 0.04 ng/mL, but CK-MB and total CK were elevated to 21.2 ng/mL and 308 U/L, respectively. Anticoagulation studies revealed an INR of 1.0, a PTT of 28, and a PT of 10.9. Following transfer to the intensive care unit, the patient was started immediately on heparin infusion for suspicion of acute coronary

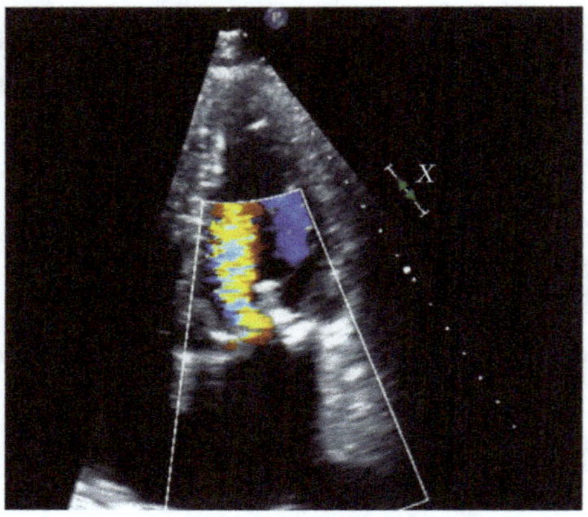

Figure 1: Severe mitral regurgitation noted on four-chamber apical view.

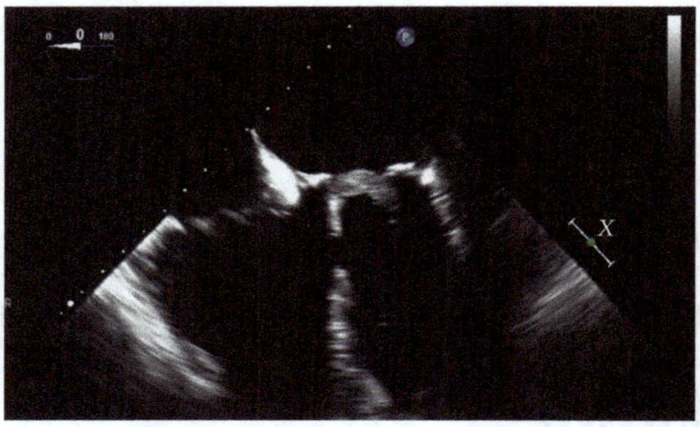

Figure 2: Four-chamber apical view of bioprosthetic mitral valve thrombosis.

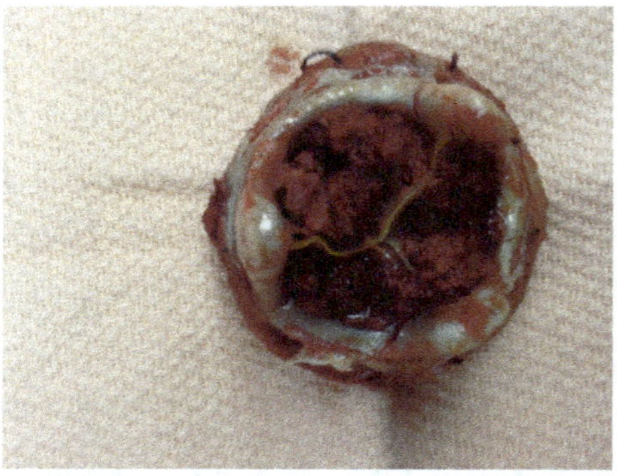

Figure 3: Massive thrombus completely obstructing the bioprosthetic valve as seen in the postoperative photo.

syndrome (ACS); computed tomography angiogram (CTA) of the chest revealed moderate patchy ground-glass and nodular airspace opacities with interstitial edema and cardiomegaly. Transesophageal echocardiogram (TEE) was performed showing an acute thrombosis of the bioprosthetic mitral valve with severe mitral stenosis and regurgitation exhibiting a mean gradient of 20.1 mmHg and valve area of 0.68 cm^2 (Figure 1). Of note, the patient had already completed 6 months of anticoagulation following his bioprosthetic mitral valve replacement and was no longer on anticoagulation. He was also found to have near complete leaflet immobility and subsequently underwent emergent redo mitral valve surgery utilizing a 33 mm St. Jude mechanical prosthesis. The valve was noted to have a massive amount of material on the ventricular side of each cusp (Figures 2 and 3) with pathology findings consistent with thrombosis. Following valve replacement, intraoperative TEE showed that the mitral valve mean gradient had improved to 4 mmHg. The procedure was well-tolerated, and the patient was successfully extubated and transitioned to warfarin for anticoagulation. Hypercoagulable workup was negative, and he was doing well on follow-up.

3. Discussion

Despite the rising popularity and efficacy of bioprosthetic valve implantation, the incidence rate of acute complications is often underreported and many patients who undergo acute intervention lack proper echocardiographic follow-up. A 2015 Mayo Clinic study identified bioprosthetic mitral valve thrombosis in 11% of explanted bioprosthetic mitral valves; in addition, this study revealed that 65% of all reoperations for bioprosthetic mitral valves occurred more than one year after implantation and up to 15% of these reoperations occurred more than five years after the initial implantation [4]. This study estimated the incidence of bioprosthetic mitral valve thrombosis at one percent, but this was based solely on a subset of the cohort of patients who had follow-up echocardiography. Almost one-half of the patients did not have proper echocardiographic follow-up [4].

Independent predictors of bioprosthetic mitral valve thrombosis include a combination of clinical and echocardiographic findings such as increased echo-doppler gradient from baseline, underlying coagulopathy, left ventricular dysfunction, prosthetic mismatch, paroxysmal atrial fibrillation, subtherapeutic International Normalized Ratio (INR), increased cusp thickness, previous Maze procedure, and abnormal cusp mobility [2, 5]. A paper by Egbe et al. recently proposed a model for diagnosing bioprosthetic valve thrombosis by combining thee echocardiographic predictors: a 50% increase in transvalvular gradient compared to baseline, increase cusp thickness (>2 mm), and abnormal cusp mobility. The study concluded that applying this model yielded a 72% sensitivity and 90% specificity [2]. Further studies addressing incidence and complication rates in patients with bioprosthetic mitral valve thrombosis will allow for the elucidation of proper follow-up intervals and treatment strategies including anticoagulation and screening intervals. Typically, the highest risk for bioprosthetic mitral valve thrombosis is within the first ten days of implantation. Our patient presented with massive bioprosthetic mitral valve thrombosis one year after transcatheter replacement with no echocardiographic follow-up following valve placement signifying that more frequent assessments in the first several years after replacement may be prudent.

It would also be beneficial to compare the effect of different antithrombotic regiments on long-term clinical outcomes after transcatheter valve replacement. Previously reported cases of bioprosthetic mitral valve thrombosis have resolved with anticoagulation therapy suggesting clot burden as a significant factor in determining optimal treatment regimens [6]. While anticoagulation is typically prescribed in the short-term setting, typically the first few months, to prevent acute complications such as thromboembolic events, cases of late valve thrombosis sometimes up to two years after valve implantation, including the above, suggest that severe complications are still possible with bioprosthetic mitral valves leading to potentially fatal outcomes [5]. The significance of establishing guidelines regarding proper screening and medical therapy is especially relevant due to recent studies supporting transcatheter valve replacement (TVR) in low-risk patients [7]. A recent 2019 meta-analysis assessing outcomes between the transcatheter versus the surgical approach of valve replacements in low-risk patients found that the transcatheter approach was associated with a significantly lower risk of all-cause death and cardiovascular death after one year [8]. The transcatheter approach for valve replacement has been of growing popularity and is slowly becoming the standard of care. However, further studies regarding optimal duration and choice of anticoagulation will be necessary in order to establish more stringent guidelines for their therapy.

References

[1] R. Puri, V. Auffret, and J. Rodés-Cabau, "Bioprosthetic valve thrombosis," *Journal of the American College of Cardiology*, vol. 69, no. 17, pp. 2193–2211, 2017.

[2] A. C. Egbe, S. V. Pislaru, P. A. Pellikka et al., "Bioprosthetic valve thrombosis versus structural failure: clinical and echocardiographic predictors," *Journal of the American College of Cardiology*, vol. 66, no. 21, pp. 2285–2294, 2015.

[3] J. G. Córdoba-Soriano, R. Puri, I. Amat-Santos et al., "Valve thrombosis following transcatheter aortic valve implantation: a systematic review," *Revista Española de Cardiología (English Edition)*, vol. 68, no. 3, pp. 198–204, 2015.

[4] S. V. Pislaru, I. Hussain, P. A. Pellikka et al., "Misconceptions, diagnostic challenges and treatment opportunities in bioprosthetic valve thrombosis: lessons from a case series," *European Journal of Cardio-Thoracic Surgery*, vol. 47, no. 4, pp. 725–732, 2014.

[5] J.-T. Kwon, T.-E. Jung, and D.-H. Lee, "Acute thrombosis of bioprosthetic mitral valve," *Journal of Cardiothoracic Surgery*, vol. 8, no. 1, p. 185, 2013.

[6] B. Thomas, F. Carreras, X. Borras, and G. Pons-Lladó, "An unusual case of bioprosthetic mitral valve thrombosis," *The Annals of Thoracic Surgery*, vol. 72, no. 1, pp. 259–261, 2001.

[7] R. Waksman, T. Rogers, R. Torguson et al., "Transcatheter aortic valve replacement in low-risk patients with symptomatic severe aortic stenosis," *Journal of the American College of Cardiology*, vol. 72, no. 18, pp. 2095–2105, 2018.

[8] D. Kolte, G. J. Vlahakes, I. F. Palacios et al., "Transcatheter versus surgical aortic valve replacement in low-risk patients," *Journal of the American College of Cardiology*, vol. 74, no. 12, pp. 1532–1540, 2019.

43

Therapeutic Dilemmas Faced when Managing a Life-Threatening Presentation of a Myocardial Bridge

Debbie Falconer,[1] **Sariha Yousfani**,[1] **Anna S. Herrey**,[1,2] **Pier Lambiase**,[1,2] **and Gabriella Captur**[1,3]

[1]*Royal Free Hospital, Pond Street, London NW3 2QG, UK*
[2]*Barts Heart Centre, W Smithfield, London EC1A 7BE, UK*
[3]*MRC Unit for Lifelong Health and Ageing at UCL, 1-19 Torrington Place, Fitzrovia, London, UK*

Correspondence should be addressed to Debbie Falconer; debbie.falconer@nhs.net

Academic Editor: Assad Movahed

Background. Myocardial bridges are congenital abnormalities, where a segment of coronary artery travels intramyocardially, rather than the typical epicardial course. The overlying muscle segment is termed "the bridge". Most myocardial bridges are asymptomatic, but some can result in myocardial ischaemia, arrhythmias, and sudden cardiac death. *Case Presentation.* A 31-year-old male with no past medical history presented to our tertiary cardiac centre following an out-of-hospital ventricular fibrillation arrest. Coronary angiography and computed tomography of the coronary arteries revealed a 2 cm myocardial bridge overlying the left anterior descending (LAD) artery. An exercise echocardiogram demonstrated severe apical ballooning and hypokinesis during peak exercise, with corresponding ST-segment elevation, resolving on rest. Options for medical therapy of a symptomatic myocardial bridge include beta blockers, calcium channel blockers, ivabradine, or a combination thereof. Surgical interventions include deroofing the bridge and revascularisation of the affected region with bypass grafting. However, a lack of trial data comparing medical regimens and surgical interventions makes it difficult to ascertain the most effective management strategy for each patient. There was disagreement between experts at different tertiary centres over the optimal management of this patient. He was treated with multiple regimes of medical therapy with ongoing ischaemia on stress testing, before undergoing a negative stress test on amlodipine, diltiazem, and isosorbide mononitrate. It was felt that no further intervention was necessary at this time given his exercise test was now negative for ischaemia. However, after seeking a second opinion, he underwent surgical intervention with bypass grafting of his left anterior descending artery, followed by implantation of an implantable cardiac defibrillator. Subsequently, an angiogram postsurgery demonstrated concomitant spasm of the LAD and he was resumed on medical therapy with calcium channel blockers and nitrates. *Discussion.* Without randomised trials, it is impossible to determine the optimal management strategy for each patient. It is possible that some patients with myocardial bridges are not being trialled on optimal medical therapy prior to undergoing invasive and irreversible interventions.

1. Introduction

Myocardial bridges are congenital abnormalities where a segment of coronary artery travels intramyocardially, rather than the typical epicardial course. The overlying segment of muscle is termed the "myocardial bridge". The commonest vessel involved is the left anterior descending (LAD) artery [1]. Estimated prevalence varies widely between studies, but one review of 1,056 patients at autopsy found bridges in 26% of subjects [2]. The vast majority of myocardial bridges are asymptomatic, but case reports indicate that bridges may clinically present as myocardial ischaemia [3], arrhythmia [4], and sudden cardiac death [5, 6].

Such complications arise from one or more of the following pathophysiological mechanisms:

(1) Systolic myocardial contraction which directly compresses the underlying artery thus limiting perfusion

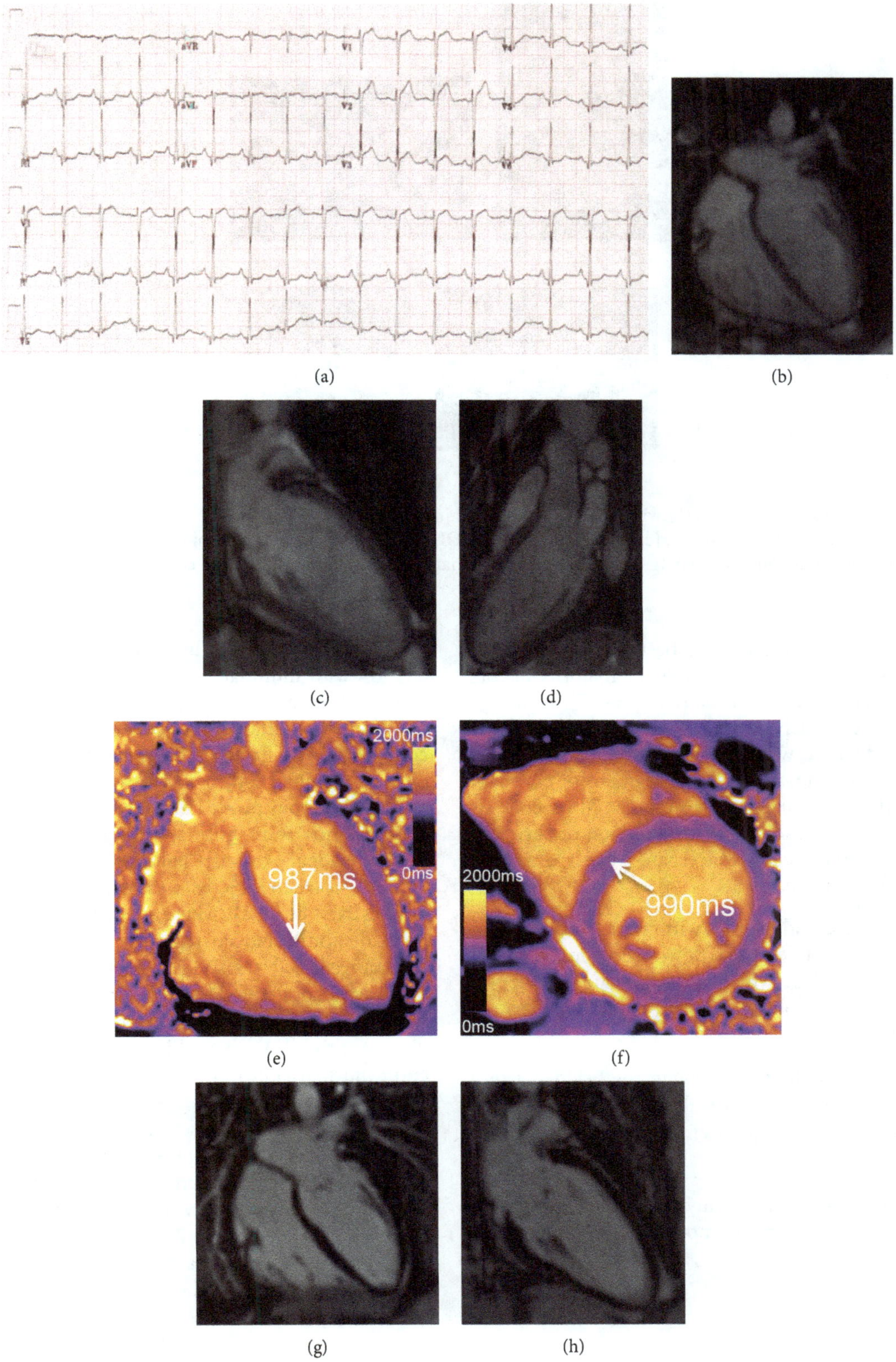

Figure 1: Continued.

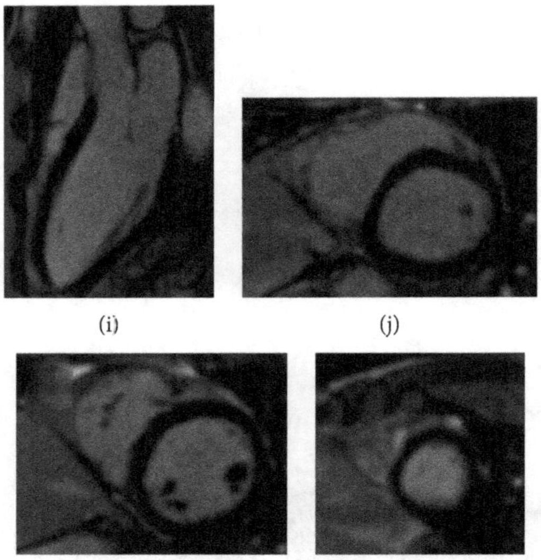

Figure 1: (a) resting ECG on admission showing early repolarization in V1-V3. (b–l) Nonperfusion cardiovascular magnetic resonance. (b–d) Cine steady-state free precession images. (e, f) T1 mapping by MOLLI 5s (3s) 3s showing normal native myocardial T1 at 1.5 T (normal reference range at our center 950-1060 ms). (g–l) Late gadolinium enhancement images with motion correction showing no focal myocardial fibrosis.

distally. This obstruction has been shown to extend from systole into diastole, where the majority of coronary artery perfusion usually occurs [7]. In tachycardic states such as exercise where diastole is shortened, there will be a further reduction in the perfusion time for the bridged segment of coronary artery, thereby worsening symptoms. Other coexisting factors such as diastolic dysfunction or coronary artery disease can exacerbate the perfusion-requirement mismatch [8]

(2) Abnormal haemodynamics within the "bridged" vessel, and reduced coronary flow reserve in the vessel distal to the bridge which can aggravate the supply-demand mismatch and result in myocardial ischaemia [9]

(3) Reversal of systolic flow through the bridged artery which leads to high shear wall stress and accelerated atherosclerosis in the segment proximal to the bridge [10]

Management of symptomatic myocardial bridges can be challenging, as there are currently no guidelines on the optimal therapeutic strategy.

2. Case Report

A 31-year-old male presented to the emergency department following an out-of-hospital ventricular fibrillation (VF) arrest, which occurred whilst running. He had no past medical history of note and no family history of heart disease or sudden death. He recalled feeling light-headed immediately before collapsing but denied chest pain or palpitations. He reported no previous episodes of loss of consciousness or dizziness with exercise.

He was rescued by a bystander's cardiopulmonary resuscitation with minimal delay, and 1 shock was administered when paramedics arrived on the scene. This was followed by return of spontaneous circulation with a normal Glasgow coma scale. His electrocardiogram (ECG; Figure 1(a)) demonstrated sinus rhythm and early repolarization in V1-V3 and his troponin peaked at 292 μg/ml. On examination, his heart sounds were normal with no added sounds. There was no evidence of heart failure clinically.

He was taken directly to the catheterization laboratory of our tertiary hospital, where a resting bedside echocardiogram demonstrated no regional wall motion abnormalities and normal left ventricular wall thickness. Angiography demonstrated a muscle bridge overlying a 2 cm portion of the LAD artery [Figure 2]. There was mild atherosclerotic disease of the LAD, felt unlikely to be the cause of the arrest, and a normal appearance of the other vessels. A nonstress cardiovascular magnetic resonance scan showed normal myocardial tissue characteristics and no focal fibrosis [Figures 1(b)–1(l)]. Computed tomography coronary angiography demonstrated 2 cm of the LAD running intramyocardially, with an overlying bridge. He was started on bisoprolol 2.5 mg, aspirin 75 mg, and atorvastatin 40 mg.

A stress echocardiogram was performed (Bruce full protocol). At peak exercise, there was ST elevation seen in V3-6, with corresponding severe apical hypokinesia of the left ventricle [Figures 3(a)–3(d)] that resolved at rest. Following discussion at the joint cardiology and cardiothoracic multidisciplinary team meeting (MDT), amlodipine 5 mg and isosorbide mononitrate 30 mg were added. On this medical therapy, his stress echocardiogram was repeated but the inducible ischaemia persisted. After further MDT discussion, it was felt he should undergo single-vessel coronary artery bypass grafting but the patient declined and opted instead for continued medical therapy.

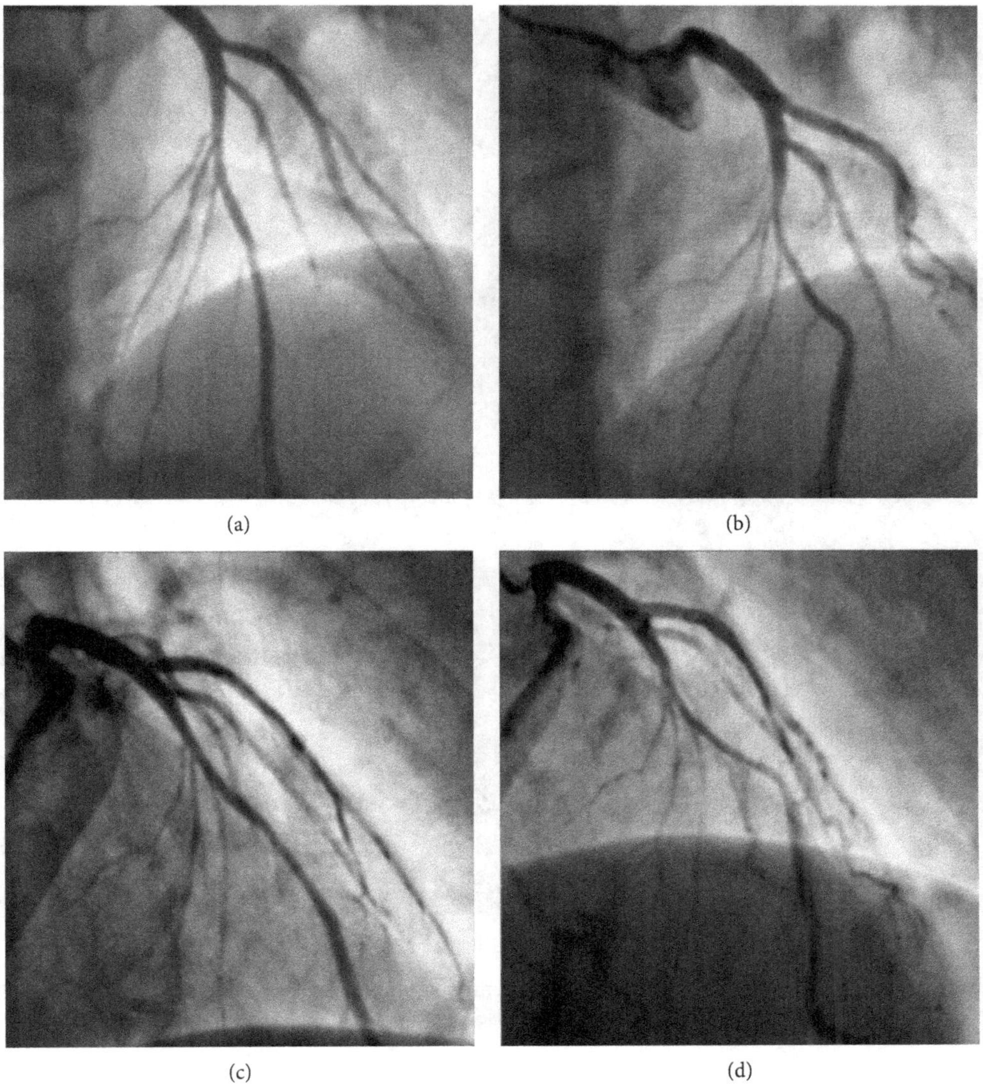

Figure 2: Angiographic images taken on admission to our tertiary centre. Panels (a) and (c) demonstrate images of the left anterior descending artery (LAD) in diastole. Panels (b) and (d) demonstrate the same views during systole with compression of the mid-LAD.

In the weeks that followed, his medical therapy was uptitrated and altered to bisoprolol 5 mg, amlodipine 20 mg, and ivabradine to 5 mg BD. The exercise stress test was repeated but this still resulted in 7 mm of anterior ST elevation that resolved with intravenous nitrates.

After further MDT discussion, he was switched to a regime consisting of amlodipine 10 mg, diltiazem 360 mg, and isosorbide mononitrate 30 mg. On this therapy, he was asymptomatic and a subsequent exercise stress test was negative for ischaemia. He was discharged on this medication regimen. Following extensive MDT discussion, it was felt that an implantable cardiac defibrillator (ICD) was not indicated given the absence of ischaemia on repeat testing, and that the VF arrest had occurred in the context of a reversible cause.

The patient sought a second opinion at another tertiary centre which led to a repeat angiogram, this time with fractional flow reserve (FFR) assessment of the LAD which was positive. He thus underwent cardiac surgery, involving unroofing of the bridge and a left inferior mammary artery (LIMA) bypass graft to the LAD. Postoperatively, an angiogram with acetylcholine provocation was performed, demonstrating spasm of the left anterior descending artery, and he was restarted on amlodipine, diltiazem, and isosorbide mononitrate. A subcutaneous ICD was also implanted at this stage.

At most recent follow-up, the patient has returned to his prior level of exercise and is asymptomatic.

3. Discussion

Difficulties in this case arose from the lack of consensus on the management of symptomatic bridges in the context of proven ischaemia. As there are no clear guidelines, management of our patient was based on multiple conflicting opinions which differed between centres and specialists.

Pharmacological therapy in the form of beta-blockers is generally first-line due to their negative chronotropic and

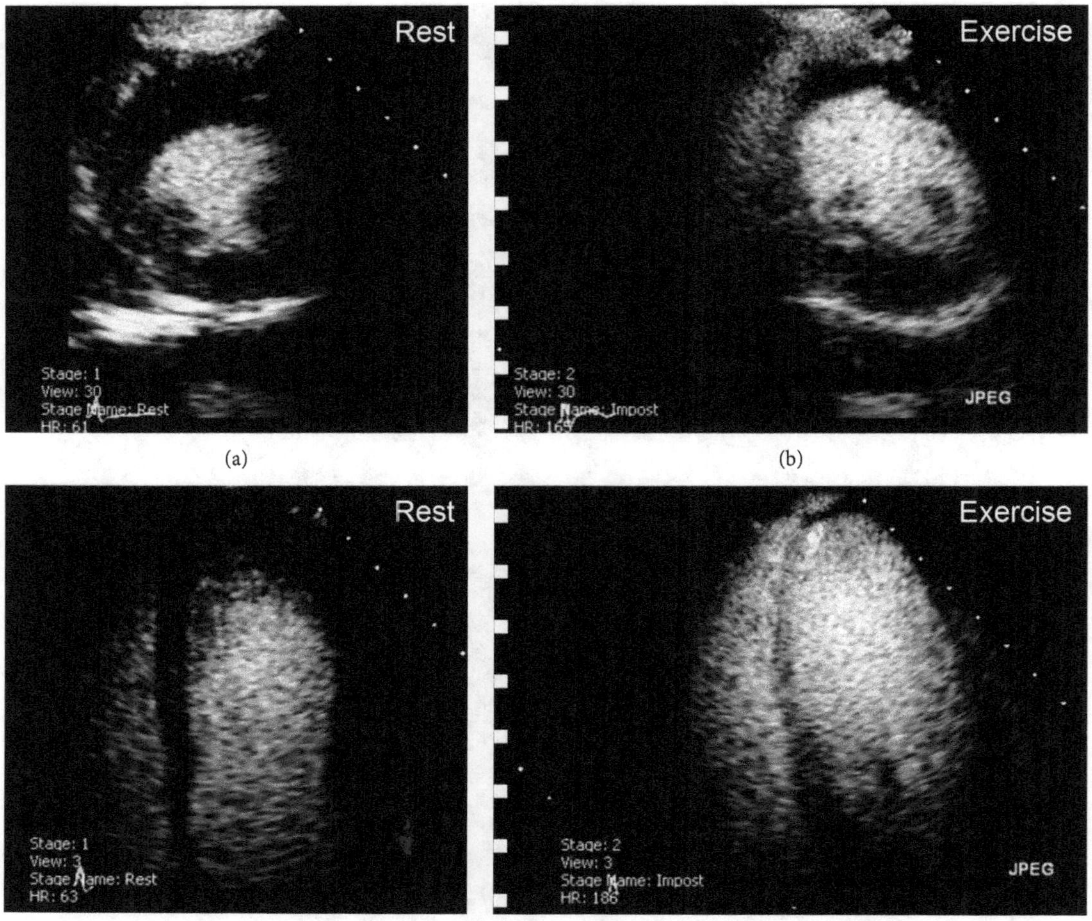

(a) (b) (c) (d)

FIGURE 3: Stress echocardiogram with contrast. Parasternal mid left ventricular short axis slices (a, b) and 4-chamber views (c, d). Images (a) and (c) are taken at rest. Images (b) and (d) are taken at peak exercise, demonstrating apical ballooning.

inotropic effects. They will reduce the arterial compression and the diastolic shortening seen in tachycardia, increasing arterial perfusion. Calcium channel blockers are often added next to reduce concomitant vasospasm [11]. Ivabradine can be used in combination with the aforementioned drugs, exerting a chrononegative effect via I_f [10]. Beta-blockers have been shown to reduce systolic compression and anginal symptoms in a small study of 15 patients [12], but no studies have demonstrated improvements in morbidity or mortality of bridge patients. Also, no trials have compared the efficacy of the aforementioned drugs. The sparsity of data makes it difficult to predict which medical regime will work best for each individual patient. Therefore, patients presenting with major adverse cardiac events may be offered surgical intervention prematurely and before an effective drug regimen is found.

Surgical or interventional approaches including myotomy, coronary artery bypass grafting and percutaneous coronary intervention are usually reserved for patients in whom medical management is unsuccessful [11]. Surgical myotomy involves resection of the overlying muscle fibres, whilst bypass grafting involves anastomosing the LIMA to the LAD. A small study of 31 patients who underwent either myotomy or bypass grafting demonstrated no ischaemia on postoperative exercise testing of any patient after a follow-up of 31 months, along with no early or late complications, suggesting surgical approaches are safe and effective in managing symptomatic bridges [13]. It is not reported, however, which medical therapies were utilised and deemed unsuccessful before proceeding to surgery. The benefit derived from surgery in our case is unclear, as he was forced to restart medical therapy postoperatively following the detection of coronary artery spasm on repeat angiogram. It is also possible that given his young age, he may require repeat surgery on the graft, re-exposing him to a substantial surgical and anaesthetic risk, whilst the benefits from the original surgery remain unknown.

In the management of our patient, opinions also differed regarding the need for an ICD. To date, no malignant ventricular arrhythmias outside the initial presentation have been detected although the device may well impact on the patient's quality of life in the long term.

It is generally accepted that nitrates are contraindicated and should not be used to treat ischaemia caused by myocardial bridges, as they may lead to proximal vessel dilatation and flow reversal, further compromising distal vessel perfusion [8]. A small study of 3 patients demonstrated that administration of intravenous nitrates exacerbated systolic compression of bridged segments of coronary arteries during angiography [14]. However, when used in combination with diltiazem and amlodipine, nitrates did not result in worsening of ischaemia on stress testing, or of our patient's symptoms. Indeed, on this regimen, his stress test was negative for ischaemia and he was asymptomatic. Given he was later diagnosed with vasospasm of the LAD, the nitrates may have been useful in preventing concomitant spasm of the bridged segment.

Another consideration is that patients may undergo repeated stress testing to determine the efficacy of medical therapy—a potentially dangerous and anxiety-inducing procedure. Our patient underwent 3 positive stress tests, each accompanied by ST elevation in the anterior leads thus risking a cardiac arrest before a successful drug combination was found. Clearer guidelines on optimal management would reduce the need for repeat testing, allowing treating teams to select the correct management the first time.

Another management strategy that can be overlooked in this group of patients is aggressive coronary artery disease risk factor modification. Given the increased risk of atherosclerosis in the area proximal to the bridge, antiplatelet and statin therapy should be considered as well as optimization of conventional risk factors.

This case highlights the urgent need for trials comparing the efficacy of different medical regimes and surgical interventions to determine which patient will benefit from which treatment strategy. All studies thus far are small, nonrandomised, and focus on the surgical or interventional treatment strategies. We also need to understand the safety of sole medical therapy in patients with a myocardial bridge following a major cardiac event, because the avoidance of surgery and device implantation may be beneficial, if at all possible.

4. Conclusion

We present the case of a patient who suffered VF arrest secondary to a myocardial bridge of the LAD. Various treatment strategies were trialled including medical therapy, surgical unroofing and bypass, and ultimately ICD implantation. Without randomised data, some patients with myocardial bridges are not being trialled on optimal medical therapy prior to undergoing invasive and irreversible interventions.

Consent

Informed consent has been sought from the patient, in accordance with COPE guidelines.

Disclosure

This research did not receive any specific grant from funding agencies in the public, commercial, or not-for-profit sectors.

References

[1] D. Cicek, N. Kalay, and H. Muderrisoglu, "Incidence, clinical characteristics, and 4-year follow-up of patients with isolated myocardial bridge: a retrospective, single-center, epidemiologic, coronary arteriographic follow-up study in southern Turkey," *Cardiovascular Revascularization Medicine*, vol. 12, no. 1, pp. 25–28, 2011.

[2] M. Risse and G. Weiler, "Coronary muscle bridge and its relations to local coronary sclerosis, regional myocardial ischemia and coronary spasm. A morphometric study," *Zeitschrift für Kardiologie*, vol. 74, no. 12, pp. 700–705, 1985.

[3] L. Rossi, B. Dander, G. P. Nidasio et al., "Myocardial bridges and ischemic heart disease," *European Heart Journal*, vol. 1, no. 4, pp. 239–245, 1980.

[4] H. Feld, V. Guadanino, G. Hollander, A. Greengart, E. Lichstein, and J. Shani, "Exercise-induced ventricular tachycardia in association with a myocardial bridge," *Chest*, vol. 99, no. 5, pp. 1295-1296, 1991.

[5] S. Zerbo, A. Lanzarone, M. Raimondi et al., "Myocardial bridge pathology and preventable accidents during physical activity of healthy subjects: a case report and a literature review," *The Medico-Legal Journal*, vol. 88, no. 4, pp. 209–214, 2020.

[6] N. Marchionni, T. Chechi, M. Falai, M. Margheri, and S. Fumagalli, "Myocardial stunning associated with a myocardial bridge," *International Journal of Cardiology*, vol. 82, no. 1, pp. 65–67, 2002.

[7] M. Bourassa, P. Bernard, G. Brevers, R. Petitclerc, and I. Dyrda, "Systolic and early diastolic coronary inflow obstruction in patients with muscular bridging of the left anterior descending artery," *Coronary artery Disease Today. Amsterdam: Excerpta Medica*, vol. 1, no. 3, pp. 380–397, 1982.

[8] M. T. Corban, O. Y. Hung, P. Eshtehardi et al., "Myocardial bridging: contemporary understanding of pathophysiology with implications for diagnostic and therapeutic strategies," *Journal of the American College of Cardiology*, vol. 63, no. 22, pp. 2346–2355, 2014.

[9] M. G. Bourassa, A. Butnaru, J. Lesperance, and J. C. Tardif, "Symptomatic myocardial bridges: overview of ischemic mechanisms and current diagnostic and treatment strategies," *Journal of the American College of Cardiology*, vol. 41, no. 3, pp. 351–359, 2003.

[10] G. Tarantini, F. Migliore, F. Cademartiri, C. Fraccaro, and S. Iliceto, "Left anterior descending artery myocardial bridging: a clinical approach," *Journal of the American College of Cardiology*, vol. 68, no. 25, pp. 2887–2899, 2016.

[11] M. S. Lee and C. H. Chen, "Myocardial bridging: an up-to-date review," *The Journal of Invasive Cardiology*, vol. 27, no. 11, pp. 521–528, 2015.

[12] E. R. Schwarz, H. G. Klues, J. vom Dahl, I. Klein, W. Krebs, and P. Hanrath, "Functional, angiographic and intracoronary Doppler flow characteristics in symptomatic patients with myocardial bridging: effect of short-term intravenous beta-blocker medication," *Journal of the American College of Cardiology*, vol. 27, no. 7, pp. 1637–1645, 1996.

[13] Q. Y. Wu and Z. H. Xu, "Surgical treatment of myocardial bridging: report of 31 cases," *Chinese Medical Journal*, vol. 120, no. 19, pp. 1689–1693, 2007.

[14] T. Ishimori, A. E. Raizner, R. A. Chahine, M. Awdeh, and R. J. Luchi, "Myocardial bridges in man: clinical correlations and angiographic accentuation with nitroglycerin," *Catheterization and Cardiovascular Diagnosis*, vol. 3, no. 1, pp. 59–65, 1977.

Management of Recurrent Pregnancy-Related Pericarditis

Michel Ibrahim,[1] **Michael Fattouh,**[2] **and Alice Jacobs**[3]

[1]*Department of Medicine, Cardiovascular Division, Temple University Hospital, Philadelphia, PA, USA*
[2]*Montefiore Medical Center, Bronx, NY, USA*
[3]*Boston University Medical Center, Boston, MA, USA*

Correspondence should be addressed to Michel Ibrahim; ibrahimichel@gmail.com

Academic Editor: Assad Movahed

The evidence on recurrent pregnancy-related pericarditis is limited, and management strategies are based on case reports and expert opinion. We describe a patient with myopericarditis complicated by cardiac tamponade presenting shortly after her first pregnancy, which was then complicated by refractory recurrent pericarditis. She was treated with standard first line therapies, such as NSAIDs, corticosteroids, and colchicine, and eventually initiated on the purine analog, azathioprine. Out of fear of teratogenicity, she self-discontinued her maintenance medications and thereafter, her course was complicated by a recurrent flare of pericarditis during a subsequent pregnancy. Our case illustrates the significant burden on our patient due to the incessant nature of her disease and on the providers due to the therapeutic dilemmas associated with family planning and pregnancy. Further data is required on this unique clinical scenario, and patient-centered management by a multidisciplinary team is critical.

1. Background

Acute pericarditis is among the most common pericardial diseases seen in pregnancy [1, 2], with recurrent disease being one of the most troublesome complications of pericarditis. The evidence on recurrent pregnancy-related pericarditis is limited, with the largest study on this topic consisting of a case series of 21 pregnancies [3]. As such, management strategies are based on case reports and expert opinion. However, in pregnant patients, the issue of pharmacotherapy is an important one, and recurrent pericarditis related to pregnancy poses a therapeutic dilemma. Our case illustrates a tailored multidisciplinary approach to the management of pregnancy-related idiopathic recurrent pericarditis (IRP), and we describe the current data surrounding this topic.

2. Case Presentation

A 25-year-old G1P1 female, originally from Brazil, developed worsening dyspnea and pleuritic chest pain immediately postpartum after a normal spontaneous vaginal delivery at an outside hospital. She was diagnosed with acute pericarditis and was successfully treated with an ibuprofen taper. Two months later, she presented to our facility with several weeks of left-sided, sharp, and pleuritic chest pain, coupled with worsening dyspnea, fever, and chills. She was hemodynamically stable and had a heart rate of 120 beat per minute (bpm). Laboratory data were notable for a C-reactive protein (CRP) level of 175 mg/L, white blood cell (WBC) 27.9K/UL, and a TnI of 5.1 ng/mL (Table 1). Electrocardiogram (ECG) showed sinus tachycardia with right bundle branch block (RBBB) (Figure 1), portable chest X-ray showed an enlarged cardio-mediastinal silhouette (Figure 2), and computed tomography (CT) chest with contrast showed a large pericardial effusion without evidence of pulmonary embolism. A subsequent transthoracic echocardiogram (TTE) confirmed the large pericardial effusion with evidence of tamponade physiology. The patient was diagnosed with pericarditis complicated by cardiac tamponade. The pericardial effusion was subsequently drained, and the patient underwent a thorough workup including thyroid testing, HIV, interferon-gamma release assay (IGRA),

Table 1: Cardiac biomarkers and inflammatory markers during disease flare.

Biomarkers	1st pregnancy				2nd pregnancy	
	1st (2 weeks postpartum)	2nd (2 months postpartum)	3rd (4 months postpartum)	4th (7 months postpartum)	1st (2 months before delivery)	2nd (2 weeks before delivery)
CRP	175	89.3	41	60.3	45	144
Troponin I	5.1	0.011	0.009	0.006	4.8	5.7

TnI: troponin I; CRP: C-reactive protein.

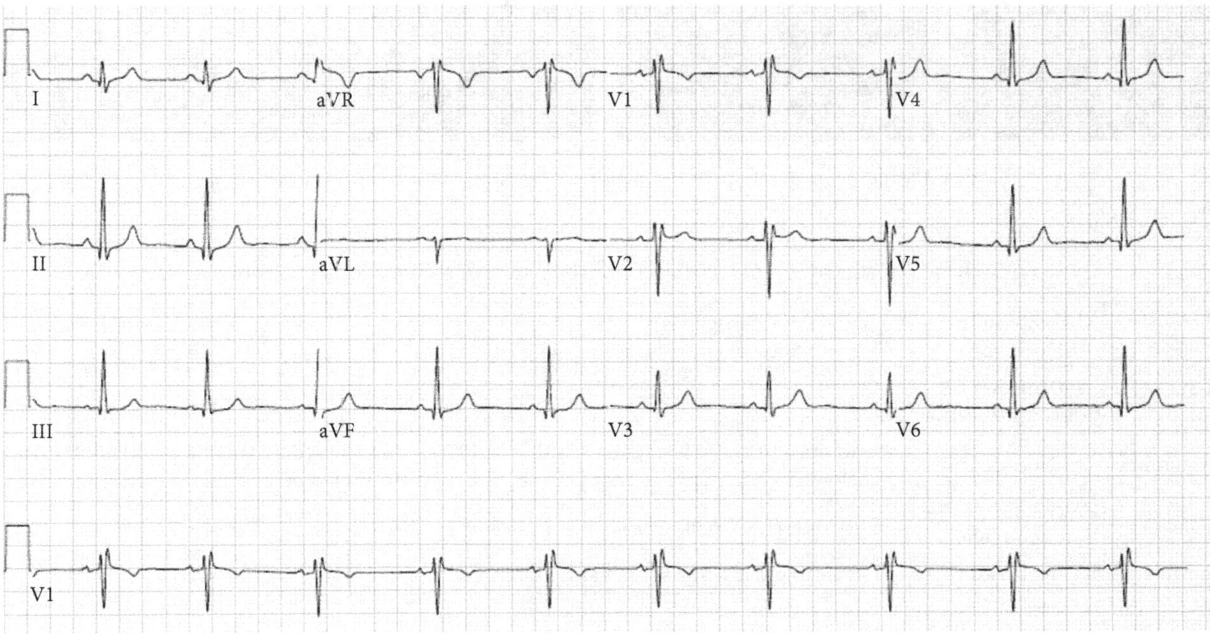

Figure 1: Normal sinus rhythm. RSR′ or QR pattern in V1 suggests right ventricular conduction delay.

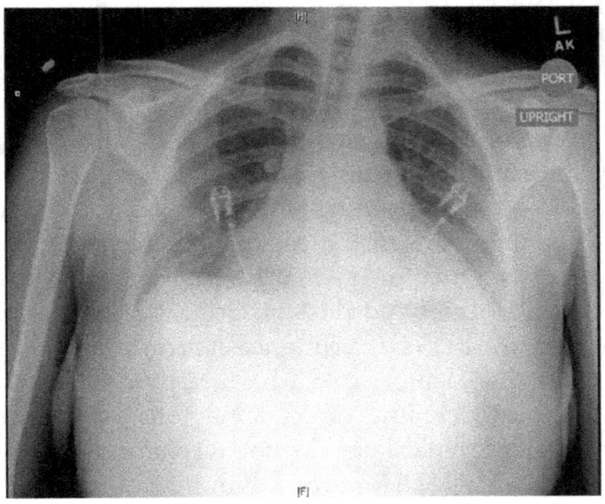

Figure 2: Enlarged cardio-mediastinal silhouette.

bacterial and viral cultures, and ANA, which only revealed elevated Coxsackie titers. For her recurrent disease with high-risk features, defined by tamponade and myocardial involvement, she was initiated on a combination of ibuprofen, a short prednisone taper, and 6 months of colchicine therapy.

Approximately 3 months following, while still on the colchicine, she had another episode of pericarditis, this time with mild to moderate pericardial effusion without tamponade physiology (Figure 3); prednisone was reinitiated.

Within another 2 months, she suffered from another relapse. This was the patient's fourth presentation since her delivery. At that point, the patient underwent another thorough but unrevealing workup including repeat thyroid testing, IGRA, HIV, and ANA in addition to double-stranded DNA, rheumatoid factor, cyclic citrullinated peptide, and genetic studies for familial Mediterranean fever (FMF). Under rheumatology's guidance, a trial of azathioprine starting at 100 mg daily was initiated in concurrence with colchicine and steroids in order to achieve complete remission. The patient was able to slowly come off the corticosteroids, while remaining on colchicine and undergoing active titration of azathioprine to 200 mg.

Over a year from her initial episode, with the disease under control, our patient hoped to conceive again, and she self-discontinued the colchicine. Reassured after several more months of disease quiescence, coupled with fears of teratogenicity, she opted to slowly come off azathioprine. She remained without evidence of recurrent disease for the next year and became pregnant during this time. Although azathioprine was deemed safe by different specialists involved in her care, including her obstetrician, cardiologist, and rheumatologist, the patient opted against taking any

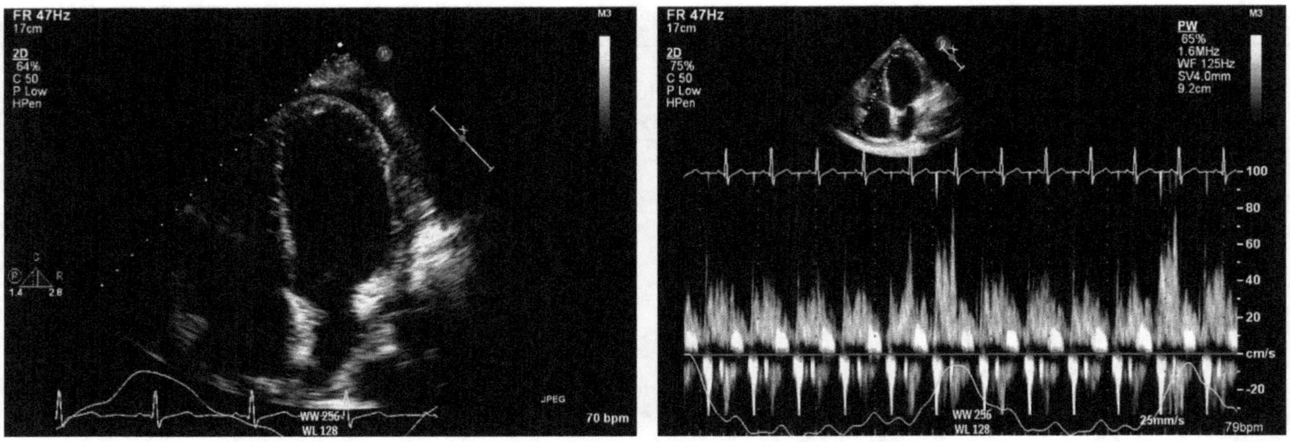

Figure 3: Mild to moderate pericardial effusion with minimal respiratory variation.

Table 2: Treatment scheme for medical therapy of pericarditis during pregnancy.

Drugs	Postpartum 1st episode	Postpartum Subsequent episodes	Pregnancy
NSAIDs (ibuprofen)	800 mg every 8 hours for 2 weeks	Not used	Not used
Corticosteroids	Not used	Prednisone 10 mg to 20 mg daily with a slow extender taper (6 months)	Prednisone 10 mg to 20 mg based on clinical response with slow taper extender taper (6 months)
Colchicine	Colchicine 0.6 mg twice daily	Colchicine 0.6 mg twice daily	Not used
Azathioprine	Not used	100 mg daily to 200 mg daily	Not used

maintenance medications during her pregnancy. Therefore, the multidisciplinary team's decision was to treat any flares during pregnancy with corticosteroids.

At 28 weeks of gestation, she presented with shortness of breath, pleuritic chest pain with elevated inflammatory markers (CRP: 120 mg/L) and cardiac biomarkers (TnI of 4.86 ng/mL) consistent with a diagnosis of myopericarditis. She had a mild pericardial effusion on TTE and no evidence of tamponade physiology. She started on prednisone 10 mg daily, and symptoms subsequently subsided with a downtrend of cardiac and inflammatory biomarkers. At that point, prednisone maintenance was initiated at a dose of 10 mg per day planned to be continued up through delivery.

Within 2 months, she presented yet again with a similar clinical picture and was diagnosed with recurrent myopericarditis. Her prednisone was increased to 20 mg daily with symptom resolution. Two weeks later, she went into labor at which pointshe received stress dose steroids and had a normal spontaneous vaginal delivery without any complications. She was discharged on prolonged and slow prednisone taper until her follow-up with rheumatology where the decision was made to reinitiate azathioprine and slowly titrate off the corticosteroids.

3. Discussion

Idiopathic recurrent acute pericarditis (IRAP) is quite prevalent, affecting 15-30% patients with a history of acute pericarditis [4]. In women of childbearing age, we aim to optimize maternal and fetal outcomes by planning pregnancy during a time of inactive disease, while also maintaining quiescence throughout the pregnancy. However, both goals come with challenges and are further complicated by the paucity of data surrounding IRAP in pregnancy.

The use of standard first-line agents is limited in pregnancy. Exposure to ASA and NSAIDs after 20 weeks' gestation can lead to premature closure of fetal ductus arteriosus, effectively contraindicating their use in the third trimester [4]. Furthermore, when used in IRAP, it is recommended that these COX-1 inhibitors are added to colchicine. Colchicine is effective in decreasing rates of recurrence of pericarditis [5], and as such, 6 months of tapered colchicine therapy is preferred. As it stands, though, because of its antimitotic mechanism of action, available guidelines do not recommend its routine use in pregnancy [4]. However, a growing body of data suggests that colchicine is probably safe in pregnancy [6], and although there are no well-controlled studies assessing its use for pericarditis specifically, a group of experts in Italy has recently supported its use [3].

Recommendations in pregnant patients continue to include corticosteroid therapy [4], which although effective in the management of symptoms and the resolution of pericarditis, come with their own set of issues. Corticosteroids increase the risk of recurrence [7], making their use somewhat counterintuitive in patients who already suffer from recurrent disease.

For patients like ours, with refractory recurrent disease, family planning is prudent. This label, "refractory" IRAP, is applied to patients who have had at least three relapses and have failed standard therapies [8]. Although data is limited, several immunosuppressive agents have emerged as promising for such patients [1]. Although their use is questionable in pregnancy, these agents can aid in achieving disease quiescence and therefore aid in family planning.

One such therapy is azathioprine, a purine analog, which acts by blocking DNA synthesis and therefore lymphocyte proliferation. Data supporting its use includes a single-center retrospective study of 46 patients with IRAP [9]. These patients were coadministered prednisone, but after 4 weeks, they began tapering off the corticosteroid. Nearly 60% of patients were able to come off both prednisone and azathioprine, while remaining in stable remission. These responders had remained on azathioprine for an average of 14.6 months (Table 2). Although no controlled trials exist regarding its use in pregnancy, data suggests that it is safe, and expert opinion regards it as such (EULAR).

Another therapeutic option in IRAP is intravenous immunoglobulin (IVIG). Data supporting its use comes from a systematic review of case series and reports of refractory recurrent pericarditis, in which just under half of the 30 patients had idiopathic disease [10]. A several day course of IVIG was administered, and this was repeated periodically based on clinical response. A promising 73% of patients were recurrent-free at a follow-up period of nearly three years. While 63% of the patients were initially on corticosteroids, only 17% remained on steroids by the end. With this, IVIG should be considered to induce remission while planning for conception in patients with IRAP. Notably, though, we may also consider its use during pregnancy for IRAP. IVIG is used during pregnancy in a number of disease states and recommended as a first-line option for immune thrombocytopenia in pregnancy [11, 12].

Perhaps most foreign among the immunosuppressive agents to consider are the ilnterleukin-1 inhibitors: anakinra, canakinumab, and rilonacept. Anakinra is a recombinant IL-1 receptor antagonist. Evidence supporting its use in pericarditis includes a small randomized controlled trial of 21 patients with recurrent, colchicine-resistant, and steroid-dependent disease [13]. All 21 patients received anakinra therapy for 60 days, at which point they were randomized to placebo or continued anakinra therapy for the year. Just 2 of the 11 patients who were randomized to receive anakinra had recurrence within the year, versus 9 of the 10 randomized to placebo. Although these data are promising in regard to the therapeutic efficacy of anakinra, they raise the concern of recurrence after discontinuation. This recurrence after anakinra therapy has also been highlighted in a systematic review of published cases [14]. The high rates of recurrence with anakinra may be attributable to its short half-life (4-6 hours), which has led to one group's experimentation with canakinumab, an antibody-based IL-1 antagonist with a half-life of approximately 28 days [15]. The safety profile of these medications in the pregnant women is unknown. However, there is growing data regarding the safety of anakinra and canakinumab in pregnancy [16]. Rilonacept is a made up of the extracellular portions of the interleukon-1 receptor bound to the constant region of an IgG1. A recent phase 3 randomized control trial supports its use in recurrent pericarditis. During an initial run-in period, all patients were treated with a loading dose of rilonacept followed by weekly maintenance dosing. They were then randomized to continue rilonacept therapy or to placebo. 74% of patients (23 of 31) in the placebo group had recurrent pericarditis, while only 7% (2 of 30) of those in the rilonacept arm suffered recurrence. To the best of our knowledge, though, there is no data available to support rilonacept's use in pregnancy, and the FDA labels this agent as pregnancy category C.

4. Conclusion

Our patient's experience underscores the necessity of well-controlled trials of therapies for IRAP in pregnancy and highlights the importance of family planning, shared decision-making, and management by an interdisciplinary team comprised of rheumatology, obstetrics/gynecology, and cardiology.

Abbreviations

CRP: C-reactive protein
TnI: Troponin I
ECG: Electrocardiogram
TTE: Transthoracic echocardiogram.

Consent

Patient referred in case has provided her consent regarding her medical history as part of the case report: "Management of Recurrent Pregnancy-Related Pericarditis."

Authors' Contributions

Dr. Michel Ibrahim, Dr. Michael Fattouh, and Dr. Alice Jacobs have participated in both the acute and long-term care of the patient. Dr. Michel Ibrahim has contributed to the skeleton of the manuscript with the guidance and mentorship of Dr. Alice Jacobs. Dr. Michael Fattouh in conjunction with Dr. Michel Ibrahim has been responsible for the first draft write-up. Dr. Michel Ibrahim and Dr. Alice Jacobs have reviewed the data relevant to the case..

References

[1] M. Imazio, A. Brucato, S. Rampello et al., "Management of pericardial diseases during pregnancy," *Journal of Cardiovascular Medicine*, vol. 11, no. 8, pp. 557–562, 2010.

[2] M. Imazio, E. Cecchi, B. Demichelis et al., "Indicators of poor prognosis of acute pericarditis," *Circulation*, vol. 115, no. 21, pp. 2739–2744, 2007.

[3] A. Brucato, N. Pluymaekers, E. Tombetti et al., "Management of idiopathic recurrent pericarditis during pregnancy," *International Journal of Cardiology*, vol. 282, pp. 60–65, 2019.

[4] Y. Adler, P. Charron, M. Imazio et al., "2015 ESC guidelines for the diagnosis and management of pericardial diseases," *European Heart Journal*, vol. 36, no. 42, pp. 2921–2964, 2015.

[5] M. Imazio, R. Belli, A. Brucato et al., "Efficacy and safety of colchicine for treatment of multiple recurrences of pericarditis (CORP-2): a multicentre, double-blind, placebo-controlled, randomised trial," *Lancet*, vol. 383, no. 9936, pp. 2232–2237, 2014.

[6] P. Indraratna, S. Virk, and D. Gurram, "Use of colchicine in pregnancy: a systematic review and meta-analysis.," *Rheumatology (Oxford)*, vol. 2, pp. 382–387, 2018.

[7] M. Lotrionte, G. Biondi-Zoccai, M. Imazio et al., "International collaborative systematic review of controlled clinical trials on pharmacologic treatments for acute pericarditis and its recurrences," *American Heart Journal*, vol. 160, no. 4, pp. 662–670, 2010.

[8] M. Imazio, G. Lazaros, A. Brucato, and F. Gaita, "Recurrent pericarditis: new and emerging therapeutic options," *Nature Reviews Cardiology*, vol. 13, no. 2, pp. 99–105, 2016.

[9] F. Vianello, F. Cinetto, M. Cavraro et al., "Azathioprine in isolated recurrent pericarditis: a single centre experience," *International Journal of Cardiology*, vol. 147, no. 3, pp. 477-478, 2011.

[10] M. Imazio, G. Lazaros, E. Picardi et al., "Intravenous human immunoglobulins for refractory recurrent pericarditis: a systematic review of all published cases," *Journal of Cardiovascular Medicine*, vol. 17, no. 4, pp. 263–269, 2016.

[11] S. Abdolmohammadi-Vahid, F. Pashazadeh, Z. Pourmoghaddam, L. Aghebati-Maleki, S. Abdollahi-Fard, and M. Yousefi, "The effectiveness of IVIG therapy in pregnancy and live birth rate of women with recurrent implantation failure (RIF): a systematic review and meta- analysis," *Journal of Reproductive Immunology*, vol. 134-135, pp. 28–33, 2019.

[12] A. Rajasekhar and T. Gernsheimer, *Clinical Practice Guide on Thrombocytopenia in Pregnancy*, American Society of Hematology, 2013.

[13] A. Brucato, M. Imazio, M. Gattorno et al., "Effect of anakinra on recurrent pericarditis among patients with colchicine resistance and corticosteroid dependence: the AIRTRIP randomized clinical trial," *Journal of the American Medical Association*, vol. 316, no. 18, pp. 1906–1912, 2016.

[14] G. Lazaros, M. Imazio, A. Brucato et al., "Anakinra," *Journal of Cardiovascular Medicine*, vol. 17, no. 4, pp. 256–262, 2016.

[15] N. Kougkas, A. Fanouriakis, I. Papalopoulos et al., "Canakinumab for recurrent rheumatic disease associated-pericarditis: a case series with long-term follow-up," *Rheumatology*, vol. 57, no. 8, pp. 1494-1495, 2018.

[16] T. Youngstein, P. Hoffmann, A. Gül et al., "International multi-centre study of pregnancy outcomes with interleukin-1 inhibitors," *Rheumatology*, vol. 56, no. 12, pp. 2102–2108, 2017.

Monitored Anesthesia Care of Two Patients with Highly Elevated Subpulmonic Ventricular Pressure Due to Adult Congenital Heart Disease

Tatsuya Kida,[1] **Tomoya Irie**,[1] **and Takahisa Goto**[2]

[1]*Department of Anesthesiology, Yokohama City University School of Medicine, 3-9 Fukuura, Kanazawa-ku, Yokohama 2360004, Japan*
[2]*Department of Anesthesiology, Yokohama City University Medical Center, 4-57 Urahune, Minami-ku, Yokohama 2320024, Japan*

Correspondence should be addressed to Tatsuya Kida; bcvn400dd@gmail.com

Academic Editor: Alfredo E. Rodriguez

Procedural sedation and analgesia for patients with adult congenital heart disease (ACHD) and highly elevated subpulmonic ventricular pressure require proper anesthesia care to prevent a pulmonary hypertensive crisis. We describe the monitored anesthesia care (MAC) of two patients with ACHD (a complete atrioventricular septal defect and congenitally corrected transposition of the great arteries) and highly elevated subpulmonic ventricular pressure. In both patients, preprocedural transthoracic echocardiography was useful for detecting severely elevated subpulmonic ventricular pressure. The MAC involved the infusion of propofol, dexmedetomidine, and fentanyl. Norepinephrine was continuously administered from the preanesthetic period. No hemodynamic instability or respiratory depression was observed during the MAC. Continuous administration of norepinephrine from the preinduction period was helpful for preventing hypotension. We added dexmedetomidine to our MAC regimen of propofol and fentanyl because it exerts both sedative and analgesic effects. Dexmedetomidine does not cause respiratory depression; thus, our MAC regimen is believed to be theoretically safe for patients with ACHD and elevated subpulmonic ventricular pressure. Our findings suggest that safe MAC for patients with ACHD and highly elevated subpulmonic ventricular pressure may require careful consideration of the anesthetic regimen and close observation by adequately trained personnel, which is best provided at regional ACHD centers.

1. Background

The population of patients with adult congenital heart disease (ACHD) has been increasing in recent years [1–3]. Therefore, physicians may encounter such patients requiring invasive procedures in their daily clinical practice. While monitored anesthesia care (MAC) provides good procedural conditions, it presents a great challenge to anesthesia providers. However, the literature is scarce with respect to the risks in patients with ACHD and highly elevated subpulmonic ventricular pressure undergoing MAC [4, 5]. Inadequate sedation and analgesia may cause an abrupt increase in pulmonary vascular resistance (PVR) in response to procedural stimuli. On the other hand, excessive use of anesthetic and analgesic agents may cause cardiorespiratory depression, which worsens pulmonary arterial pressure, causing subpulmonic ventricular failure. Thus, patients with ACHD and elevated subpulmonic ventricular pressure have a very narrow margin of safety with regard to sedation and analgesia. In this report, we describe the successful MAC of two patients with ACHD and highly elevated subpulmonic ventricular pressure. Figure 1 provides a schematic demonstration of the circulation in each patient. The authors confirm that written informed consent for submission and publication of this report has been obtained from both patients.

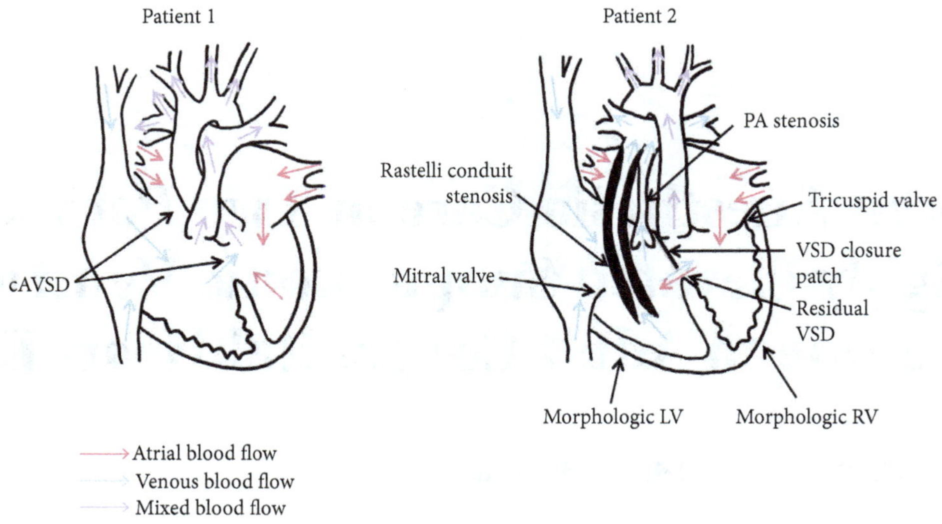

FIGURE 1: Illustrations of the cardiac anatomy and physiology of two patients with adult congenital heart disease (ACHD) and highly elevated ventricular pressure circulating to the pulmonary artery (PA). cAVSD, complete atrioventricular septal defect; PA: pulmonary artery; VSD: ventricular septal defect; LV: left ventricle; RV: right ventricle.

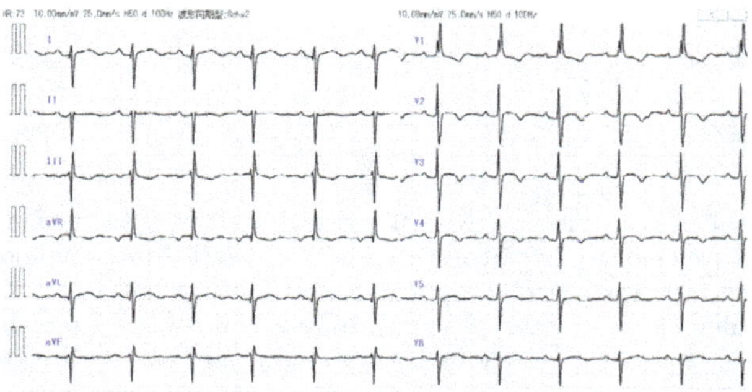

FIGURE 2: The preprocedural electrocardiogram of patient 1 shows sinus rhythm, northwest axis, incomplete right bundle branch block pattern, and biphasic QRS complexes in V2-5 and deep *S* waves in V5-6.

2. Case Presentation

2.1. Patient 1. A 22-year-old woman with Down syndrome and Eisenmenger syndrome due to a complete atrioventricular septal defect (cAVSD) that was diagnosed at birth was scheduled for central venous catheter (CVC) placement for acute myelocytic leukemia management. The patient was prescribed tadalafil and furosemide, and her condition was classified as New York Heart Association (NYHA) class II. The preprocedural brain natriuretic peptide (BNP) level was 22.6 pg/mL. Her electrocardiogram (ECG) showed sinus rhythm, northwest axis, incomplete right bundle branch block pattern, and biphasic QRS complexes in V2-5 and deep S waves in V5-6 (Figure 2). Transthoracic echocardiography (TTE) showed mild common atrioventricular valve regurgitation and persistently elevated right ventricular pressure (RVP), which was estimated to be equal to or higher than the left ventricular pressure (LVP) indicated by interventricular septal (IVS) motion. Right ventricular function was preserved with a tricuspid annular plane systolic excursion (TAPSE) of 23.5 mm and E/A 0.94; E/e' 4.9. Left ventricular function was also preserved with a fraction area change (FAC) of 56% and E/A 0.97; E/e' (septal) 20; E/e' (lateral) 11. Since central venous catheter placement is an invasive procedure, MAC or general anesthesia with tracheal intubation (GETA) was required in this patient to avoid sudden increases in PVR because of noncooperation, crying, screaming, or struggling. Since MAC is less invasive than GETA, we scheduled the patient for CVC placement under MAC.

The anesthesia record is shown in Figure 3. Her preprocedural vital signs in the operating room were as follows: blood pressure (BP)—98/52 mmHg; heart rate (HR)—54 beats/min; and oxygen saturation measured by pulse oximetry (SpO_2)—80% in room air. During MAC, 5 L/min of 100% oxygen was administered via face mask. End-tidal carbon dioxide ($EtCO_2$) was monitored with capnography. Before the induction of anesthesia, a continuous peripheral venous infusion of norepinephrine was initiated at 0.1 μg/kg/min and maintained at 0.02–0.1 μg/kg/min to maintain the systolic systemic arterial blood pressure (sSABP) above 100 mmHg (her resting sSABP). MAC was provided with a continuous infusion of propofol (2 mg/kg/h), dexmedetomidine (a loading dose of 1 μg/kg over 10 minutes followed by a 0.5 μg/kg/h infusion), and fentanyl (total dose: 75 μg) to achieve optimal sedation and analgesia. Local anesthesia was obtained by a superficial injection of 1% lidocaine. During MAC, glossoptosis occurred temporarily and was easily rectified by a jaw lift. The CVC was placed successfully without hemodynamic instability, respiratory depression, or oxygen desaturation. The infusion of norepinephrine was tapered according to sSABP and discontinued after 30 minutes of the procedure. The level of consciousness was arousable on calling, and no airway obstruction was observed at the end of the MAC. The postprocedural course was uneventful. Chemotherapy was started on postprocedural day 4.

2.2. Patient 2. A 39-year-old woman presented for transesophageal echocardiography (TEE) to rule out intracardiac

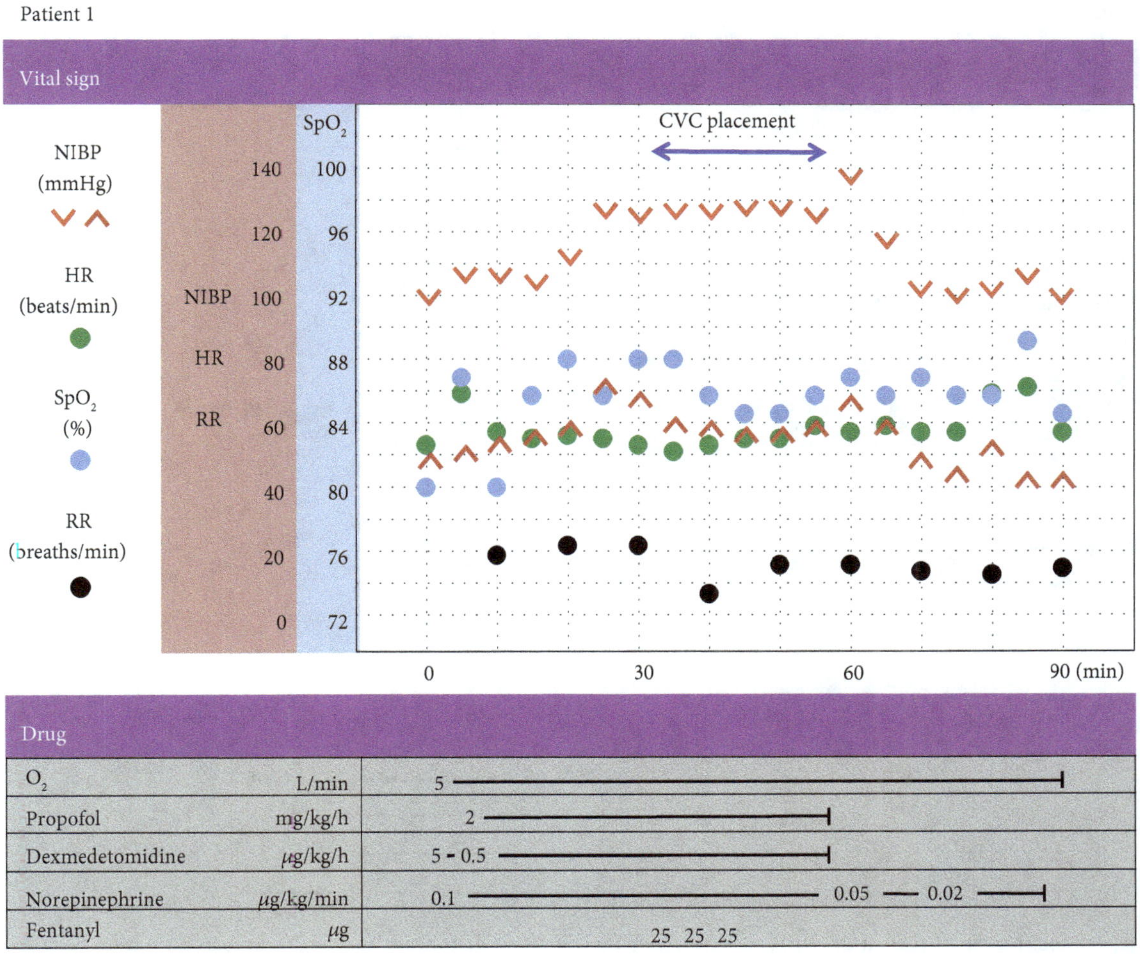

Figure 3: Anesthesia record of patient 1. NIBP: noninvasive blood pressure; HR: heart rate; SpO_2: oxygen saturation measured by pulse oximetry; RR: respiratory rate; CVC: central venous catheter.

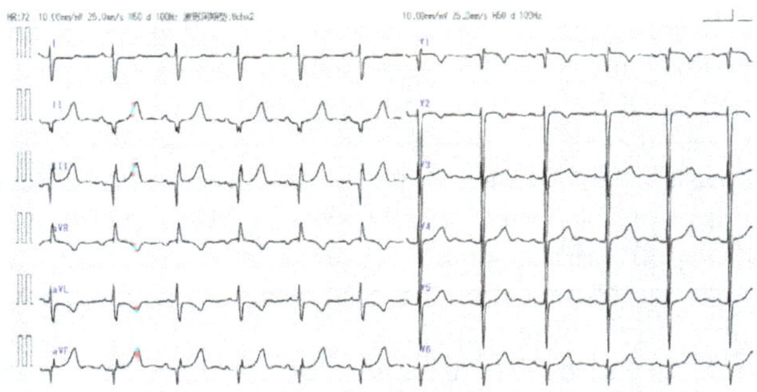

Figure 4: The preprocedural electrocardiogram of patient 2 shows sinus rhythm, northwest axis, notched *P* wave, and Qr pattern in V1.

thrombus. She had chronic cough and progressive dyspnea, and a history of a ventricular septal defect (VSD), pulmonary artery (PA) stenosis, and congenitally corrected transposition of the great arteries (ccTGA). At 8 years of age, she underwent the Rastelli procedure only, which connected the morphologic left ventricle (LV) to the PA via a conduit graft for PA stenosis. She did not undergo anatomic repair of the corrected transposition, in which an atrial inversion procedure (Senning or Mustard) is combined with either an arterial (arterial switch) or ventricular (Rastelli procedure) level repair. The patient was not prescribed any medications and was NYHA class II. The preprocedural BNP level was 50.1 pg/mL. The ECG showed sinus rhythm, northwest axis, notched *P* wave, and Qr pattern in V1 (Figure 4). TTE showed persistently elevated morphologic LVP, which was estimated to be equal to morphologic RVP. The suspected morphologic LV volume overload was indicated by a residual VSD with bidirectional shunting (diameter: 18 mm), mild mitral regurgitation, mild tricuspid regurgitation, and a suspected thrombus in the right atrium. Morphologic right ventricle (RV) function was preserved with an ejection fraction (EF) of 61% and E/A 1.59; E/e' 12.4. Morphologic LV function was also preserved with an FAC of 49%, mitral annular plane systolic excursion (MAPSE) of 20.9 mm, and E/A 1.91; E/e' (septal) 11; E/e' (lateral) 10. Although TTE could not detect the Rastelli conduit, progression of conduit stenosis was suspected from her clinical course and other echocardiography data. She was scheduled for TEE under MAC for a detailed observation of the thrombus.

The anesthesia record is shown in Figure 5. Her preprocedural vital signs in the operating room were as follows: BP—126/72 mmHg; HR—80 beats/min; and SpO_2—82% in room air. During MAC, 3 L/min of 100% oxygen was administered via a nasal cannula. Her $EtCO_2$ was

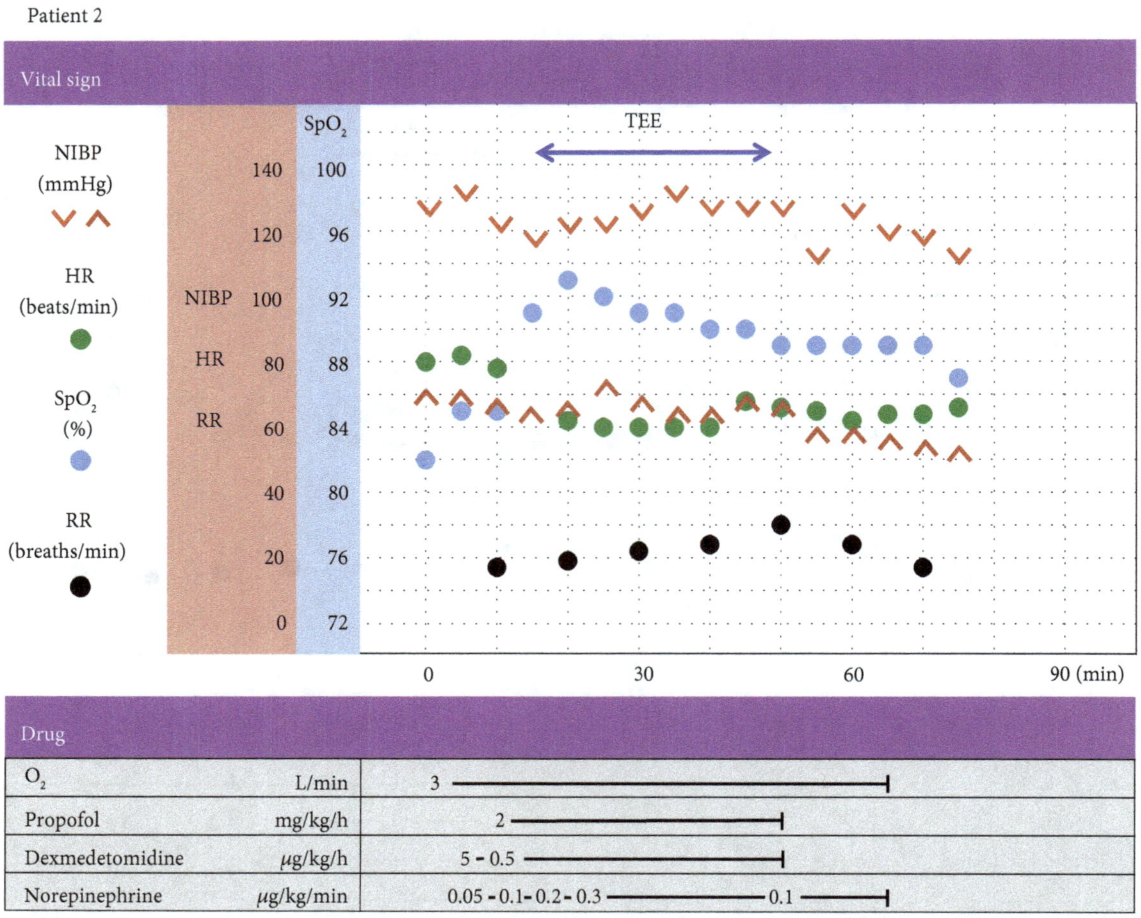

Figure 5: Anesthesia record of patient 2. NIBP: noninvasive blood pressure; HR: heart rate; SpO_2: oxygen saturation measured by pulse oximetry; RR: respiratory rate; TEE: transesophageal echocardiography.

monitored with capnography. Before the induction of anesthesia, a continuous peripheral venous infusion of norepinephrine was initiated at 0.05 μg/kg/min and maintained at 0.05–0.3 μg/kg/min to maintain the sSABP above 110 mmHg (her resting sSABP). MAC was provided with a continuous infusion of propofol (2–2.3 mg/kg/h) and dexmedetomidine (a loading dose of 1 μg/kg over 10 minutes followed by a 0.5 μg/kg/h infusion) to achieve optimal sedation and analgesia. For local anesthesia, 2% viscous lidocaine was used on the pharynx and larynx. No hemodynamic instability, respiratory depression, or oxygen desaturation was observed during MAC. The infusion of norepinephrine was tapered according to sSABP and discontinued after 20 minutes of the procedure. The level of consciousness was arousable on calling, and no airway obstruction was observed at the end of the MAC. The postprocedural course was uneventful. The patient was discharged on postprocedural day 1.

3. Discussion

We successfully provided MAC to two patients with ACHD and elevated subpulmonic ventricular pressure with an intracardiac shunt. The clinical courses of these two patients suggest several important points for anesthesia providers.

First, we found that a continuous infusion of norepinephrine from the preinduction period was helpful in maintaining hemodynamic stability in these patients. Many agents commonly used for sedation and anesthesia, such as propofol, decrease the systemic vascular resistance (SVR), which may increase the right-to-left shunt flow and cause oxygen desaturation [6, 7]. Moreover, perfusion of the coronary artery that supplies the subpulmonic ventricle is dependent on a pressure gradient between the aorta and the subpulmonic ventricle. When the subpulmonic ventricular pressure is elevated, decreased SVR reduces coronary blood flow to the subpulmonic ventricle for pulmonary circulation, leading to subpulmonic ventricular dysfunction. Furthermore, the morphologic RV was a ventricle for systemic circulation in patient 2. In ACHD patients with ccTGA that have not undergone anatomic repair of the corrected transposition, the morphological RV is forced to generate the pressure required to overcome the systemic afterload. However, the morphologic RV is not anatomically suited to withstand the systemic pressure, unlike the morphologic LV. Therefore, increased or decreased SVR directly correlates with deterioration of morphologic RV systolic function, which causes a further decrease in the cardiac output. A titrated infusion of vasopressors from the preinduction period effectively counteracts anesthesia-induced vasodilation. According to a review of 33 patients with Eisenmenger syndrome or a similar pathology, the use of a vasopressor significantly decreased the incidence of hypotension during anesthetic induction [8]. In both of our patients, norepinephrine was peripherally infused before anesthesia induction and titrated to maintain the sSABP above the resting level throughout the procedure. Other vasopressors such as phenylephrine, dopamine, and vasopressin may also be used to raise the sSABP. Norepinephrine is preferred over phenylephrine because of the $\beta 1$ effect of the former, which increases ventricular contractility and helps counteract the increase in PVR. Dopamine titration is more complicated than that of norepinephrine because of the dose-dependent shift in the predominant effects of dopamine. Vasopressin is a nonsympathomimetic vasopressor, which has the possibility of decreasing PVR without decreasing SVR [9, 10]. However, because of its much longer half-life (10–30 min) than that of norepinephrine (1–2.5 min), vasopressin is difficult to titrate in response to rapid changes in the sSABP. A continuous basal infusion of vasopressin may be used as an adjunct to norepinephrine.

Second, an increase in PVR also should be prevented. Any catecholamine surge caused by pain, agitation, or anxiety will abruptly increase PVR, so judicious doses of sedatives and analgesics should be provided to prevent it. Propofol is an intravenous sedative drug that provides effective sedation and rapid recovery from anesthesia. Owing to its extensive usage in anesthesia patients, we chose propofol as the first-choice sedative. Fentanyl is a commonly used analgesic for MAC, but may cause dose-dependent hypercarbia, which may increase PVR. To avoid this problem, we used local anesthetics and also added dexmedetomidine to our anesthetic regimen. Dexmedetomidine is a selective $\alpha 2$ adrenergic agonist with sedative, analgesic, and anxiolytic properties but does not promote respiratory depression [11]. Dexmedetomidine may help to reduce the propofol and fentanyl requirements and thereby may lower the risk of hypercarbia [12, 13]. A pilot study of 22 pediatric patients following congenital heart disease surgery demonstrated that dexmedetomidine did not increase pulmonary arterial pressure [14]. We did not observe substantial respiratory depression in either of our cases as indicated by a reduced respiratory rate and/or elevated $EtCO_2$ compared with baseline levels.

Third, continuous and careful observation of airway patency is of paramount importance during MAC. We chose MAC with spontaneous breathing over general anesthesia with endotracheal intubation and positive pressure ventilation because we believe that the former might be more advantageous in lowering PVR compared with the latter. However, once the airway is compromised, hypoxia may ensue and increase PVR. Therefore, in both cases, we always had at least one designated anesthesiologist at the bedside who continuously monitored the $EtCO_2$ and other clinical signs of adequate airway patency who could intervene if airway obstruction occurred.

Procedural sedation and analgesia without careful consideration of the anesthetic regimen can be harmful to patients with ACHD and highly elevated subpulmonic ventricular pressure. In fact, we suppose that these patients have periprocedural risks similar to those observed in patients with severe pulmonary arterial hypertension [15]. There are many sedative and analgesic drug choices for MAC [16]. However, there is no conclusive evidence for the most effective drug. Although MAC with a combination of propofol, dexmedetomidine, and fentanyl provides safe and effective sedation and analgesia, drug interactions among these three anesthetics complicate anesthetic management. Patients with ACHD and highly elevated subpulmonic ventricular pressure may receive better anesthetic care at an appropriately equipped regional ACHD center with an experienced cardiac anesthesiologist.

4. Conclusion

In the anesthetic management of patients with ACHD and highly elevated subpulmonic ventricular pressure, it is most important to prevent a pulmonary hypertensive crisis. Most anesthetic agents have a hypotensive effect, which causes poor coronary perfusion, right-to-left shunting, and subpulmonic ventricle dilation/failure. Continuous administration of adequate norepinephrine from during the preanesthetic period is crucial for the prevention of sudden systemic hypotension. Although MAC with a combination of propofol, dexmedetomidine, and fentanyl provides safe and effective sedation and analgesia, it may be better performed by a trained anesthesiologist. Patients with ACHD and highly elevated subpulmonic ventricular pressure may be treated at a regional ACHD center.

References

[1] A. J. Marelli, A. S. Mackie, R. Ionescu-Ittu, E. Rahme, and L. Pilote, "Congenital heart disease in the general population: changing prevalence and age distribution," *Circulation*, vol. 115, no. 2, pp. 163–172, 2007.

[2] Y. Shiina, T. Toyoda, Y. Kawasoe et al., "Prevalence of adult patients with congenital heart disease in Japan," *International Journal of Cardiology*, vol. 146, no. 1, pp. 13–16, 2011.

[3] A. J. Marelli, R. Ionescu-Ittu, A. S. Mackie, L. Guo, N. Dendukuri, and M. Kaouache, "Lifetime prevalence of congenital heart disease in the general population from 2000 to 2010," *Circulation*, vol. 130, no. 9, pp. 749–756, 2014.

[4] B. G. Maxwell, J. K. Wong, C. Kin, and R. L. Lobato, "Perioperative outcomes of major noncardiac surgery in adults with congenital heart disease," *Anesthesiology*, vol. 119, no. 4, pp. 762_769, 2013.

[5] E. Foster, T. P. Graham Jr., D. J. Driscoll et al., "Task force 2: special health care needs of adults with congenital heart disease," *Journal of the American College of Cardiology*, vol. 37, no. 5, pp. 1176–1183, 2001.

[6] M. Cannesson, M. G. Earing, V. Collange, and J. R. Kersten, "Anesthesia for noncardiac surgery in adults with congenital heart disease," *Anesthesiology*, vol. 111, no. 2, pp. 432–440, 2009.

[7] C. T. Gan, J. W. Lankhaar, J. T. Marcus et al., "Impaired left ventricular filling due to right-to-left ventricular interaction

in patients with pulmonary arterial hypertension," *American Journal of Physiology-Heart and Circulatory Physiology*, vol. 290, no. 4, pp. H1528–H1533, 2006.

[8] J. M. Bennett, J. M. Ehrenfeld, L. Markham, and S. S. Eagle, "Anesthetic management and outcomes for patients with pulmonary hypertension and intracardiac shunts and Eisenmenger syndrome: a review of institutional experience," *Journal of Clinical Anesthesia*, vol. 26, no. 4, pp. 286–293, 2014.

[9] D. A. Currigan, R. J. Hughes, C. E. Wright, J. A. Angus, and P. F. Soeding, "Vasoconstrictor responses to vasopressor agents in human pulmonary and radial arteries: an in vitro study," *Anesthesiology*, vol. 121, no. 5, pp. 930–936, 2014.

[10] S. L. Siehr, J. A. Feinstein, W. Yang, L. F. Peng, M. T. Ogawa, and C. Ramamoorthy, "Hemodynamic effects of phenylephrine, vasopressin, and epinephrine in children with pulmonary hypertension: a pilot study," *Pediatric Critical Care Medicine*, vol. 17, no. 5, pp. 428–437, 2016.

[11] R. Gertler, H. C. Brown, D. H. Mitchell, and E. N. Silvius, "Dexmedetomidine: a novel sedative-analgesic agent," *Baylor University Medical Center Proceedings*, vol. 14, no. 1, pp. 13–21, 2001.

[12] K. N. Kim, H. J. Lee, S. Y. Kim, and J. Y. Kim, "Combined use of dexmedetomidine and propofol in monitored anesthesia care: a randomized controlled study," *BMC Anesthesiology*, vol. 17, no. 1, p. 34, 2017.

[13] B. Scheinin, L. Lindgren, T. Randell, H. Scheinin, and M. Scheinin, "Dexmedetomidine attenuates sympathoadrenal responses to tracheal intubation and reduces the need for thiopentone and peroperative fentanyl," *British Journal of Anaesthesia*, vol. 68, no. 2, pp. 126–131, 1992.

[14] J. P. Lazol, S. E. Lichtenstein, E. H. Jooste et al., "Effect of dexmedetomidine on pulmonary artery pressure after congenital cardiac surgery: a pilot study∗," *Pediatric Critical Care Medicine*, vol. 11, no. 5, pp. 589–592, 2010.

[15] M. L. Bernier, A. I. Jacob, J. M. Collaco, S. A. McGrath-Morrow, L. H. Romer, and C. C. Unegbu, "Perioperative events in children with pulmonary hypertension undergoing non-cardiac procedures," *Pulmonary Circulation*, vol. 8, no. 1, p. 204589321773814, 2017.

[16] J. D. Tobias and M. Leder, "Procedural sedation: a review of sedative agents, monitoring, and management of complications," *Saudi Journal of Anaesthesia*, vol. 5, no. 4, pp. 395–410, 2011.

Permissions

All chapters in this book were first published by Hindawi Publishing Corporation; hereby published with permission under the Creative Commons Attribution License or equivalent. Every chapter published in this book has been scrutinized by our experts. Their significance has been extensively debated. The topics covered herein carry significant findings which will fuel the growth of the discipline. They may even be implemented as practical applications or may be referred to as a beginning point for another development.

The contributors of this book come from diverse backgrounds, making this book a truly international effort. This book will bring forth new frontiers with its revolutionizing research information and detailed analysis of the nascent developments around the world.

We would like to thank all the contributing authors for lending their expertise to make the book truly unique. They have played a crucial role in the development of this book. Without their invaluable contributions this book wouldn't have been possible. They have made vital efforts to compile up to date information on the varied aspects of this subject to make this book a valuable addition to the collection of many professionals and students.

This book was conceptualized with the vision of imparting up-to-date information and advanced data in this field. To ensure the same, a matchless editorial board was set up. Every individual on the board went through rigorous rounds of assessment to prove their worth. After which they invested a large part of their time researching and compiling the most relevant data for our readers.

The editorial board has been involved in producing this book since its inception. They have spent rigorous hours researching and exploring the diverse topics which have resulted in the successful publishing of this book. They have passed on their knowledge of decades through this book. To expedite this challenging task, the publisher supported the team at every step. A small team of assistant editors was also appointed to further simplify the editing procedure and attain best results for the readers.

Apart from the editorial board, the designing team has also invested a significant amount of their time in understanding the subject and creating the most relevant covers. They scrutinized every image to scout for the most suitable representation of the subject and create an appropriate cover for the book.

The publishing team has been an ardent support to the editorial, designing and production team. Their endless efforts to recruit the best for this project, has resulted in the accomplishment of this book. They are a veteran in the field of academics and their pool of knowledge is as vast as their experience in printing. Their expertise and guidance has proved useful at every step. Their uncompromising quality standards have made this book an exceptional effort. Their encouragement from time to time has been an inspiration for everyone.

The publisher and the editorial board hope that this book will prove to be a valuable piece of knowledge for researchers, students, practitioners and scholars across the globe.

List of Contributors

Bandar Al-Ghamdi
Heart Centre, King Faisal Specialist Hospital and Research Centre (KFSH&RC), Riyadh, Saudi Arabia
Alfaisal University, Riyadh, Saudi Arabia

Andres Cordova Sanchez and Suman Rao
Department of Medicine, SUNY Upstate Medical University, Syracuse, NY 13210, USA

Ryan Murphy
College of Medicine, SUNY Upstate Medical University, Syracuse, NY 13210, USA

Fidel Martinez
Division of Cardiology, SUNY Upstate Medical University, Syracuse, NY 13210, USA

Stephanie Bryant
Department of Pathology, SUNY Upstate Medical University, Syracuse, NY 13210, USA

Aniket S. Rali, Nilay Patel, Benjamin Wiele, Zubair Shah and Jayant Nath
Department of Cardiovascular Diseases, University of Kansas Medical Center, Kansas City, KS, USA

Mejalli Al-Kofahi
Department of Internal Medicine, University of Kansas Medical Center, Kansas City, KS, USA

Bashar Khiatah, Sam Jazayeri, John Wilde and Mathew Westfall
Department of Internal Medicine, Community Memorial Hospital, 147 N Brent St, Ventura, CA 93003, USA

Thomas Q. Kong Jr.
Ventura Cardiology Consultants, 100 North Brent Street, Suite 301, Ventura, CA 93003, USA

Amanda Frugoli
Department of GME Internal Medicine, GME Internal Medicine of Community Memorial Hospital of Ventura, 147 N Brent St, Ventura, CA 93003, USA

Sakae Takenaka, Takao Konishi, Tomoya Sato, Atsushi Tada, Takuya Koizumi, Yoshifumi Mizuguchi, Takahide Kadosaka, Ko Motoi, Yuta Kobayashi, Hirokazu Komoriyama, Yoshiya Kato, Miwa Sarashina, Kazunori Omote, Shingo Tsujinaga, Takuma Sato, Rui Kamada, Kiwamu Kamiya, Hiroyuki Iwano, Toshiyuki Nagai and Toshihisa Anzai
Department of Cardiovascular Medicine, Faculty of Medicine and Graduate School of Medicine, Hokkaido University, Sapporo, Japan

Tatsuya Orimo, Hirofumi Kamachi and Akinobu Taketomi
Department of Gastroenterological Surgery I, Faculty of Medicine and Graduate School of Medicine, Hokkaido University, Sapporo, Japan

Muhammad Shabbir Rawala
Department of Internal Medicine, WVU-Charleston Division, Charleston, WV, USA

Alex Munoz
Department of Radiology, University of Kentucky, Louisville, KY, USA

Mohammad Hassan Pervaiz
Department of Cardiology, WVU-Charleston Division, Charleston, WV, USA

Osayi Lawani
University of Houston College of Medicine/HCA Houston Healthcare, USA

Mark Winter
Southeast Texas Poison Center, University of Texas Medical Branch, USA

Naji Maaliki, Michael Omar, Aleem Azal Ali and Amy Roemer
Internal Medicine, University of Florida College of Medicine, Jacksonville, USA

Jose Ruiz and Edin Sadic
Cardiology, University of Florida College of Medicine, Jacksonville, USA

Florian Appenzeller, Meinrad Gawaz and Iris Müller
University Hospital, Department of Cardiology and Cardiovascular Medicine, Eberhard Karls University Tübingen, 72076 Tübingen, Germany

Jun Muneuchi, Yuichiro Sugitani, Masaru Kobayashi, Hiroki Ezaki, Hiromu Yamada and Mamie Watanabe
Department of Pediatrics, Kyushu Hospital, Japan Community Healthcare Organization, Kitakyushu, Japan

Christian Birner, Matthias Gasche, Rainer Voisard and Christian Neumann
Joint Medical Service (Germany), Department of Internal Medicine, Military Hospital Ulm, 89081 Oberer Eselsberg 40 Ulm, Germany

James Keeton
University of Texas Health Science Center, San Antonio, Texas, USA

Pedro Engel Gonzalez, Robert M. Morlend, Alpesh A. Amin, Pradeep P. A. Mammen, Lynn C. Huffman and Faris G. Araj
University of Texas Southwestern Medical Center, Dallas, Texas, USA

Julie Cox
Baylor Scott and White Health, Dallas, Texas, USA

John S. Dayco
PGY-I, Internal Medicine, Department of Internal Medicine, Detroit Medical Center, USA

Shaun Cardozo
Division of Cardiology, Physician, Division of Cardiology, Detroit Medical Center, Wayne State University, Wayne State University Physician Group, USA

Alisha Khan, Thu Thu Aung and Debanik Chaudhuri
State University of New York Upstate University Hospital, USA

Vijay Chander Vinod, Zuhair Eltayeb Yousif, Najat Omer Salim and Talib Majwal
Mediclinic City Hospital, Dubai, UAE

Chika-Nwosuh Ogechukwu, Nnaoma Christopher, Sossou Christoph, Okundaye Etinosasere and Bustillo Jose
Department of Medicine, Newark Beth Israel Medical Center, Robert Wood Johnson Barnabas Health, Newark, NJ, USA

Lauren Giudicatti, Xiao-Fang Xu and Anthony Putrino
Department of Cardiology, Fiona Stanley Hospital, Perth, Australia

Benjamin Silbert, Felicity Lee, Amit Shah and Kaitlyn Lam
Advanced Heart Failure and Cardiac Transplantation Unit, Fiona Stanley Hospital, Perth, Australia

Robert Larbalestier and Karim Slimani
Department of Cardiothoracic Surgery, Fiona Stanley Hospital, Perth, Australia

Andrew Laycock
PathWest, Fiona Stanley Hospital, Perth, Australia

Ankit Agrawal
Division of Internal Medicine Rutgers Robert Wood, Johnson Medical School/Saint Peter's University Hospital, New Jersey, USA

Maria Cardinale
Division of Pharmacy, Saint Peter's University Hospital, New Jersey, USA
Ernest Mario School of Pharmacy, Rutgers University, New Jersey, USA

Douglas Frenia
Division of Pulmonary and Critical Care Medicine, Rutgers Robert Wood Johnson Medical School/Saint Peter's University Hospital, New Jersey, USA

Tarun Dalia
Division of Internal Medicine, University of Kansas Medical Center, Kansas, USA

Chirag Shah
Division of Cardiovascular Sciences Rutgers, Robert Wood Johnson Medical School/Saint Peter's University Hospital, New Jersey, USA

Yohei Numasawa, Souichi Yokokura, Yasuhiro Hitomi, Shohei Imaeda, Makoto Tanaka, Ryota Tabei and Masaki Kodaira
Department of Cardiology, Japanese Red Cross Ashikaga Hospital, Ashikaga, Japan

John Ning and Nunzio Gaglianello
Medical College of Wisconsin, 8701 West Watertown Plank Road Milwaukee, WI 53226, USA

James Livesay, Emmanuel Isang, Jeffrey Johnson and Hassan Tahir
Department of Medicine, University of Tennessee Graduate School of Medicine, Knoxville, TN, USA

Raj Baljepally
Department of Medicine, University of Tennessee Graduate School of Medicine, Knoxville, TN, USA
Heart Lung Vascular Institute, University of Tennessee Medical Center, Knoxville, TN, USA

Habtewold Shibru, Ermias shenkutie Greffie and Zenahbezu Abay
Department of Internal Medicine, University of Gondar, Gondar, Ethiopia

Oumer Abdu Muhie
Department of Internal Medicine, GAMBY Teaching General Hospital, Bahir Dar, Ethiopia

Saeki Watanabe, Yuki Ichihara, Kozo Morita, Satoshi Saito and Hiroshi Niinami
Tokyo Women's Medical University, Department of Cardiovascular Surgery, Kawada-cho 8-1, Shinjuku ku, Tokyo, Japan

James L. Laws
Department of Internal Medicine, Vanderbilt University Medical Center, Nashville, Tennessee, USA

Esther Kim, Rebecca Hung and JoAnn Lindenfeld
Department of Cardiovascular Medicine, Vanderbilt University Medical Center, Nashville, Tennessee, USA

Richa Gupta
Department of Cardiovascular Medicine, MedStar Washington Hospital Center, Washington, DC, USA

Siddhant Dogra, Asha M. Mahajan, Albert Jung, Michael Attubato, Muhamed Saric and Alan Shah
Leon H. Charney Division of Cardiology, Department of Medicine, New York University School of Medicine, 530 First Avenue, Skirball 9U, New York, NY10016, USA

Nikolaos Iakovis, Andrew Xanthopoulos , Aikaterini Chamaidi, Michail Papamichalis, Apostolos Dimos, Filippos Triposkiadis and John Skoularigis
Department of Cardiology, University General Hospital of Larissa, Larissa, Greece

Garly Saint-Croix
Department of Internal Medicine, Jackson Memorial Hospital/University of Miami Hospital, Miami, FL, USA

Rosario Colombo
Department of Cardiovascular Medicine, Jackson Memorial Hospital, Miami, FL, USA

Ramy Mando
Department of Internal Medicine, Beaumont Health System, Royal Oak, MI, USA

Robert Gemayel
Michigan State University College of Osteopathic Medicine, Lansing, MI, USA

Ashish Chaddha, Julian J. Barbat and Elvis Cami
Department of Cardiovascular Medicine, Beaumont Health System, Royal Oak, MI, USA

Jessica O'Neil
Department of Medicine, Massachusetts General Hospital, Massachusetts, USA

Soumyaa Mazumder
Harvard Medical School, Massachusetts, USA

Danita Yoerger Sanborn
Department of Medicine, Massachusetts General Hospital, Massachusetts, USA
Department of Cardiology, Massachusetts General Hospital, Massachusetts, USA

Samantha Wu
Department of Medicine, Massachusetts General Hospital, Massachusetts, USA
Hospital Medicine Unit Massachusetts General Hospital, Massachusetts, USA

Parth J. Sampat, Sana Riaz and Maneesh Bisen
Department of Medicine, SUNY Upstate Medical University, Syracuse, NY, USA

Robert Carhart
Department of Cardiology, SUNY Upstate Medical University, Syracuse, NY, USA

Diego H. González-Bravo, Sergio Alegre-Boschetti, Richard Silva-Cantillo, Joshua Mercado-Maldonado and Josue Mercado-Crespo
Cardiovascular Division, Department of Medicine, VA Caribbean Healthcare System, San Juan, Puerto Rico

Reyshley Ramos-Márquez and Gabriel Torres-Rivera
Internal Medicine Division, Department of Medicine, VA Caribbean Healthcare System, San Juan, Puerto Rico

Carlos Cortés
Internal Medicine and Nephrology Division, Department of Medicine, VA Caribbean Healthcare System, San Juan, Puerto Rico

Tejas Raxwal and Dipak Parekh
Access Health Care Physicians, Hudson, Florida, USA

Cauvery Balhara
Regional Medical Center Bayonet Point, Hudson, Florida, USA

Erind Gjermeni, Andreas Bollmann, Gerhard Hindricks and Andreas Müssigbrodt
Department of Electrophysiology, Heart Center University of Leipzig, Strümpellstraße 39, 04289 Leipzig, Germany

Arnold Nongmoh Forlemu
Creighton University School of Medicine-Phoenix/ Maricopa Integrated Health System, Department of Internal Medicine-Cardiology, 2601 E Roosevelt St., Phoenix, AZ 85008, USA

Muhammad Ajmal
University of Arizona College of Medicine-Tucson, Sarver Heart Center, Department of Cardiology, 750 W Orange Grove Road, Tucson, AZ 85704, USA

Mehrdad Saririan
Creighton University School of Medicine-Phoenix/ Maricopa Integrated Health System, Department of Cardiology, 2601 E Roosevelt St., Phoenix, AZ 85008, USA

Wytch Rigger
Department of Medicine, Medical College of Georgia at Augusta University, Augusta, GA, USA

Sean P. Javaheri, Gyanendra K. Sharma and Neal L. Weintraub
Division of Cardiology, Medical College of Georgia at Augusta University, Augusta, GA, USA

Norris Stanley Nahman Jr.
Division of Nephrology, Medical College of Georgia at Augusta University, Augusta, GA, USA

Mark Sheynshteyn
Division of Endocrinology, Diabetes and Metabolism, Medical College of Georgia at Augusta University, Augusta, GA, USA

Preeti Singhal
Department of Internal Medicine, Keck School of Medicine of USC, Los Angeles, CA, USA
Los Angeles County + University of Southern California Medical Center, Los Angeles, CA, USA

Somsupha Kanjanauthai and Wilson Kwan
Los Angeles County + University of Southern California Medical Center, Los Angeles, CA, USA
Department of Cardiovascular Medicine, Keck School of Medicine of USC, Los Angeles, CA, USA

Shashikanth Ambati, Javier Sanchez and Adnan Bakar
Division of Pediatric Critical Care, Department of Pediatrics, Bernard & Millie Duker Children's Hospital, Albany, New York, USA

Michael Colon
Pediatric Cardiology, Capital District Pediatric Cardiology Associates, Albany, New York, USA

Maya Mihic
Department of Pediatrics, Bernard & Millie Duker Children's Hospital, Albany, New York, USA

Mariann Al-Jehani and Jomanah Shahbaz
King Saud bin Abdulaziz University for Health Sciences, Jeddah, Saudi Arabia

Faisal Al-Husayni
King Abdullah International Medical Research Center, Jeddah, Saudi Arabia
Department of Internal Medicine, National Guard Hospital, Jeddah, Saudi Arabia

Ahmed Almaqati
Department of Internal Medicine, National Guard Hospital, Jeddah, Saudi Arabia

Saad Albugami
King Saud bin Abdulaziz University for Health Sciences, Jeddah, Saudi Arabia
King Abdullah International Medical Research Center, Jeddah, Saudi Arabia
Department of Cardiac Sciences, King Faisal Cardiac Center, National Guard Hospital, Jeddah, Saudi Arabia

Wail Alameen
Department of Cardiac Sciences, King Faisal Cardiac Center, National Guard Hospital, Jeddah, Saudi Arabia

Lance Alquran and Ankita Patel
Department of Internal Medicine, Hackensack Meridian Health Mountainside Medical Center, Montclair, New Jersey 07028, USA

Lucy Safi
Department of Cardiology, Hackensack University Medical Center, Hackensack, New Jersey 07601, USA

Ankitkumar Patel
Department of Internal Medicine, Hackensack Meridian Health Mountainside Medical Center, Montclair, New Jersey 07028, USA
Department of Cardiology, Hackensack University Medical Center, Hackensack, New Jersey 07601, USA

Kazuhiro Kurisu, Hiroshi Mitsuo and Yasutaka Ueno
Department of Cardiovascular Surgery, Shimonoseki City Hospital, Shimonoseki, Japan

Zeid Nesheiwat, Pinang Shastri, Rohit Vyas and Cameron Burmeister
Department of Internal Medicine, The University of Toledo College of Medicine, 3000 Arlington Avenue, Toledo, Ohio 43614, USA

Robert Grande and Hazem Malas
Division of Cardiovascular Medicine, Toledo Hospital, 2142 N Cove Boulevard, Toledo, Ohio 43606, USA

Debbie Falconer and Sariha Yousfani
Royal Free Hospital, Pond Street, London NW3 2QG, UK

Anna S. Herrey and Pier Lambiase
Royal Free Hospital, Pond Street, London NW3 2QG, UK
Barts Heart Centre, W Smithfield, London EC1A 7BE, UK

Gabriella Captur
Royal Free Hospital, Pond Street, London NW3 2QG, UK
MRC Unit for Lifelong Health and Ageing at UCL, 1-19 Torrington Place, Fitzrovia, London, UK

Michel Ibrahim
Department of Medicine, Cardiovascular Division, Temple University Hospital, Philadelphia, PA, USA

Michael Fattouh
Montefiore Medical Center, Bronx, NY, USA

Alice Jacobs
Boston University Medical Center, Boston, MA, USA

Tatsuya Kida and Tomoya Irie
Department of Anesthesiology, Yokohama City University School of Medicine, 3-9 Fukuura, Kanazawa -ku, Yokohama 2360004, Japan

Takahisa Goto
Department of Anesthesiology, Yokohama City University Medical Center, 4-57 Urahune, Minami-ku, Yokohama 2320024, Japan

Index